1989
YEAR BOOK OF
NEUROLOGY AND
NEUROSURGERY®

The 1989 Year Book® Series

Year Book of Anesthesia®: Drs. Miller, Kirby, Ostheimer, Roizen, and Stoelting

Year Book of Cardiology®: Drs. Schlant, Collins, Engle, Frye, Kaplan, and O'Rourke

Year Book of Critical Care Medicine®: Drs. Rogers and Parrillo

Year Book of Dentistry®: Drs. Rose, Hendler, Johnson, Jordan, Moyers, and Silverman

Year Book of Dermatology®: Drs. Sober and Fitzpatrick

Year Book of Diagnostic Radiology®: Drs. Bragg, Hendee, Keats, Kirkpatrick, Miller, Osborn, and Thompson

Year Book of Digestive Diseases®: Drs. Greenberger and Moody

Year Book of Drug Therapy®: Drs. Hollister and Lasagna

Year Book of Emergency Medicine®: Dr. Wagner

Year Book of Endocrinology®: Drs. Bagdade, Braverman, Halter, Horton, Korenman, Kornel, Metz, Molitch, Morley, Rogol, Ryan, Sherwin, and Vaitukaitis

Year Book of Family Practice®: Drs. Rakel, Avant, Driscoll, Prichard, and Smith

Year Book of Geriatrics and Gerontology: Drs. Beck, Abrass, Burton, Cummings, Makinodan, and Small

Year Book of Hand Surgery®: Drs. Dobyns, Chase, and Amadio

Year Book of Hematology®: Drs. Spivak, Bell, Ness, Quesenberry, and Wiernik

Year Book of Infectious Diseases®: Drs. Wolff, Barza, Keusch, Klempner, and Snydman

Year Book of Infertility: Drs. Mishell, Lobo, and Paulsen

Year Book of Medicine®: Drs. Rogers, Des Prez, Cline, Braunwald, Greenberger, Wilson, Epstein, and Malawista

Year Book of Neurology and Neurosurgery®: Drs. DeJong, Currier, and Crowell

Year Book of Nuclear Medicine®: Drs. Hoffer, Gore, Gottschalk, Sostman, Zaret, and Zubal

Year Book of Obstetrics and Gynecology®: Drs. Mishell, Kirschbaum, and Morrow

Year Book of Oncology®: Drs. Young, Coleman, Longo, Ozols, Simone, and Steele

Year Book of Ophthalmology®: Dr. Laibson

Year Book of Orthopedics®: Dr. Sledge

Year Book of Otolaryngology–Head and Neck Surgery®: Drs. Bailey and Paparella

Year Book of Pathology and Clinical Pathology®: Drs. Brinkhous, Dalldorf, Grisham, Langdell, and McLendon

Year Book of Pediatrics®: Drs. Oski and Stockman

Year Book of Perinatal/Neonatal Medicine: Drs. Klaus and Fanaroff

Year Book of Plastic, Reconstructive, and Aesthetic Surgery®: Drs. Miller, Bennett, Haynes, Hoehn, McKinney, and Whitaker

Year Book of Podiatric Medicine and Surgery®: Dr. Jay

Year Book of Psychiatry and Applied Mental Health®: Drs. Talbott, Frances, Freedman, Meltzer, Schowalter, and Weiner

Year Book of Pulmonary Disease®: Drs. Green, Ball, Michael, Peters, Terry, Tockman, and Wise

Year Book of Rehabilitation®: Drs. Kaplan, Frank, Gordon, Lieberman, Magnuson, Molnar, Payton, and Sarno

Year Book of Sports Medicine®: Drs. Shepard, Sutton, and Torg, Col. Anderson, and Mr. George

Year Book of Surgery®: Drs. Schwartz, Jonasson, Peacock, Shires, Spencer, and Thompson

Year Book of Urology®: Drs. Gillenwater and Howards

Year Book of Vascular Surgery®: Drs. Bergan and Yao

1989

The Year Book of NEUROLOGY AND NEUROSURGERY®

"Published without interruption since 1902"

Neurology

Editors

Russell N. DeJong, M.D.
Professor Emeritus of Neurology,
The University of Michigan Medical School

Robert D. Currier, M.D.
Professor and Chairman, Department of Neurology, University of Mississippi
Medical Center, Jackson

Neurosurgery

Editor

Robert M. Crowell, M.D.
Professor and Head, Department of Neurological Surgery, University of
Illinois at Chicago, College of Medicine

Year Book Medical Publishers, Inc.
Chicago · London · Boca Raton

Editorial Director, Year Book Publishing: Nancy Gorham
Sponsoring Editor: Judy L. Plazyk
Manager, Medical Information Services: Laura J. Shedore
Assistant Director, Manuscript Services: Frances M. Perveiler
Associate Managing Editor, Year Book Editing Services: Elizabeth Griffith
Production Manager: H.E. Nielsen
Proofroom Manager: Shirley E. Taylor

Table of Contents

Journals Represented

Year Book Medical Publishers subscribes to and surveys more than 700 U.S. and foreign medical and allied health journals. From these journals, the Editors select the articles to be abstracted. Journals represented in this YEAR BOOK are listed below.

Acta Cytologica
Acta Medica Scandinavica
Acta Neurochirurgica
Acta Neurologica Scandinavica
Alabama Journal of Medical Sciences
American Journal of Clinical Pathology
American Journal of Diseases of Children
American Journal of Medicine
American Journal of Neuroradiology
American Journal of Roentgenology
American Surgeon
Annales D'Oto-Laryngologie
Annals of Emergency Medicine
Annals of Neurology
Annals of Surgery
Archives of Disease in Childhood
Archives of Internal Medicine
Archives of Neurology
Archives of Surgery
Biological Psychiatry
Brain—Journal of Neurology
Canadian Journal of Neurological Sciences
Cancer
Cleveland Clinic Journal of Medicine
Clinical Orthopaedics and Related Research
Diabetic Medicine
Epilepsia
Experimental Neurology
Geriatrics
Headache
IEEE Transactions on BioMedical Engineering
International Rehabilitation Medicine
Italian Journal of Neurological Sciences
Journal of the American Geriatrics Society
Journal of the American Medical Association
Journal of Bone and Joint Surgery (American vol.)
Journal of Computer Assisted Tomography
Journal of Immunology
Journal of Laboratory and Clinical Medicine
Journal of Neurological Sciences
Journal of Neurology
Journal of Neurology, Neurosurgery, and Psychiatry
Journal of Neurosurgery
Journal of Nuclear Medicine
Journal of Pediatric Orthopedics
Journal of Pediatrics
Journal of Surgical Research
Journal of Trauma

Journal of Vascular Surgery
Laboratory Investigation
Lancet
Laryngoscope
Life Sciences
Magnetic Resonance in Medicine
Mayo Clinic Proceedings
Medicine
Movement Disorders
Nervenarzt
Neurochirurgia
Neurochirurgie
Neurology
Neuropediatrics
Neuroradiology
Neurosurgery
New England Journal of Medicine
New York State Journal of Medicine
Otolaryngology—Head and Neck Surgery
Pain
Pediatric Neurology
Pediatrics
Plastic and Reconstructive Surgery
Postgraduate Medical Journal
Postgraduate Medicine
Quarterly Journal of Medicine
Radiology
Revue Neurologique
Rofo: Fortschritte auf dem Gebiete der Rontgenstrahlen und der
Nuklearmedizin
S.A.M.J./S.A.M.T.—South African Medical Journal
Science
Semaine des Hopitaux
Southern Medical Journal
Spine
Stroke
Surgical Neurology
Virchows Archiv A: Pathological Anatomy and Histopathology

NEUROLOGY

———

RUSSELL N. DE JONG, M.D.

———

ROBERT D. CURRIER, M.D.

———

Introduction

The YEAR BOOK that dealt with neurology in 1909, 80 years ago, was titled *Nervous and Mental Diseases* and was Volume 10 of the Practical Medicine Series under the general editorial direction of Gustavus P. Head, Professor of Laryngology and Rhinology at the Chicago Postgraduate Medical School. It was edited by Hugh T. Patrick, Professor of Neurology in the Chicago Polyclinic, and Charles L. Mix, Professor of Physical Diagnosis at Northwestern. In those days the editorial offices were at 40 Dearborn Street. The volumes were smaller, 237 pages, with a single column of type and few illustrations. Information on mental diseases occupied 10 pages at the very end. The rest of the book dealt with neurology and included a fair amount of new information on diagnostic testing and the neurologic examination, including comments on the plantar reflex. Did this reflect the relative importance of the two fields, or the editors' interests? Nearly 30 pages contained information on the neuroses: hysteria, neurasthenia, epilepsy, migraine, ambulatory automatism, and chorea. The last section in the main body of the text was entitled "Miscellaneous Nervous Diseases," which included tic, torticollis, Raynaud's disease, myopathy, myatonia, myasthenia, acromegaly, and other organic diseases. The difference between the neuroses and this last category of disease is something that I have difficulty with. The term *neuroses* did not have the same meaning then. But hysteria and neurasthenia were neurotic manifestations then, as now. Why epilepsy and migraine were included with the neuroses escapes me. It seems obvious that they were considered organic diseases, as shown by the choice of articles selected on organic treatments.

As I mentioned in last year's YEAR BOOK OF NEUROLOGY in my comments about the 1908 volume, one of the most impressive things about that volume is the nearly total lack of any comment on stroke as a disease; this is true of the 1909 volume as well. There are a few pages on cerebral hemorrhage and hemiplegia, but no speculation as to the causes of stroke per se, no comment on treatment, and no pathologic study except for hemorrhages. Another similarity is the total absence of comments on the disease we call amyotrophic lateral sclerosis in the 1909 (and the 1949) YEAR BOOK.

The few pages on mental disease include just a single note on schizophrenia (dementia praecox), a review of a paper by Kanavel, Pollock, and Eustace (*Illinois Medical Journal*, September 1909) on thyroidectomy for dementia praecox. Following the lead of Berkley and Follis, who found improvement in 5 of 8 thyroidectomized schizophrenics, Kanavel et al. operated on 11 patients with schizophrenia, 8 of them catatonic. They removed seven eighths of either the right or the left lobe and in 3 cases also the parathyroid glands. The outcome is unstated and the summary does not conclude that thyroidectomy is a treatment for schizophrenia, but only that continuation of the investigation seems justifiable in early cases.

Considerable space is occupied with discussion of aphasia, based on an article by Moutier in the *Gaz. des Hop.*, Oct. 1, 1908.

No introduction to the 1909 YEAR BOOK was provided. Forty years ago, however, when Roland Mackay took over from Hans Reese the editing of the neurologic portion of the YEAR BOOK OF NEUROLOGY, PSYCHIATRY AND NEUROSURGERY (1949), he provided a well-balanced introduction. I never met Dr. Mackay, but his fame was general 40 years ago in the Midwest. He was a thorough, thoughtful, and painstaking man. He once told my father to send me over for training sometime, but I never made it. Perhaps I should have.

Much of his introduction as a new editor was devoted to the relationship between neurology and psychiatry and his pleasure at the fact that the two are joined and that persons training in one or the other are required to know something of the sister specialty.

It was absolutely impossible to predict 40 years ago the direction neurology has taken. Neurology now is a rugged specialty. It is demanding both intellectually and emotionally and the rewards are not outstanding.

Years ago when neurology was a division of Internal Medicine at the University of Mississippi, the head of Medicine, Bob Snavely, a wonderful man, found me one late afternoon gloomily staring into a corner. When he asked what the trouble was, I replied that the patients were ill and, no matter what we did, not infrequently died and I couldn't fathom what we were doing wrong. He said, "Hmmmm, yes" and went on his way.

The next day he came by and said, "Currier, you know, you are in a tough racket." His comment cheered me considerably, and I have often taken solace from it over the years when backed into a corner by that one particular law of nature. I have come to agree with his assessment of neurology more and more completely. The diseases we deal with as neurologists are treacherous and often subject to irregular recurrent disequilibrium. Since the passing of the time when neurologists could reap financial rewards from doing arteriograms, neurology has not been a highly paid specialty. The neurologist must respond at all times of the day or night, so neurology cannot be practiced in its completeness in a 40-hour week. In short, it is a tough, demanding, punishing, highly intellectual field that is not attractive to the majority of medical students in spite of being "the Queen of the Arts," as Bert Sprofkin says. Recruiting has never filled the slots in training programs. In addition, neurology now requires a greater knowledge of internal medicine than of psychiatry.

Thus, should we not give credit for neurology board purposes for internal medicine training time to those who have had a change of heart and wish to become neurologists? Internists do, after all, make excellent neurologic physicians, and to tell them that they must undergo the entire neurologic 3 years of training, allowing no credit for internal medicine, is a mistake. We are missing many good people who could otherwise be included in our brotherhood. Therefore, why don't we allow a year of credit for neurology board eligibility if full training in medicine has been completed in the last 5 years? Our closest allies are, after all, not the neurosurgeons and not the psychiatrists, but the internists. Let us openly acknowledge that fact and open the door to neurologic training of internists. All right now, all you defenders of psychiatry, rise up and smite me.

The YEAR BOOK of 1949 contains, amazingly enough, a review of an article by Dewey Ziegler on familial periodic paralysis. Dr. Ziegler, still in his prime, has an article on headache reviewed in this YEAR BOOK (Abstract 8–5). Is this a record for continued YEAR BOOK reviewed productivity? Maybe not, since Macdonald Critchley is still going strong. But a startling discovery is also in the 1949 edition: Clara Torda and Harold Wolff reported in July 1949 (*Proc Soc Exp Biol Med* 71:432–435, July 1949) on the treatment of 5 women with myasthenia gravis. They gave 20 mg of ACTH every 6 hours for a total dose of 400 mg. The patients gradually became weaker until the second day after completion of the injections (the seventh day after starting the injections), and then went into a period of partial improvement, which at the time of writing had lasted 3 months.

Although they did not understand that they were treating an immune disease, I believe that this comment precedes any other report of steroid or ACTH treatment of myasthenia gravis.

Dr. Armin Haerer, Dr. DeJong, and I would like to make special mention of the colleagues we have lost in the last year.

After a long illness, Torben Fog died at his home in Copenhagen on April 19, 1987. A founding editor of *Acta Neurologica Scandinavica,* he was also for many years secretary of the World Federation of Neurology's Research Group on Multiple Sclerosis. The work of this Research Group will continue under the leadership of the co-chairmen, Reginald Kelly, Byron H. Wachsman, and Y. Kuroiwa.—R.N. DeJong, M.D.

On February 11, 1988, American neurology suffered a significant loss with the death of Dr. Thomas Richard Johns II. Born in West Virginia, he studied at Harvard Medical School and trained with Drs. Alpers and Merritt. Known as T.R. by his friends, he made major contributions to the field of neuromuscular disease, especially myasthenia gravis. As chairman of Neurology at the University of Virginia Medical Center since 1967, he was a fine leader and teacher. He held numerous important advisory positions in neurology; his advice was sought and appreciated by many. He had a history of heart disease, but kept on working until he died at his desk at the age of 63. We will all miss him.

Bruce Schoenberg, M.D., Dr. P.H., died on July 14, 1987, after a short illness. As Director of Neuroepidemiology at NINCDS, Dr. Schoenberg was in a unique position to promote international understanding of neurologic disorders by promoting cooperative studies of incidence and prevalence. At the time of his death he had helped to coordinate projects in many parts of the developed and undeveloped world. He was persistent and adamant in demanding the attention of neurologists and other health care professionals toward proper epidemiologic assessments. He was a major contributor to the latest revision of the ICD, was interested in the history of neurology, and was active in many other areas. Almost to the day of his untimely death he continued to write papers and advise colleagues on directions for present and future research. Although he was a true whirlwind of activity, he was always calm, friendly, and kind. He will be sorely missed.—A.F. Haerer, M.D.

Dr. Bruce Schoenberg was an amazing individual and a good friend to both Armin and me. In his own epidemiologic teams he was at least 4 to 5 SD from the mean. He had his hand in everything, or so it seemed. At meetings there he would be, illuminating all at the conference table both with his smile of greeting and his balanced, thoughtful common sense.—R.D. Currier, M.D.

Dr. A.B. Baker died on January 18, 1988, after a long illness. He was a first-rate example of the right man at the right time. He stimulated and prodded neurology, ignoring or bypassing those who impeded its growth, until he formed the larger than most believed possible, some say larger than life, neurologic establishment now existing in the United States.

Most didn't believe his predictions of growth or need. I didn't. But he was right and I wrong. He did other things, too.

When I was in medical school, my father one Sunday afternoon mused that "some of the young fellas down at French Lick were starting a new society." I suspect that he thought it was a good thing. Earlier, in the 1930s, he had written to the American Neurologic Association requesting a membership application and was duly notified that admission was by invitation only. There was no other neurologic organization in this country then.

Dr. Baker, Frank Forster, Ady Sahs, Russell DeJong, Pearce Bailey, Howard Fabing, and with the help of many others, started a new organization, the American Academy of Neurology. They, with Baker at the lead, stimulated the federal government to finance training programs in neurology. He and they are in a true sense, our founders. They fostered and promoted our growth. We owe them much.

Dr. Baker was known as a teacher, investigator, organizer, writer, and leader. He was prominent in the development of American neurology. Our sympathy goes to his wife and family.—R.D. Currier, M.D. and R.N. DeJong, M.D.

Ray Bauer, a good friend from Michigan days, died in March. Ray was a happy, friendly, competent neurologist at Wayne State University and when I first knew him, he was very interested in cerebrovascular disease. He developed a chronic illness in spite of which he in his later years founded the Michigan Parkinson Foundation, thus activating a situation of mutual regard and respect.

He was an exceptionally clear-thinking and honest man whose loss is felt by all who knew him.—R.D. Currier, M.D.

Robert D. Currier, M.D.

1 Diagnosis

The Utility of Cerebrospinal Fluid Examination in Patients With Partial Epilepsy
Thompson J, Salinsky M (Univ of Wisconsin, Madison)
Epilepsia 29:195–197, 1988   1–1

Computed tomography (CT) is especially effective in evaluating patients with partial seizure disorders, but the value of cerebrospinal fluid (CSF) analysis is uncertain. Of 95 patients with adult-onset partial epilepsy whose initial assessment included both CSF analysis and CT scanning, 24 had a CSF abnormality not temporally related to seizures. In 4 patients, CSF study confirmed subarachnoid hemorrhage; 19 patients had an isolated mild rise in CSF protein, 8 of whom had a structural lesion on CT. Follow-up of the other 11 patients for a mean of 5 years showed no evidence of a focal lesion or more frequent seizures.

The clinical significance of mildly elevated CSF protein in patients with partial seizure disorders is not clear. Examination of CSF does not appear to be necessary in the routine evaluation of new adult-onset partial seizure disorders as long as CT is performed. In none of the present patients did CSF analysis provide added diagnostic information unless it was specifically indicated, such as for suspected bleeding or multiple sclerosis.

▶ Here we find that a routine spinal fluid examination in patients with partial epilepsy is not helpful unless there are signs that would lead you to suspect subarachnoid hemorrhage or tumor. I can remember years ago having sharp discussions with a fellow resident, who had received part of her training elsewhere, about the necessity of spinal fluid examination as part of an epileptic work-up. She thoroughly believed in it.— R.D. Currier, M.D.

Neuro-Ophthalmological Complications of Coronary Artery Bypass Graft Surgery
Shaw PJ, Bates D, Cartlidge NEF, Heaviside D, French JM, Julian DG, Shaw DA (Univ. of Newcastle-upon-Tyne; Freeman Hosp, Newcastle-upon-Tyne, England)
Acta Neurol Scand 76:1–7, July 1987   1–2

Visual disorders are among the neurologic complications of heart surgery, but they are seldom reported. Because postoperative visual dysfunction is likely to distress the patient, it is important to identify the range of visual disorders that may develop after heart surgery. This study describes the postoperative ophthalmologic abnormalities that occurred in a series of 312 patients who had undergone coronary artery bypass graft (CABG) surgery.

Patients were assessed preoperatively by fundoscopy, confrontation visual field examination, Jaeger chart measurement of visual acuity, examination of eye movements, and evaluation of cortical aspects of visual function. Patients were assessed postoperatively and at 1 month and 6 months after operation. A control group of 50 patients scheduled for major peripheral vascular surgery were also evaluated preoperatively and postoperatively.

In approximately 25% of the study group postoperative neuro-ophthalmologic complications developed, including areas of retinal infarction, retinal emboli, visual field defects, reduction of visual acuity, and Horner's syndrome. In the control group that did not undergo extracorporeal circulation during surgery, there were no ophthalmologic complications. At 6 months, 10 patients still had detectable neuro-ophthalmologic abnormalities, but only those with persistent visual field defects had functional disability.

Because findings indicate that neuro-ophthalmologic complications can occur after CABG surgery, patients should be advised that they are at risk for these problems. Improvements in CABG procedures may make it possible to prevent the formation of microemboli.

▶ This study reveals that in one fourth of the patients who undergo CABG surgery some type of neuro-ophthalmologic complication develops. They should be informed of this possibility before surgery. Prolonged duration of heart disease and a major drop in hemoglobin level during surgery predispose to such complications.—R.N. DeJong, M.D.

Cerebral Blood Velocity in Subarachnoid Haemorrhage: A Transcranial Doppler Study

Compton JS, Redmond S, Symon L (Inst of Neurology, London)
J Neurol Neurosurg Psychiatr 50:1499–1503, 1987   1–3

Since radiologically identifiable spasm of the major intracranial arteries after subarachnoid hemorrhage (SAH) was first described in 1915, controversy has surrounded its prognosis, relationship to neurologic state, and effect on investigation and treatment. A study was done to examine the relationship between cerebral blood velocity, appearance of the cerebral vasculature on angiogram, cerebral blood flow, and patients' clinical condition and progress to determine its efficacy in confirming the presence of vasospasm.

Transcranial Doppler ultrasound was used to determine cerebral vasospasm after SAH in 20 patients. In addition, a control group of 21 healthy persons and a group of 26 patients with other intracranial pathologies were studied. The Doppler flow velocity was significantly higher when vasospasm was present. If it was higher than 100 cm/second, 80% of the patients had vasospasm. If it was lower than 100 cm/

second, fewer than 10% of patients had spasm. Doppler flow velocity did not increase after craniotomy in patients who did not have SAH. In patients with SAH there was a trend toward increased Doppler flow velocity, especially in patients in whom neurologic deficits developed. Doppler flow velocity and initial slope index (ISI) by xenon clearance did not correlate with clinical grade. The ISI/DFV quotient, which can be mathematically demonstrated to be related to vessel diameter, correlated well with clinical grade.

Transcranial Doppler ultrasonography is a noninvasive means of predicting the presence of angiographic vasospasm. Patients with preangiography Doppler flow velocities of greater than 100 cm/second are likely to have angiographic spasm.

▶ If an indirect method of finding vasospasm such as transcranial Doppler should in the long run prove to be useful in the management of those with SAH, then all we need is some way to combat the vasospasm when the Doppler picks it up.

The vasospasm of SAH increases the flow rate, but a decreased rate in the middle cerebral artery in unconscious children was a predictor of brain-stem death (Kirkham et al: *J Neurol Neurosurg Psychiatry* 50:1504–1513, 1987).—R.D. Currier, M.D.

Amaurosis Fugax in Teenagers: A Migraine Variant
Appleton R, Farrell K, Buncic JR, Hill A (Univ. of British Columbia; British Columbia's Children's Hosp, Vancouver; Univ of Toronto; The Hosp for Sick Children, Toronto)
Am J Dis Child 142:331–333, March 1988   1–4

Amaurosis fugax is sudden transient monocular loss of vision that disappears over several minutes. It is associated with atherosclerotic disease in adults, and cerebral angiography is often performed. The authors described amaurosis fugax in 5 teenagers.

Girl, 16, had a 1-year history of episodic right eye visual loss. She drew the pattern of expanding islands of visual loss (Fig 1–1). The episodes lasted for

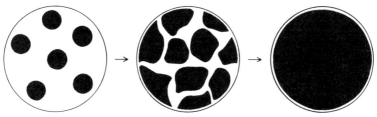

Fig 1–1.—Artist's impression of drawing by patient of pattern of visual loss that evolved over 2–3 minutes. (Courtesy of Appleton R, Farrell K, Buncic JR, et al: *Am J Dis Child* 142:331–333, March 1988.)

about 10 minutes. The patient had migraine headaches at other times. Examination, laboratory, and radiologic findings were all normal.

In these teenagers with amaurosis fugax, no underlying pathophysiologic basis could be determined. The characteristic pattern of visual loss suggested ischemia of the choroid. Prognosis was excellent. Therefore, in teenagers with amaurosis fugax and the characteristic pattern of visual loss, cerebral angiography is not indicated.

▶ These investigators express the belief that transient amaurosis fugax in adolescence is a migraine variant rather than an evidence of the presence of atherosclerosis, and that cerebral angiography should not be carried out in such patients.— R.N. DeJong, M.D.

Magnetic Resonance Imaging of Periventricular Hyperintensity in a Veterans Administration Hospital Population

Sarpel G, Chaudry F, Hindo W (Univ of Health Sciences/Chicago Med School)
Arch Neurol 44:725–728, July 1987   1–5

Magnetic resonance (MR) imaging is useful for the detection of pathologic alterations of the CNS, such as areas of periventricular hyperintensity (PVH). The MR studies of 60 male patients (most of them white) were retrospectively evaluated. Grades were assigned to MR patterns: 0, no PVH; 1, punctate hyperintense foci (caps); 2, only a thin band of PVH (stripes); 3a, caps and stripes less than 2 mm thick (Fig 1–2); 3b, caps and stripes more than 2 mm thick (Fig 1–3); 4, thick, irregular caps and stripes (Fig 1–4).

Of the 60 patients, 80% had PVH. Of the patients who were older than 50 years, 90% had PVH; of the younger patients, only 50% had PVH. Patterns 3b and 4 predicted abnormal neurologic examinations. The presence of PVH did not correlate with serum cholesterol level or a history of smoking, alcohol or drug use, hypertension, diabetes, transient ischemic attacks, or stroke. Diagnoses of atherosclerotic cardiovascular disease and malignant conditions both correlated with PVH.

Although the numbers in this study were too small to be conclusive, several clinical implications of PVH could be seen. The incidence of PVH is high in white men and increases with age. Only atherosclerotic disease and extracranial malignancy were correlated with PVH. Pattern 3a is the pattern most frequently seen. Patterns 0–3a were associated with normal neurologic examinations, while patterns 3b and 4 were associated with abnormal neurologic examination findings; however, those findings were relatively nonspecific.

▶ It seems that periventricular hyperintensity is quite common in older patients but not significant until it becomes severe (the 3b and 4 patterns), when it then is associated with cardiovascular disease and malignancy. The pathologic substrate is so far undefined.— R.D. Currier, M.D.

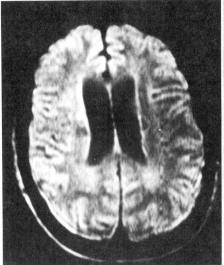
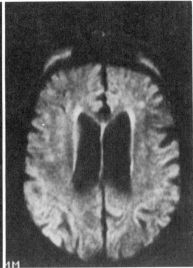
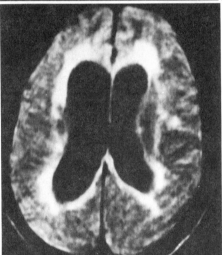

Fig 1–2 (above left).—Spin-echo image (echo time, 48 msec; relaxation time, 1800 msec) demonstrating pattern 3a. Diffuse, continuous, smooth, thin line of hyperintensity is seen along ventricles.

Fig 1–3 (above).—Spin-echo image (echo time, 56 msec; relaxation time, 1842 msec) demonstrating pattern 3b. Diffuse, smooth, thick line of hyperintensity is seen at ventricular border.

Fig 1–4 (left).—Spin-echo image (echo time, 56 msec; relaxation time, 1842 msec) demonstrating pattern 4. Diffuse, thick periventricular hyperintensity with irregular border is seen.

(Courtesy of Sarpel G, Chaudry F, Hindo W, et al.: *Arch Neurol* 44:723–728, July 1987.)

Do White Matter Changes on MRI and CT Differentiate Vascular Dementia From Alzheimer's Disease?

Erkinjuntti T, Ketonen L, Sulkava R, Sipponen J, Vuorialho M, Iivanainen M (Univ of Helsinki)
J Neurol Neurosurg Psychiatry 50:37–42, 1987   1–6

Twenty-nine patients with vascular dementia and 22 patients with Alzheimer's disease were assessed with magnetic resonance imaging (MRI) and computed tomography (CT) to evaluate white-matter changes as a method of discriminating between these two types of dementia. Vascular dementia was defined as dementia referable to disturbances in cerebral circulation, often associated with elevated blood pressure, abrupt onset, and stepwise deterioration. Alzheimer's disease was defined as progressive deterioration without findings referable to any other cause.

Moderate to severe white-matter changes were detected with MRI in all vascular dementia patients, while mostly mild white-matter changes were detected in 8 Alzheimer's patients. Infarcts were seen on MRI in 19 of the vascular dementia patients and on CT in 18. Infarcts were not seen on MRI or CT in any of the Alzheimer's patients. White-matter changes or infarcts detected by CT had a 97% sensitivity and a 96% specificity for a diagnosis of vascular dementia. White-matter changes detected with MRI had a 100% sensitivity and a 63% specificity.

White-matter changes seen on MRI and CT appear to be useful in the differential diagnosis of vascular and Alzheimer's dementia.

▶ Significant white-matter change observed on MRI scanning differentiates vascular dementia from Alzheimer's disease. The changes in Alzheimer's were mild, whereas changes with vascular dementia were in the 3b and 4 category of the previous article (see Abstract 1–5).

The diagnoses were made clinically, of course, but probably are valid, and one expects that this will in the long run be a useful laboratory test for differentiation of the two entities.—R.D. Currier, M.D.

Magnetic Resonance Imaging of the Central Nervous System
Council on Scientific Affairs
JAMA 259:1211–1222, Feb 26, 1988
1–7

Magnetic resonance imaging (MRI) has had a major impact on neurologic diagnosis. It now somewhat reduces the need for diagnostic computed tomography (CT). The applications of MRI of the brain and spinal cord were reviewed.

Magnetic resonance imaging can often visualize hypoxic lesions producing transient ischemic attacks and reversible ischemic neurologic deficits that were frequently missed by CT. Peri-infarct parenchyma that appears normal on CT scans often yields a pattern of abnormality on MRI that may relate to ischemic demyelinization or the ischemic penumbra surrounding the lesions. In a proportion of patients with systemic lupus erythematosus, lesions are seen on MRI that may be vasculitis or microinfarctions missed on CT. Both MRI and CT demonstrate intracerebral hemorrhages well; however, the MRI appearance depends on the age and size of the hemorrhage. In trauma, MRI can reveal most of the lesions seen on CT, except those of bone, and can demonstrate lesions missed by CT. A broad spectrum of intracranial tumors can be seen on MRI and CT; however, MRI often shows more extensive involvement than CT, particularly in cases of low-grade gliomas. Computed tomography detects meningiomas better than MRI. Such tumors may be missed by T_2-weighted MRI pulse sequences, but their extra-axial location, vascularity, and mass effect are usually visualized on T_1-weighted images. Magnetic resonance imaging is much better than CT in identifying all types of posterior fossa tumors and is the study of choice for brain-stem gliomas. It is also far superior to CT in identifying the lesions of multiple sclerosis and assessing patients with isolated optic neuritis. Magnetic resonance imaging should replace CT in evaluating patients with demyelinating disorders, and it has shown that Binswanger's disease may be a relatively common cause of adult-onset dementia. Abnormal patterns not well understood are visualized by MRI and not CT in patients with normal-pressure hydrocephalus. Otherwise, MRI is not superior to CT in evaluating demented patients. Because direct sagittal and coronal sections can be made, a wide spectrum of pathology of the cervicomedullary junction and cervical spinal cord is clearly seen on MRI.

Magnetic resonance imaging is the study of choice in assessing cervicomedullary and cervical spinal cord regions and will probably replace myelography of these areas. Its shortcomings include its expense, poor visualization of cortical bone, complicated hemorrhage images, its inability to differentiate edema from tumor, the relatively thick sections obtained, long scan times, contraindication in patients with cardiac pacemakers, and the complexity of its scan theory and interpretation.

Magnetic resonance imaging has had a major impact on the practice of neurology. It is superior to CT for imaging many diseases of the brain and spine, although it still has some shortcomings.

▶ Since its introduction in the early 1980s, magnetic resonance imaging has made a major impact into the practice of neurology. It has largely replaced computed tomography in diagnosing many diseases of the brain and spinal cord and may replace myelography as well.

A "Consensus Conference" on magnetic resonance imaging was published in the April 8, 1988 *Journal of the American Medical Association (JAMA* 259:2132–2138, 1988). The conference was cosponsored by the Division of Research Resources, the National Cancer Institute, the National Heart, Lung, and Blood Institute, the National Institute on Aging, the National Institute of Neurological and Communicative Disorders and Stroke of the National Institutes of Health, the Food and Drug Administration, and the National Institute of Mental Health. The investigators discussed the safety and efficacy of the technique, its contraindications and risks, its advantages and limitations, its indications, and the directions for future research. This is one of the most detailed and comprehensive reviews of magnetic resonance imaging available at this time.— R.N. DeJong, M.D.

Nuclear Magnetic Imaging in Multiple Sclerosis: Cystic Plaques and Prognosis

Weihe W, Manke A, Gowin W, Marisz G, Welter FL (Hardtwaldklinik, Zwesten, West Germany)
Nervenarzt 59:14–18, January 1988   1–8

Nuclear magnetic resonance (NMR) imaging is capable of visualizing cystic or lacunar defects in the walls of the lateral ventricle of patients with multiple sclerosis (MS). The lacunar defects appear as periventricular plaques of increased signal intensity with centers of decreased signal intensity. Other abnormal NMR findings characteristic of MS include a marked tendency to bilateral symmetry; multiple, round, oval, or band-shaped isolated lesions that show some preference for sites near the medullary layer but that can be found in all areas of the brain; more or less clearly marked inner and outer atrophy; and secondary degeneration of the corpus callosum (Fig 1–5).

In this study, 175 patients with a clinical diagnosis of MS underwent NMR imaging to determine whether the presence or absence of these lacunar defects has prognostic significance. The study population consisted of 52 (30%) men and 123 (70%) women with MS, with a mean age at MS onset of 31.4 years, a mean duration of MS of 10.4 years, and a mean disability score of 4.1 on a standard 10-point neurologic impairment rating scale. Patients in acute MS exacerbation were excluded from the study.

The clinical diagnosis of MS was confirmed by NMR imaging in 170 (97%) of the 175 patients. T_1-weighted images showed lacunar defects in

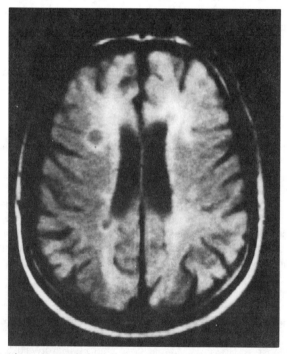

Fig 1–5.—Axial tomogram at the level of the ventricle (spin-echo 1600/35) of a 53-year-old woman (duration of illness, 3 years; disability score, 6). Cross-section of a lacunar defect with a central area of decreased signal intensity at the left anterior horn, the right posterior horn, and in the medullary layer, right. (Courtesy of Weihe W, Manke A, Gowin W, et al: *Nervenarzt* 59:14–18, January 1988.)

59 (34%) patients, whereas the other 116 (66%) patients met some of the NMR criteria of MS but had no evidence of lacunar defects. Of 116 patients without lacunar defects on NMR, 79 (68%) were still able to walk unassisted, 25 (22%) required assistance such as canes or walkers, and 12 (10%) needed a wheelchair to get around. In comparison, only 22 (37%) of the 59 patients with lacunar defects were still able to walk unassisted; 21 (36%) required assistance and 16 (27%) were wheelchair-bound. Within 10 years of MS onset, about one third (35%) of all patients with lacunar defects had become wheelchair-bound, and 58% had become so disabled that they could no longer walk unassisted. Conversely, of all 18 patients who became wheelchair-dependent within 10 years of MS onset, 11 (61%) had lacunar defects, while only 4 (13%) of 30 patients who were still ambulatory without assistance 11—20 years after MS onset had lacunar defects. Thus, a finding of lacunar defects was strongly prognostic for decreased ambulation.

Nuclear magnetic resonance examination to determine the presence or absence of lacunar defects in MS patients is strongly prognostic for neurologic disability at an early stage of the disease.

▶ If the MS patient has a round hole on MRI scan it is probably cystic degeneration and, according to the authors, the patient has highly active disease and a poor prognosis. One would have no argument with their findings.—R.D. Currier, M.D.

Predictive Testing for Huntington's Disease With Use of a Linked DNA Marker

Meissen GJ, Myers RH, Mastromauro CA, Koroshetz WJ, Klinger KW, Farrer LA, Watkins PA, Gusella JF, Bird ED, Martin JB (Massachusetts Gen Hosp, Harvard Univ, Boston Univ, McLean Hosp, Boston; Integrated Genetics Inc, Framingham, Mass)
N Engl J Med 318:535–542, March 3, 1988   1–9

The probability of carrying the gene for Huntington's disease can sometimes be estimated in the children of affected persons by identifying a specific DNA marker genetically linked to the gene. A study was done to develop and assess appropriate procedures for administering and following up the predictive test for Huntington's disease.

The series included 47 individuals at 50% risk of inheriting Huntington's disease who requested a presymptomatic or prenatal genetic-linked test between 1986 and 1988. All underwent pretest counseling and psychological and neurologic examinations. Nineteen persons later voluntarily withdrew from the study. Three D4S10 restriction-fragment-length polymorphisms produced by the *Hind*III, *Eco*RI, and *Bgl*I enzymes were used for all testing. The probability that an individual was a Huntington's disease carrier was then calculated. The test accuracy was compromised by a 4% recombination frequency between D4S10 and the Huntington's disease gene. Of 15 presymptomatic tests and 1 prenatal test completed, 4 yielded positive results; 7, negative; and 5, uninformative. Seven persons are awaiting test results. Those with positive test results experienced intermittent depression, but none required hospitalization or threatened to commit suicide. Five had a diagnosis of Huntington's disease on the basis of the neurologic examination.

Administering predictive tests for Huntington's disease is a complex, lengthy process. All persons in this study, regardless of their test results, indicated that they did not regret having had the test. Those whose test results were negative expressed profound relief.

▶ Although dabbling in the linkage business a bit myself, I still struggle to understand how DNA linkage marker research works.

After reading this article twice I am beginning to understand, and those of you who are still struggling are advised to look at this careful analysis, read it twice, and think about it.

Predictive testing by this method for Huntington's disease is not an easy task. It is complex, cumbersome, expensive, time-consuming, and useful in only a minority of families. The lay press, of course, has been misleading in their announcements of "a test" for Huntington's over the last several years. Some test.

For those looking for a reference on peroxisomal disorders (which Huntington's is not), we can recommend the review by Naidu, Moser, and Moser in *Pediatric Neurology* (4:5–12, 1988).—R.D. Currier, M.D.

Electroencephalographic Activity After Brain Death
Grigg MM, Kelly MA, Celesia GG, Ghobrial MW, Ross ER (Loyola Univ, Maywood, Ill)
Arch Neurol 44:948–954, September 1987   1–10

The reliability of the electroencephalogram (EEG) to confirm brain death continues to be controversial. A study was done to determine how often EEG activity persists in patients who fulfill all clinical criteria for brain death.

From January 1984 through May 1986, 56 patients were given the clinical diagnosis of brain death at 1 institution. All 56 had at least 1 EEG recording after this diagnosis. Eleven (20%) were found to have EEG activity after the diagnosis of brain death. The duration of the observed EEG activity was 2 to 168 hours, with a mean of 36.6 hours. Three patterns of EEG activity were noted. Low-voltage, 4 to 20 μV, theta or beta activity was recorded for 9 patients (16%) for as long as 72 hours after brain death. In 1 of these patients, neuropathologic studies revealed hypoxic-ischemic neuronal changes involving all cell layers of the cerebral cortex, basal ganglia, brain stem, and cerebellum. The second pattern noted was a sleep-like activity—a mixture of synchronous 30 to 40 μV theta and delta activity and 60 to 80 μV, 10 to 12 Hz spindle-like potentials. This was observed in 2 patients (3.6%) for as long

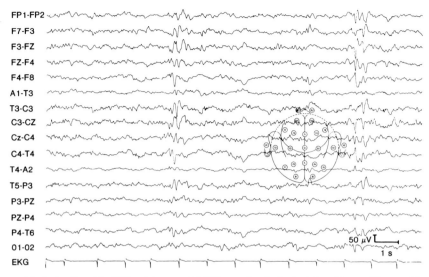

FP1-FP2
F7-F3
F3-FZ
FZ-F4
F4-F8
A1-T3
T3-C3
C3-CZ
Cz-C4
C4-T4
T4-A2
T5-P3
P3-PZ
PZ-P4
P4-T6
O1-O2
EKG

50 µV
1 s

Fig 1–6.—Sleep-like EEG activity recorded 56 hours after brain death in a 63-year-old man with brain stem infarction. Note medium voltage 20 to 50 µV, 4-Hz to 5-Hz theta, and 2-Hz to 3-Hz delta activity interrupted by frequent paroxysmal bursts of bilaterally synchronous, medium-to-high voltage 60 to 80 µV spindle-like potentials that resemble stage II sleep. No reactivity was noted. (Courtesy of Grigg MM, Kelly MA, Celesia GG, et al: *Arch Neurol* 44:948–954, September 1987.)

as 168 hours after brain death (Fig 1–6). Pathologic studies in both patients demonstrated ischemic necrosis of the brain stem with relative preservation of the cerebral cortex. The third pattern was an alpha-like activity—monotonous, unreactive, anteriorly predominant, 25 to 40 µV, 2 to 12 Hz activity—noted in 1 patient 3 hours after brain death. No patients recovered, irrespective of EEG activity. Using EEG activity after brain death as a confirmatory test of brain death may be of questionable value.

► It is clear now that the EEG criteria for brain death are not really helpful. These patients fulfilled all criteria for brain death with the exception of a lack of EEG activity. In 1 patient with EEG activity, autopsy showed complete necrosis of the brain stem and cerebellum.

Elimination of the EEG criterion for brain death, it seems, would be logical at this time. The British have not paid it much attention all along.—R.D. Currier, M.D.

Outcome Prediction in Comatose Patients: Significance of Reflex Eye Movement Analysis

Mueller-Jensen A, Neunzig H-P, Emskötter T (Univ of Hamburg)
J Neurol Neurosurg Psychiatry 50:389–392, 1987   1–11

Analysis of the oculomotor system is important in the diagnosis of brain-stem disorders. The oculocephalic response was compared with the

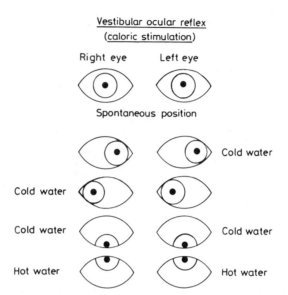

Fig 1–7.—Vestibulo-ocular reflex in horizontal and vertical directions after caloric stimulation. (Courtesy of Mueller-Jensen A, Neunzig H-P, Emskötter T: *J Neurol Neurosurg Psychiatry* 50:389– 392, 1987.)

vestibulo-ocular reflex (VOR) in 81 comatose patients to evaluate the usefulness of these variables in predicting patient outcome (Fig 1–7).

In 25 patients without an oculocephalic response or with inconclusive evidence of a response, VOR response was maintained. In general, VOR response provided more information than oculocephalic response. Of the patients without VOR, 92% died. Patients with a normal response had a

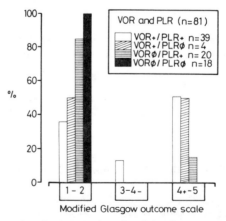

Fig 1–8.—Vestibulo-ocular reflex (VOR) and pupillary light reflex (PLR) responses in 81 patients, as measured on modified Glasgow outcome scale (Ø indicates absent response; +, preserved response). (Courtesy of Mueller-Jensen A, Neunzig H-P, Emskötter T: *J Neurol Neurosurg Psychiatry* 50:389– 392, 1987.)

good recovery in 67% of the cases. All patients without VOR and pupillary light reflex died (Fig 1–8).

These results indicate that in comatose patients with a VOR response, the assumption of a good outcome is justified. Loss of VOR indicates a poor outcome. Absent VOR and pupillary light reflex predicts a negative outcome in 100% of the cases, indicating the importance of these 2 brain-stem reflexes.

▶ So, the combination of an absent VOR (or caloric reflex) and a lost pupillary light reaction in a comatose patient is invariably fatal. I suppose one cannot hope yet for any such acceptable simplification of the rules regarding brain death, but this certainly is simpler to use than isotope flow studies, EEG, and arteriography.— R.D. Currier, M.D.

2 Cerebral Localization and Neurology of Behavior

The Frenchay Aphasia Screening Test: A Short, Simple Test for Aphasia Appropriate for Non-Specialists
Enderby PM, Wood VA, Wade DT, Hewer RL (Frenchay Hosp, Bristol, England)
Int Rehabil Med 8:166–170, 1987   2–1

Assessing whether and to what extent a patient is dysphasic is important in diagnosis and management. The Frenchay Aphasia Screening Test (FAST) is purported to be brief and simple to administer, useful on busy wards, reliable when used by nonspecialists, and reliable in identifying patients with aphasia. It does not differentiate different types of aphasia; rather, it is a clinical aid to be interpreted in light of other relevant information. The first studies on the validity and reliability of FAST were reviewed.

The FAST evaluates comprehension, expression, reading, and writing. It was developed for use with patients within days or weeks of an acute stroke. In an abbreviated version of the test, the reading and writing sections are omitted. Normative data were obtained by administering the FAST to 123 normal subjects. The provisional cutoff values of 27 points for those up to age 60 years and 25 points for those older than 60 years were derived; any score below these cutoff points was considered abnormal. The FAST was given to 50 stroke victims an average of 8 days after the stroke occurred to validate cutoff values. Based on cutoffs derived from normative data, there were 20 true positives, 14 false positives, 16 true negatives, and no false negatives. On the abbreviated version, these values were 20, 7, 23, and 0, respectively. Based on cutoff values derived from aphasic patients, there were 20 true positives, 7 false positives, 23 true negatives, and no false negatives. These values for the abbreviated version were 20, 3, 27, and 0, respectively. The test was also found to be valid when measuring severity. Interobserver reliability was statistically and clinically strong.

The FAST, which takes 3 to 10 minutes to administer, was found to be a valid and sensitive method of detecting aphasia in its full and abbreviated versions. Its 3 particular uses are to detect language disturbance when this may help localize a neurologic lesion, to detect aphasia when it is known to be a potential consequence of an identified lesion, and to screen for aphasia before giving other tests that rely on good linguistic function.

▶ The Frenchay Aphasia Screening Test is simple and easy to administer, and it can be administered by students, house officers, and other nonspecialists. It is valid and reliable. It may help to localize a neurologic lesion, to detect aphasia, and to screen for aphasia before administering other tests for language dysfunction.— R.N. DeJong, M.D.

A Short Test of Mental Status: Description and Preliminary Results
Kokmen E, Naessens JM, Offord KP, (Mayo Clinic, Rochester, Minn)
Mayo Clin Proc 62:281–288, April 1987   2–2

It is often desirable to assess the mental status of a patient in the course of a medical examination. A practical, short mental test was designed that can be administered and scored by any practitioner and can be given on an outpatient basis in about 5 minutes.

The test has 8 sections. The orientation section asks questions of a name and address nature. The attention section asks the patient to recall and repeat a series of 5 to 7 numbers. The learning section requires the recall of 4 words. The arithmetic calculation section poses one relatively simple problem each in multiplication, subtraction, division, and addition. The abstraction section measures the ability to interpret similarities in word pairs. The information section asks 4 common knowledge questions such as the number of weeks in a year. The construction section requires drawing a clock face showing 11:15 as the time, and copying a 3-dimensional cube (Fig 2–1). The final section tests recall of the 4 words originally introduced in the learning section. The scoring is simple, with 38 points being the highest possible score. The test must be given in the patient's native language.

The efficacy of the test was determined by administering it to 93 consecutive neurologic outpatients who were not suffering dementia, 67 outpatients who had Alzheimer-type dementia, and 20 outpatients with other types of dementia. The mean scores for the whole test, as well as for individual sections, were considerably higher for the group in which

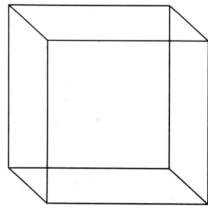

Fig 2–1.—Three-dimensional cube that patients are asked to copy in construction component of short test of mental status. (Courtesy of Kokman E, Naessens JM, Offord KP: *Mayo Clin Proc* 62:281–288, April 1987.)

dementia was not a problem. A total score of 29 of the possible 38 points was used as a screen for dementia. This criterion demonstrated a sensitivity of 92% and a specificity of 91%. In patients aged older than 60 years, a score below 30 resulted in 95% sensitivity and 88% specificity.

Although this test obviously should not be used as the sole means for diagnosing dementia, it can serve a valuable preliminary screening function. It is recommended that any score under 30 warrants further testing of mental stability. In some cases, the test profile may provide even more important diagnostic information than the total test score.

▶ We sorely need a short, reliable mental status test. This one, which can be performed in about 5 minutes in an outpatient setting, is said to have a high degree of specificity and sensitivity in screening for dementia. These authors should be congratulated for presenting this test to us. They warn that it should not be used as the sole means of diagnosing dementia.—R.N. DeJong M.D.

Clinical Determination of Mental Competence: A Theory and a Retrospective Study
Alexander MP (Boston Univ)
Arch Neurol 45:23–26, January 1988   2–3

Questions of competence frequently arise in the setting of rehabilitation neurology. A model was developed that defines the mental functions required for competent behavior. The first general property is the ability to recognize that a purposeful decision-making response is required. This is implicit in the capacity to understand all basic areas of human communication. In addition, a person must be able to activate the cognitive mechanisms underlying decision processing, and to implement competent behavior.

Ninety-two consecutive patients on a neurobehavioral service were studied for mental competence. Only 9 patients lacked functional limitations to competence, and 36 patients had multiple defects. The chief deficit was operational in 25 instances and general in 58. In only 11 cases were legal issues of competence raised, and these often were secondary to social factors rather than to intrinsically neurologic ones. The combination of profoundly disruptive emotional disturbance with aphasia was a frequent observation.

The model of competence based on analysis of individual cognitive operations will be clinically useful. Both general features of competence, cutting across all domains, and operational competence limited to a single cognitive domain are taken into account.

▶ In spite of its importance from a medicolegal point of view in assessing the results of rehabilitation, there are few published, organized tests for mental competence available. This study approaches the problem, but does not give a complete answer.—R.N. DeJong, M.D.

Traveler's Amnesia: Transient Global Amnesia Secondary to Triazolam

Morris HH III, Estes ML (Cleveland Clinic Found)
JAMA 258:945–946, Aug 21, 1987

2–4

Transient global amnesia (TGA) consists of a nontraumatic episode of anterograde amnesia that lasts several hours and then spontaneously clears. Triazolam is a benzodiazepine that has been reported to minimize jet lag. Transient global amnesia occurred in 3 neuroscientists who took triazolam, 0.5 mg, during a transatlantic flight to minimize jet lag. All also consumed alcohol.

All 3 individuals, aged 43, 45, and 33 years, respectively, experienced TGA that lasted for 8–11 hours. Because of their ages and health it is reasonable to attribute the TGA to the triazolam.

These episodes of TGA appeared secondary to the triazolam or to the combination of triazolam and alcohol. Caution should be exercised if triazolam is to be taken to avoid jet lag, especially if alcohol is consumed.

▶ Triazolam (Halcion), a rapidly acting benzodiazepine hypnotic, has recently been used to minimize the effects of "jet lag." When used in major dosage (0.5 mg), especially if taken at the same time as ethyl alcohol, it has been found to produce transient global amnesia. It should be used with caution, especially if alcoholic beverages are also to be consumed.—R.N. DeJong, M.D.

Rapid Eye Movement Sleep Behavior Disorder: A Treatable Parasomnia Affecting Older Adults

Schenck CH, Bundlie SR, Patterson AL, Mahowald MW (Minnesota Regional Sleep Disorders Ctr, Hennepin County Med Ctr, Univ of Minnesota, Minneapolis)
JAMA 257:1786–1789, Apr 3, 1987

2–5

In a previous study, 5 patients were described with rapid eye movement (REM) sleep behavior disorder (RBD), which is a behavioral deviation from the state of muscular flaccid paralysis characteristic of normal REM sleep. Individuals become physically active, sometimes violent, in their attempts to act out REM sleep dreams; RBD is easily misdiagnosed as obstructive sleep apnea, psychiatric disturbance, or nocturnal epilepsy. Five additional such patients with RBD were seen. Cumulative experience with all 10 patients was reviewed.

Each patient underwent a comprehensive neuropsychological evaluation. Sleep laboratory data were collected by monitors including videotape, electrooculogram, electroencephalogram, electromyography, electrocardiogram, and nasal air flow measurement. All patients but 1 were male, and the mean age at which RBD became troublesome was 62 years. A typical case is described.

Man, 57, began talking, yelling, moving about, and sitting up while asleep after 52 years of sleeping normally. After 2 years, his behavior escalated to punch-

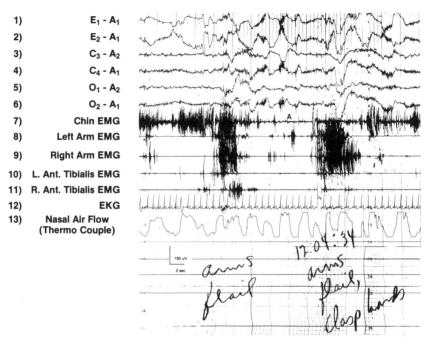

1)	$E_1 - A_1$
2)	$E_2 - A_1$
3)	$C_3 - A_2$
4)	$C_4 - A_1$
5)	$O_1 - A_2$
6)	$O_2 - A_1$
7)	Chin EMG
8)	Left Arm EMG
9)	Right Arm EMG
10)	L. Ant. Tibialis EMG
11)	R. Ant. Tibialis EMG
12)	EKG
13)	Nasal Air Flow (Thermo Couple)

Fig 2–2.—Polygraphic correlates of complex movements during rapid eye movement (REM) sleep. Rapid eye movements (1 and 2) and activated electroencephalogram (3–6) are present. Chin (7) electromyogram (EMG) has augmented tone except for intermittent suppression *(A)* between bursts of limb twitching (8–11) (*L Ant* indicates left anterior; *R Ant,* right anterior). Premature ventricular contractions are present on the electrocardiogram (12). Air flow (13) has characteristic REM irregularity. Paper speed, 10 mm/s. (Courtesy of Schenck CH, Bundlie SR, Patterson AL, et al: *JAMA* 257:1786–1789, Apr 3, 1987.)

ing, kicking, and leaping from bed, sometimes every night of the week. The episodes always happened at least 2 hours after falling asleep, and were attempted enactments of vivid and threatening dreams. On various occasions, he hurt himself or his wife, and once put his fist through a wall. He finally resorted to using a sleeping bag, particularly when traveling on business. His waking behavior was relatively placid, and neurologic and psychiatric examination results were normal. However, his extraordinary REM sleep activities were well-documented in the sleep laboratory (Fig 2–2). This man and the other patients in the study were treated with 0.50 mg of clonazepam at bedtime, which effectively controlled both disturbing dreams and RBD.

A brief screening for abnormal sleep behavior should be a part of routine medical history taking, particularly for older adults and anyone with disorders of the central nervous system. Practitioners should be aware of RBD and refer possible patients to a sleep disorders center that is equipped to differentiate RBD from other sleep abnormalities.

► About 2 decades ago the existence and significance of REM sleep was just being recognized. About 1 decade ago sleep disorders laboratories and centers were just being established. Now we are told of a new syndrome, the manifestations of which occur during REM sleep and the clinical-pathologic features of which become apparent in a sleep disorders laboratory. In this condition, intermittent loss of electromyographic atonia occurs during REM sleep and is accompanied by complex and vigorous behavior such as punching, kicking, leaping from bed, and sometimes inflicting injury on oneself or others. Polysomnographic studies confirmed the diagnosis. This disturbed sleep syndrome often was associated with various neurologic, but not psychiatric, disorders. Fortunately, treatment with clonazepam induced rapid and sustained improvement in 7 patients, as did desipramine hydrochloride in another.—R.N. DeJong, M.D.

Mood Disorder and Multiple Sclerosis
Joffe RT, Lippert GP, Gray TA, Gordon Sawa G, Horvath Z (St Michael's Hosp, Toronto; Univ of Toronto)
Arch Neurol 44:376–378, April 1987   2–6

Several studies have described an association between multiple sclerosis (MS) and mood disorders. One hundred patients with MS were examined for the features and occurrence of affective disorder.

A lifetime history of depression was found in 42% of the patients. According to Research Diagnostic Criteria, 13% of the patients had a diagnosis of bipolar disorder (table), significantly higher than the 1% prevalence in the general population. Only 28 patients were completely free from psychiatric disorders, and these patients were more functionally impaired.

A high prevalence of affective disorders was found in this series of patients with MS. There appears to be no direct relation between functional impairment and mood disorder. Further studies are necessary to evaluate the use of antidepressives in the treatment of mood disorders associated with MS.

Prevalence of Current and Past
Psychiatric Disorders in Patients With
Multiple Sclerosis*

Disorder	Current	Past
Major depression	14	47
Minor depression	1	9
Intermittent depression	1	4
Hypomania	1	2
Bipolar disorder	0	13
Generalized anxiety	2	3
Panic anxiety	1	5
Schizophrenia	0	0

*Based on Research Diagnostic Criteria.
(Courtesy of Joffe RT, Lippert GP, Gray TA, et al: Arch Neurol 376–378, April 1987.)

▶ This interesting study of the psychiatric evaluation of patients with multiple sclerosis shows a very high prevalence of affective illness, both recurrent depression and bipolar affective disorder, in patients with multiple sclerosis. The association between mood disorder and multiple sclerosis suggests that these disorders may share common neurologic and biochemical mechanisms. There are very little data on the use of antidepressants in the treatment of depression associated with the disease except for many studies by Schiffer et al. (*Am J Psychiatry* 143:94–95, 1986). Further studies would be of benefit.—R.N. DeJong, M.D.

Mamillary Body Atrophy in Wernicke's Encephalopathy: Antemortem Identification Using Magnetic Resonance Imaging
Charness ME, DeLaPaz RL (Univ of California, San Francisco)
Ann Neurol 22:595–600, November 1987   2–7

Wernicke's encephalopathy, occurring commonly in alcoholics, results from thiamine deficiency. It is diagnosed in fewer than 0.04%–0.13% of hospitalized patients, yet its unique neuropathologic lesions are found at autopsy in 0.8%–2.8% of the population and in up to 12.5% of alcoholics. Those patients with Wernicke's encephalopathy who currently elude diagnosis may be identified by imaging techniques. Magnetic resonance imaging (MRI) was used to determine the volume of the mamillary bodies in 3 groups of patients.

Patients were selected by chart review at 2 institutions. Nine patients with chronic Wernicke's encephalopathy, 7 patients with presumed Alzheimer's disease, and 37 control subjects were studied. All measurements were made with T_1-weighted images. The mean mamillary body volume in patients with Wernicke's encephalopathy was 21.3 ± 5.8 mm^3; in patients with Alzheimer's disease, 40.1 ± 3.7 mm^3; and in control subjects, 51.7 ± 2.5 mm^3. Seventy-eight percent of the patients with Wernicke's encephalopathy had smaller mamillary bodies than 36 of the 37 control subjects and all of the patients with Alzheimer's disease. The decrease in mamillary body volume was not related to patient age or the degree of ventricular enlargement. It most likely reflects the mamillary body atrophy grossly apparent at autopsy in up to 81% of patients with Wernicke's encephalopathy. The MRI technique provides a means of identifying the most specific macroscopic lesion of Wernicke's encephalopathy.

▶ With the right MRI cut it seems that Wernicke's encephalopathy can be diagnosed and differentiated from Alzheimer's disease. How reliable this is remains to be determined.

One of the questions unanswered in stroke risk analysis is, What is it about alcoholism that predisposes to stroke? Helzer (*J Consult Clin Psychol* 55:284–292, 1987) recently has summarized the epidemiology of alcoholism rather well, and Tabakoff et al. (*N Engl J Med* 318:135–139, 1988) have found a higher inhibition of monamine oxidase by ethanol in the platelets of alcoholics.—R.D. Currier, M.D.

3 Dementia

Zinc Selectively Blocks the Action of *N*-Methyl-D-Aspartate on Cortical Neurons
Peters S, Koh J, Choi DW (Stanford Univ)
Science 236:589–593, May 1, 1987   3–1

Zinc may have a signaling function in mammalian central excitatory neurotransmission. Large amounts of zinc are present in synaptic vesicles of excitatory boutons. To determine the function of zinc in this setting, the effect of zinc on cultures of dissociated mouse cortical cells in a zinc-free buffer was examined.

Pressure ejection of N-methyl-D-aspartate (NMDA), quisqualate, or kainate produced depolarizing responses. Zinc alone, in concentrations up to 1 mM, produced no response. However, zinc produced a concentration-dependent, rapid-onset, reversible attenuation of the membrane response to NMDA, homocysteate, and quinolinate. Zinc potentiated the membrane response to quisqualate and to α-amino-3-hydroxy-5-methyl-4-isoxazolepropionate. Zinc did not affect the cellular response to kainate. Zinc attenuated NMDA receptor-mediated neurotoxicity, but not quisqualate or kainate toxicity.

Zinc appears able to modulate the postsynaptic response to excitatory amino acid transmitters. It is likely that corelease of zinc and glutamate would lower the proportion of NMDA channels activated, which could alter neurotransmission. Zinc may be involved in regulating lasting synaptic changes. Endogenous zinc might also serve to protect against NMDA neurotoxicity. A defect in this system would then produce the pattern of neural death seen in Huntington's disease.

▶ Dr. Stephen E. Nadeau, Assistant Professor of Neurology, Department of Neurology, University of Mississippi School of Medicine, Jackson, comments on this interesting study.—R.D. Currier, M.D.

▶ Localization of the genetic defect in Huntington's disease to the short arm of chromosome 4 has raised the hope of ultimately determining the pathogenesis of this disease through DNA mapping. However, this prospect remains several years in the future and in the meantime, work proceeds apace on other approaches to the problem. One of the most promising avenues of investigation has focused on the possible role of excitatory amino acid neurotransmitters in the neuronal destruction of Huntington's disease. The remarkable findings reported by Choi and colleagues constitute a major advance in this area and provide strong support for the validity of this investigatory approach.—S.E. Nadeau, M.D.

Huntington's Disease: Correlations of Mental Status With Chorea

Webb M, Trzepacz PT (Univ of Pittsburgh)
Biol Psychiatry 22:751–761, June 1987   3–2

Huntington's disease (HD) causes progressive deterioration of the brain. Psychiatric symptoms are common. The authors studied 10 patients with HD using the Choreometer, a simple instrument to objectively detect chorea, as well as several psychiatric assessments, including the Schedule for Affective Disorders and Schizophrenia, the Mini-Mental State examination, the Wechsler Memory Scale, and the Booklet Categories Test.

The patients were divided into 3 groups: psychiatric onset, chorea onset, and mixed onset. The mean age of the chorea-onset group was 22 years at onset, and mean age of the other 2 groups was older than 40 years at onset. In the early course of the disorder, personality disorders, explosive disorders and organic affective disorders were common; later, dementia was the most common diagnosis. An abnormal Wechsler Memory Quotient was found in 80% of patients, and 80% were severely impaired in the Categories Test. Only 50% of patients demonstrated abnormal results on the Mini-Mental State examination. On the Choreometer, 80% of patients had scores in the abnormal range. There was a significant correlation between Choreometer score and the duration of chorea, as well as the Wechsler Memory Quotient and the Categories Test score.

This study related chorea to psychological disturbance, and showed that the psychological manifestations of HD change over time. There appears to be an association between chorea severity and cognitive/behavioral change, which implies that the deterioration of the basal ganglia may directly relate to the psychiatric complications of HD.

▶ It has long been assumed that there is no relationship between the severity of the chorea and the degree of psychiatric involvement, especially memory impairment, in patients with Huntington's disease. These investigators, however, find that there is a close relationship between these 2 separate manifestations of the disorder.—R.N. DeJong, M.D.

Clinical and Neuropathologic Assessment of Severity in Huntington's Disease

Myers RH, Vonsattel JP, Stevens TJ, Cupples LA, Richardson EP, Martin JB, Bird ED (Boston Univ, Massachusetts Gen Hosp, Harvard Univ, Boston)
Neurology 38:341–347, March 1988   3–3

The extent of the neuropathologic involvement of the striatum of patients with Huntington's disease varies widely. The factors associated with this variation have not been defined. A study was done to examine the relationship of the extent of neuropathologic involvement with 4 variables in the clinical expression of Huntington's disease: age at onset,

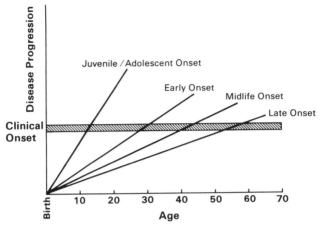

Fig 3–1.—The close association between age at onset and rate of disease progression produces a model for expression of the HD gene whereby a single mechanism determines both age at onset and rate of progression. By this model, a cumulative effect of the gene may proceed at different rates, thereby reaching a threshold for toxic effects and clinical onset at different ages. A rapid process of accumulation produces both earlier onset and a rapid course; a slow process of accumulation results in a late onset and slow course. This model suggested that the gene for HD is expressed at an early age and that the clinical manifestation is delayed. (Courtesy of Myers RH, Vonsattel JP, Stevens TJ, et al: *Neurology* 38:341–347, March 1988.)

sex of affected parent, degree of functional disability, and duration of illness.

Postmortem brain specimens from 163 persons with the clinical diagnosis of Huntington's disease were studied. The specimens were graded on a 5-point scale for degree of neuropathologic involvement in the striatum. Disease onset between the ages of 4 and 19 years of age was associated with a very severe neuropathologic involvement produced by an apparent rapid degenerative process. Cases of early onset—between 20 and 34 years of age—and midlife onset—between 35 and 49 years of age—had respectively less severe striatal involvement, which suggests a slower degenerative progression. There were high correlations among the grade of neuropathologic involvement, cell counts of neurons, and a rating of physical disability, which suggests that each represents a common underlying degenerative process of the disease. The relationship between age at disease onset and extent of neuropathologic involvement implies that a single mechanism may determine both onset and rate of degenerative disease progression (Fig 3–1).

In this study, the degree of neuropathologic severity of striatal involvement was found to be related to age of onset, sex of affected parent, disease duration, and clinical physical disability rating. It was proposed that a single mechanism determined both the age at disease onset and the rate of neuropathologic progression of the disease.

▶ These investigators, in a careful study comparing neuropathologic involvement with clinical symptomatology in patients with Huntington's disease, found a high correlation between the grade of neuropathologic involvement and the severity and rate of progression of disease. In patients with juvenile or adolescent onset (4 to 19 years of age), there were severe neuropathologic changes in the striatum and a rapid degenerative process. In early and mid-adult life (20 to 49 years), there was less severe striatal involvement and slower degenerative progression. The relationship between age of onset and extent of neuropathologic involvement suggests that a single mechanism may determine both onset and rate of degenerative disease progression.—R.N. DeJong, M.D.

Types of Multi-Infarct Dementia

Erkinjuntti T, (Univ of Helsinki)
Acta Neurol Scand 75:391–399, June 1987   3–4

Vascular dementia is the second most common cause of dementia. Because it can be caused by more than 1 pathophysiologic mechanism, there have been attempts to subdivide this syndrome. Data were reviewed on 79 patients with multiinfarct dementia (MID) and an attempt made to categorize them as having cortical or subcortical MID on the basis of computed tomographic (CT) scans.

Cortical MID was characterized by multiple strokes, sensory/motor hemiparesis, severe aphasia, and abrupt cognitive failure. Atrial fibrillation and coronary disease were more common in the cortical MID group (table). Subcortical MID was characterized by lacunar strokes, dysarthria, motor hemiparesis, depression, and emotional lability. White-matter low attenuation was seen in all patients in the subcortical MID group and in more than 60% of all patients in the cortical MID group.

Frequency of Cardiovascular Disorders, A History
of Stroke and Other Cerebrovascular Episodes in
Patients With Cortical and Subcortical Multiinfarct
Dementia (Percentages in Parentheses)

	Cortical MID N=65	Subcortical MID N=14
Coronary heart disease	32 (49.2)	3 (21.4)
Myocardial infarct	21 (32.3)	2 (14.3)
Cardiac failure	42 (64.6)	7 (50.0)
Arterial hypertension	36 (55.4)	9 (64.3)
All cardiac arrhythmias	33 (50.8)	6 (42.9)
Atrial fibrillation	26 (40.0)	1 (7.1) *
Stroke	57 (87.7)	10 (71.4)
Other acute cerebrovascular episodes	25 (38.5)	5 (35.7)

Cortical MID vs. subcortical MID: *= $p < 0.05$.

(Courtesy of Erkinjuntii T: *Acta Neurol Scand* 75:391–399, June 1987.)

Computed tomographic scans showed the same number of deep infarcts in both groups.

There were no differences between these 2 groups in stroke risk, ischemia, and CT findings. Thus, it is not clear that subcortical and cortical MID are really 2 distinct syndromes.

▶ Because patients with cortical multi-infarct dementia (repeated atherothrombotic and cardiogenic strokes, hemiparesis, severe aphasia, and cognitive failure) and those with subcortical multi-infarct dementia (history of lacunal strokes, bulbar signs, depression, and emotional lability) overlap with each other in ischemic scores and findings on neurologic examination, the authors think that it is still an open question that these 2 varieties of multi-infarct and Binswanger's disease are different or merely represent biological variations having the same etiopathogenesis.—R.N. DeJong, M.D.

Vacuolar Change in Alzheimer's Disease
Smith TW, Anwer U, DeGirolami U, Drachman DA (Univ of Massachusetts, St Vincent Hospital, Worcester, Mass)
Arch Neurol 44:1225–1228, December 1987   3–5

Several Alzheimer's disease patients were seen in whom neuropathologic examination revealed a striking vacuolar change, in addition to the usual histologic changes in Alzheimer's disease. This vacuolar change was essentially morphologically identical to the spongiform change observed in Creutzfeldt-Jakob disease and was almost wholly confined to the medial temporal cortex. These observations prompted a retrospective neuropathologic study of 66 cases of histologically confirmed Alzheimer's disease to determine the frequency, anatomical distribution, and intensity of vacuolar change.

Histologic sections from the brains of these patients, aged 55 to 94 years, were retrieved from autopsy files. None had a clinical diagnosis of Creutzfeldt-Jakob disease. Ten nondemented patients comprised a comparison group. In 50 (76%) of the 66 brains with Alzheimer's disease, vacuolar change was seen. In all 50, the change was observed in the medial temporal isocortex, primarily the parahippocampal and fusiform gyri, and also frequently in the amygdala (Fig 3–2). Vacuolar change was also seen in the insula in a few cases. Vacuole distribution was throughout layers 2 to 6 of the cortex in these regions. The intensity of the vacuolar change ranged from slight in 54% of the patients, to moderate in 24%, to severe in 22%. None of the aged control brains had vacuolar changes. In a combined group of Alzheimer's disease and nondemented aged brain specimens, a strong correlation was seen between the presence of vacuolar change and large numbers of grade 3 to 4+ neuritic plaques and neurofibrillary tangles. Also, an association was seen between vacuolar change and the presence of gliosis.

This study demonstrated that a vacuolar change virtually identical in light microscopic appearance to the spongiform change characterizing

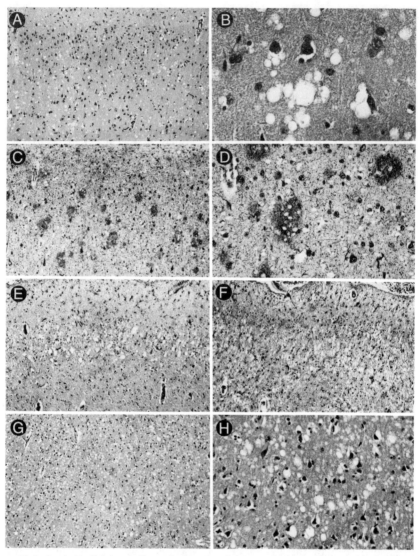

Fig 3–2.—A–D, Alzheimer's disease. Section of medial temporal lobe showing vacuolar change and neuritic plaques in cortex [hematoxylin-eosin, (original magnification, ×60 (**A**), original magnification, ×230 (**B**), Bielschowsky, original magnification, ×60 (**C**), original magnification, ×140 (**D**)]. **E,** Alzheimer's disease. Microvacuolation in upper layers of isocortex (hematoxylin-eosin, original magnification, ×60). **F,** Alzheimer's disease. Status spongiosus (hematoxylin-eosin, original magnification, ×60). **G** and **H,** Creutzfeldt-Jakob disease. Section of frontal cortex showing characteristic spongiform change [hematoxylin-eosin, original magnification, ×60 (**G**), original magnification, ×140 (**H**)]. (Courtesy of Smith TW, Anwer U, DeGirolami U, et al: *Arch Neurol* 44:1225–1228, December 1987.)

Creutzfeldt-Jakob disease may be seen in Alzheimer's disease. Since vacuolar change does not invariably occur in Alzheimer's disease, it may represent a subtype of this disorder or a variant of the pathologic change that can occur. Its relationship to Creutzfeldt-Jakob disease and other slow virus disorders is not known.

▶ The etiology of Alzheimer's disease is still unknown. This article demonstrates that in some cases of Alzheimer's disease, there are vacuolar changes similar to those found in Creutzfeldt-Jakob disease. This latter disease has been found to be caused by a slowly acting viral infection. Further studies are needed to determine whether Alzheimer's is also of viral origin.— R.N. DeJong, M.D.

Alzheimer's Disease and Other Dementing Illnesses in a Defined United States Population: Incidence Rates and Clinical Features
Schoenberg BS, Kokmen E, Okazaki H (Mayo Clinic, Rochester, Minn)
Ann Neurol 22:724–729, December 1987   3–6

Although dementia has long been recognized as a common symptom among the elderly, this condition has only recently received epidemiologic investigation. Because of problems involved in surveying dementia, incidence data are only available for a few selected populations. A study was done to determine the incidence rates and clinical features of dementia in the entire population of Rochester, Minnesota.

A unique records-link system available for residents of this small city was used. This system comprised medical data sources inside and outside of the Mayo Clinic and involved all medical facilities in the area, including nursing homes, state medical institutions, and private practitioners. The records of Rochester residents with a diagnosis suggestive of dementia were reviewed. In an average annual at-risk population of 18,991 people older than age of 29 years, in 178 dementia developed between 1960 and 1964. Thus, the average annual incidence rate in this population was 187.5 new cases per 100,000 per year. Alzheimer's disease was the most common cause of dementia in this community. The corresponding rate for clinically or pathologically diagnosed Alzheimer's disease or both was 123.3 new cases per 100,000 per year, based on 117 cases. The incidence rates for dementia in general and Alzheimer's disease in particular increased markedly with age. All patients were followed until they died or until 1982. Median survival was 63 months.

This study is the first to document all new cases of Alzheimer's disease and other dementing illnesses in a well-defined U.S. community. Although the data include only those who came to medical attention, the incidence rates found were higher than in studies from Scandinavia.

▶ This is the first reliable study of the incidence of dementia in a well-defined American community. The incidence rate for dementia in general was 187.5 new cases per 100,000 per year, and for Alzheimer's disease, the most common type encountered currently, 123.3 new cases per 100,000 per year. This is an important investigation, and it gives essential statistical information.—R.N. DeJong, M.D.

Early-Onset Alzheimer's Disease: Clinical Predictors of Institutionalization and Death

Heyman A, Wilkinson WE, Hurwitz BJ, Helms MJ, Haynes CS, Utley CM, Gwyther LP (Duke Univ)

Neurology 37:980–984, June 1987

3–7

Studies were made of 92 noninstitutionalized patients with early-onset Alzheimer's disease whose diagnoses were based on a history of progressive dementia and impairment in several areas of cognitive function. Follow-up for 2 years or longer was possible for 79 patients, and 39 patients were followed for 5 years.

The mean patient age at admission to the study was 61 years for the 30 men and 63 years for 62 women. Symptoms had begun at an estimated age of 58 years. Mortality at 5 years was 24%, compared with an expected rate for an age- and sex-matched United States population of 9.5%. Fifty-four patients were admitted to nursing homes during follow-up. Language ability at entry into the study was predictive of later institutionalization and death. Scores on a brief screening test of cognitive function and overall clinical dementia ratings also were predictive of institutional care and mortality. Younger patients with severe cognitive impairment were at the highest risk of both death and the need for institutionalization.

These patients with early-onset Alzheimer's disease followed a rapidly progressive course. Nearly two thirds of such patients can be expected to enter a nursing home within 8 years of the first manifestations of dementia, and one third can be expected to die within 3 years of institutionalization. It remains unclear whether the course is more rapid than that of patients having late-onset disease.

▶ This is a study of the demographic, clinical, and neuropsychological features of early-onset Alzheimer's disease. The language ability of patients on admission to the study, their scores on a test of cognitive functions, and their overall rating on tests for dementia were found to predict their subsequent institutional care and death. Age had a significant modifying effect on these predicting factors: the younger patients with more cognitive impairment had an earlier institutional age and earlier death.—R.N. DeJong, M.D.

The Genetic Defect Causing Familial Alzheimer's Disease Maps on Chromosome 21

St George-Hyslop PH, Tanzi RE, Polinsky RJ, Haines JL, Nee L, Watkins PC, Myers RH, Feldman RG, Pollen D, Drachman D, Growdon J, Bruni A, Foncin J-F, Salmon D, Fromme HP, Amaducci L, Sorbi S, Piacentini S, Stewart GD,

Hobbs WJ, Conneally PM, Gusella JF (Harvard Univ; Natl Inst of Neurological and Communicative Disorders and Stroke, Bethesda, Md; Indiana Univ; Integrated Genetics Inc; Boston Univ, et al)
Science 235:885–890, Feb 20, 1987   3–8

Alzheimer's disease (AD) is a degenerative disorder of the human CNS, characterized by progressive impairment of memory and intellectual function. There is no known treatment effective in preventing or arresting the neurodegenerative process of AD. An understanding of the biochemical basis of the disorder would clearly facilitate attempts to develop useful therapies.

The occasional observation of more than 1 affected member in a single family does not necessarily imply that AD is inherited. However, it has been documented that several large families display autosomal dominant transmission of the disorder. In these pedigrees, the familial form of AD (FAD) is clearly the result of a genetic defect. Using genetic linkage to DNA markers on chromosome 21, the chromosomal location of this defective gene has been discovered. Importantly, the localization on chromosome 21 provides an explanation for the occurrence of Alzheimer's disease–like pathology in Down's syndrome.

Isolation and characterization of the gene at this locus may provide new insights into the nature of the defect causing FAD and possibly into the etiology of all forms of AD.

▶ Several families have been described in which Alzheimer's disease is caused by an autosomal dominant gene defect located on chromosome 21. The defect was found by using DNA markers. This localization on chromosome 21 provides an explanation for the Alzheimer's disease–like pathology in Down's syndrome. The isolation and localization of the gene on this locus may yield new insights into the nature of the defect causing familial Alzheimer's disease.—R.N. DeJong, M.D.

Dementia of the Alzheimer Type: Clinical and Family Study of 22 Twin Pairs

Nee LE, Eldridge R, Sunderland T, Thomas CB, Katz D, Thompson KE, Weingartner H, Weiss H, Julian C, Cohen R (Natl Inst of Communicative Disorders and Stroke, Natl Cancer Inst, Bethesda, Md; Brigham and Women's Hosp, Boston; Natl Inst of Mental Health, Bethesda, Md; Albert Einstein School of Medicine, et al)
Neurology 37:359–363, March 1987   3–9

The familial form of Alzheimer's disease may account for 33% of all affected patients. Twin studies might provide information on the relationship between genetic and environmental factors in the etiology of this disease. If genetic factors are the most important, higher concordance in monozygotic (MZ) than in dizygotic (DZ) twins would be expected.

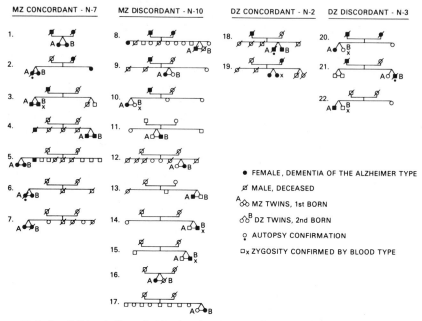

Fig 3–3.—Alzheimer's disease in 22 twin pairs. (Courtesy of Nee LE, Eldridge R, Sunderland T, et al: *Neurology* 37:359–363, March 1987.)

Twenty-two twin pairs in which at least 1 twin had Alzheimer's disease were studied.

Of 17 MZ pairs, 7 were concordant. Of 5 DZ pairs, 2 were concordant (Fig 3–3). The concordance rates were 41% for MZ and 40% for DZ twins. Females had a significantly older mean age at onset.

The incidence of Alzheimer's disease in this series cannot be explained fully by a single autosomal dominant gene. Disease expression seems to be delayed in females. Further study of more sets of twins is necessary to verify these findings.

▶ This study supports the belief that, etiologically, Alzheimer's disease cannot be accounted for by a single autosomal dominant gene. Under certain genetic circumstances, disease expression may be delayed in women.—R.N. DeJong, M.D.

4 Stroke

Risk Factors for Ischemic Stroke: A Prospective Study in Rochester, Minnesota
Davis PH, Dambrosia JM, Schoenberg BS, Schoenberg DG, Pritchard DA, Lilienfeld AM, Whisnant JP (Natl Inst of Neurological and Communicative Disorders and Stroke, Bethesda, Md.; Univ of Queensland, Australia; Mayo Clinic and Found, Rochester, Minn)
Ann Neurol 22:319–327, September 1987   4–1

Major risk factors of stroke have been shown to include hypertension, cardiovascular disease such as coronary heart disease (CHD), congestive heart failure (CHF), left ventricular hypertrophy on EKG, and diabetes mellitus. A study was done to elucidate the relative importance of these stroke risk factors and to explore their relationship to time-to-stroke occurrence using a time-dependent multivariate regression model.

A cohort of 1,804 residents of Rochester, Minnesota, was followed for 13 years. The participants were at least 50 years old, were free of stroke, and underwent an initial examination at the Mayo Clinic in 1960. One hundred ten first ischemic strokes and 616 deaths without stroke occurred during the follow-up period. The time of onset or the time of diagnosis of potential risk factors was determined for all patients. Using these data, a proportional hazards model of time to occurrence of stroke with time-dependent risk factors was constructed. The model considered 2 fixed and 6 time-dependent risk factors. Individual relative risks for each were 1.6 for age (per 10 years), 2.0 for men, 4.0 for definite hypertension, 3.9 for transient ischemic attacks, 2.2 for hypertensive heart disease, 2.2 for coronary heart disease, 1.7 for congestive heart failure, and 1.7 for diabetes mellitus. Atrial fibrillation was found not to be a significant risk factor using time-dependent multivariate analysis.

The important time-dependent risk factors in this series were found to be, in descending order by relative risk: definite hypertension, transient ischemic attacks, hypertensive heart disease, CHD, CHF, and diabetes mellitus.

▶ I was unable to find anywhere in this superb study a mention of smoking or alcohol as risk factors and must conclude that smoking and drinking histories were not considered important at the time the patients were interviewed.

The Mayo Clinic group (*N Engl J Med* 317:669–674, 1987) have shown also that lone uncomplicated atrial fibrillation under the age of 60 is associated with a low risk of stroke and suggest that routine anticoagulation is not indicated. Recently Baum and Manton (*Gerontologist* 27:293–300, 1987) have studied the decreasing stroke mortality data with great care and suggest that the decline in stroke is more apparent than real and may be because the patients' other stroke-related diseases (as listed on death certificates) are less lethal. They think that perhaps stroke occurs at the same rate but is not as fatal. There is some confirmation in 2 related studies by Garraway and Whisnant (*JAMA* 258:214–217, 1987) and Homer, Whisnant, and Schoenberg (*Ann Neurol* 22:245–251, 1987), who have shown in the Rochester area that there is a close association of stroke to the changing pattern of hypertension and that this probably is responsible for lessening of stroke rates in recent decades.

For those who feel that they need to learn about the genetic causes of stroke, the recent summary "Mendelian etiologies of stroke" by Natowicz and Kelley (*Ann Neurol* 22:175–192, 1987) is a book in itself. A remarkable job and a great reference to keep around.

Also in the *Annals* (22:72–76, July 1987) an ANA committee on health care issues has, wonder of wonders, come up with a statement on the value of carotid endarterectomy which actually says something. "Carotid endarterectomy may be of value, provided the procedures are performed with a very low surgical complication rate. No clinical trial has addressed adequately the benefit or lack of benefit of the procedure. It is possible that the net effect of carotid endarterectomy in patients with carotid TIAs in the United States is unfavorable. Even the best surgical results that have been published probably have produced about a 33% reduction in stroke in 5 years."—R.D. Currier, M.D.

▶ The following three abstracts (Abstracts 4–2 to 4–4) further evaluate risk factors for stroke, particularly smoking, hypertension, and oral contraceptives.—R.D. Currier, M.D.

Cigarette Smoking as a Risk Factor for Stroke: The Framingham Study
Wolf PA, D'Agostino RB, Kannel WB, Bonita R, Belanger AJ (Boston Univ; Univ of Auckland, New Zealand)
JAMA 259:1025–1029, Feb 19, 1988   4–2

Data on the impact of cigarette smoking on stroke victims have been inconclusive or variable. To elucidate further, the impact of cigarette smoking on stroke incidence was assessed in the Framingham Heart Study cohort of 4,225 men and women who were aged 36 to 68 years and free of stroke and transient ischemic attacks.

During 26 years of follow-up, stroke or transient ischemic attacks developed in 459 patients. The average annual incidence of stroke was 4.15 per 1,000, and it was 23.3% greater in men than in women. Atherothrombotic brain infarction accounted for 243 (52.9%) of all strokes, and it was 32.3% greater in men than in women. Regardless of smoking status and in each sex, hypertensive patients had twice the incidence of stroke. The Cox proportional hazard regression method showed that the relative risks for stroke were significantly increased in smokers, even after age and definite hypertension were accounted for. Even after controlling for other major cardiovascular risk factors, such as total serum cholesterol level, relative weight, left ventricular hypertrophy on ECG, and glucose intolerance in the Cox regression model, cigarette smoking continued to make a significant independent contribution to the risk of stroke generally and brain infarction specifically. The relative risk of stroke in heavy smokers (>40 cigarettes per day) was nearly twice that of persons smoking fewer than 10 cigarettes per day. Lapsed smokers developed stroke at the same time level as nonsmokers soon after quitting. Stroke risk decreased significantly by 2 years after quitting and reverted to the level of nonsmokers within 5 years after stopping.

Cigarette smoking is a risk factor for stroke in both normotensive and hypertensive patients. The risk of stroke increases as the number of cigarettes smoked increases. The rapid reduction in risk after quitting smoking suggests that cigarette smoking acts by precipitating the clinical event, increasing fibrinogen levels in the blood, and adversely affecting hemorrheologic factors that promote thrombus formation.

Analysis of Risk Factors for Stroke in a Cohort of Men Born in 1913
Welin L, Svärdsudd K, Wilhelmsen L, Larsson B, Tibblin G (Gothenburg Univ, Gothenburg, Sweden; Uppsala Univ, Uppsala, Sweden)
N Engl J Med 317:521–526, Aug 27, 1987   4–3

The incidence of stroke and potential risk factors for stroke were analyzed in 789 men born in 1913. All men were initially examined at age 54 years.

The men were followed for 18.5 years. During this time, 57 men (7.2%) had strokes. Risk factors that correlated significantly with stroke by univariate analysis included increased systolic and diastolic blood pressure, larger waist circumference, higher waist/hip ratio, increased plasma fibrinogen level, lower vital capacity, and maternal history of death from stroke (Fig 4–1). Potential risk factors that were not correlated with stroke were body-mass index, serum cholesterol level, hematocrit, blood glucose level, smoking, heart disease, left ventricular hypertrophy, and paternal history of stroke death. By multivariate analysis,

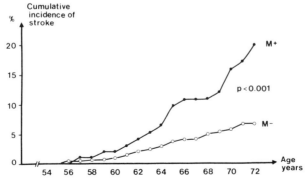

Fig 4–1.—Cumulative incidence of stroke among men with (M+) and without (M−) mothers who died of stroke (principal cause of death). (Courtesy of Welin L, Svärdsudd K, Wilhelmsen L, et al: *N Engl J Med* 317:521–526, Aug 27, 1987.)

increased blood pressure, abdominal obesity, increased plasma fibrinogen level, and maternal history of stroke were correlated with stroke risk.

These results confirm the previously reported association of high blood pressure, abdominal obesity, and increased plasma fibrinogen level with an increased risk of stroke. A maternal history of stroke was also associated with a risk of stroke in middle-aged men. The maternal history can be used to identify patients at high risk to motivate them to reduce other risk factors.

Cerebrovascular Deaths Before and After the Appearance of Oral Contraceptives
Lidegaard Ø (Copenhagen County Hosp, Gentofte, Denmark)
Acta Neurol Scand 75:427–433, June 1987   4–4

The annual vital statistics from 1953 to 1980 in Denmark were examined to look for an association between oral contraceptives (OC) and thrombogenic risk. Cerebrovascular diseases were divided into 3 groups: subarachnoidal hemorrhages, intracerebral hemorrhages, and cerebral thromboembolism.

During the 28 years, 1,670 deaths were recorded in the registry. The female incidence of cerebrovascular death increased by 19%, whereas the male incidence was unchanged. There was a 33% increase in female deaths from cerebral thromboembolic attacks and a 14% decrease in male deaths. This increase in female deaths was most prominent in the 15–34 year age group. This group has the highest OC use. A relative risk of 3.3–4.5 for OC users vs. nonusers could explain the cerebrovascular death rate difference between women and men.

The only currently identifiable factor that might explain the gender difference in cerebrovascular death seen in this longitudinal study is the use of OC.

Alcohol and Stroke
Gorelick PB (Michael Reese Hosp and Med Ctr, Chicago)
Stroke 18:268–271, January–February 1987   4–5

The acute and chronic effects of alcohol on the brain are well known. The evidence linking stroke and alcohol consumption were reviewed.

Alcohol consumption can contribute to stroke in several ways. It induces cardiac arrhythmias and wall motion abnormalities, which can predispose to cerebral embolism. Heavy alcohol consumption is linked to hypertension. Alcohol causes platelet hyperaggregation and activates the clotting cascade. Alcohol also alters cerebral metabolism and causes vasospasm, both of which reduce cerebral blood flow.

Epidemiologic evidence also suggests a link between alcohol and stroke. Regular alcohol ingestion is associated with hypertension, intracranial hemorrhage, cerebral infarction, and increased risk of death from stroke. Further studies are required to expand and substantiate these findings.

▶ This is a general discussion of the acute and chronic effects of alcohol on cerebrovascular disease and its action in altering disturbances of cardiac rhythm, blood pressure, coagulation and platelet disorders, and cerebral blood flow. The article is good reading and contains much important information.—R.N. DeJong, M.D.

The Relationship Between Carotid Plaque Composition and Neurologic Symptoms

Seeger JM, Klingman N (Univ of Florida; VA Med Ctr, Gainesville, Fla)
J Surg Res 43:78–85, July 1987   4–6

Because "soft" atherosclerotic plaques may contain increased amounts of lipid, whereas dense or calcified plaques have more collagen and calcium, plaque composition may be an important factor in the occurrence of plaque-related neurologic symptoms. Lipid-laden plaques are expected to be unstable and prone to embolization, thrombosis, and intraplaque hemorrhage. Thirty-five plaques from 31 patients undergoing carotid endarterectomy were analyzed for either symptomatic carotid bifurcation disease or asymptomatic stenosis exceeding 80%.

Plaques from symptomatic patients contained more total lipid and cholesterol than those from asymptomatic patients, and less collagen and calcium. They also were lighter. More collagen in symptomatic plaques could be solubilized by pepsin digestion. Serum cholesterol and plasma low-density lipoprotein cholesterol were higher in symptomatic patients, but these values could not be correlated with plaque cholesterol values.

Plaque lipid and cholesterol levels are associated with ipsilateral neurologic symptoms in patients undergoing carotid endarterectomy. A high plaque lipid concentration may be a marker of a plaque at high risk of embolization or intramural hemorrhage. A reduction in plasma lipids in animals can reduce plaque lipid content, and it is possible that treatment could alter the risk of ischemic neurologic symptoms in patients with carotid atherosclerosis.

▶ These workers suggest that the type of plaque that can be guessed by ultrasound carotid imaging relates to the resulting symptomatology, a minor clue that may slightly improve our treatment of cerebrovascular disease.—R.D. Currier, M.D.

The Cerebral Ischemic Penumbra

Hakim AM (McGill Univ)
Can J Neurol Sci 14:557–559, 1987   4–7

Between the dense ischemic region and normally perfused brain tissue is an intermediate zone where blood flow is reduced to interrupt neuronal function, but membrane pumps continue to work and ion gradients are preserved. The interrupted function characterizing the "ischemic penumbra" is reversible, but only for a limited time.

Electrically the ischemic penumbra is the paraischemic zone that loses electrical excitability, as measured by EEG and sensory evoked potentials (SEP) recording, while maintaining neuronal membrane potential. Reversibility may continue for several hours if cerebral blood flow is near the upper limit of the penumbra range. The positron emission tomography (PET) studies show an area consistent with penumbra, where function deteriorates over time and which may be a target of therapeutic intervention.

Further studies are needed to determine the predictability of the metabolic and histologic sequelae of stroke and the role of hyperemia in the outcome of the penumbra. In addition, the events involved in metabolic deterioration of the penumbra zone require clarification. Drugs with therapeutic potential such as calcium channel blockers and N-methyl-D-aspartate receptor antagonists are under study in PET-based trials.

▶ This paper and 1 at about the same time in the *Annals* (Leblanc et al: *Ann Neurol* 22:707–713, 1987) point out that there is an area around the permanently infarcted area that is ischemic and shows up on scanning and blood flow testing, but is not dead, although it is nonfunctional. Hakim points out that the interruption of clinical function is fundamentally reversible but that the reversibility is time limited.

The concept, of course, has always been in the minds of those who treat strokes and look at their scans. In the article by Leblanc et al. mentioned above, PET scanning was used to measure cerebral perfusion and metabolism in patients with severe carotid stenosis but no infarction. Anterior border zone ischemia was shown to be present in that situation, which is not unexpected.

While we are on the subject of cerebral circulation, the recent aspirin study preliminarily reported in the *New England Journal of Medicine* 318:262–264, Jan 28, 1988) shows a clear advantage to physicians taking 1 aspirin a day for the prevention of myocardial infarction. There was also a clear disadvantage in the aspirin group for the occurrence of moderate, severe, or fatal hemorrhagic brain infarction— 10 occurrences in the aspirin group and 2 in the placebo group ($P = .02$). The authors do not mention any other details about that subgroup; we will wait to hear in later publications whether the hemorrhagic stroke group might have had mild or intermittent hypertension, a fact that would not have excluded them from the study. (See also *N Engl J Med* 318:922–925, April 7, 1988).—R.D. Currier, M.D.

The Risk of Perioperative Stroke in Patients With Asymptomatic Carotid Bruits Undergoing Peripheral Vascular Surgery
Gutierrez IZ, Barone DL, Makula PA, Currier C (VA Med Ctr, Buffalo; State Univ of New York, Buffalo)
Am Surg J 53:487–489, September 1987   4–8

Perioperative stroke after peripheral vascular reconstruction in patients without previous neurologic symptoms is a dreaded complication. Asymptomatic internal carotid artery disease that may predispose a patient to this complication may be manifested by carotid bruit. A study was done to determine the incidence of perioperative stroke in patients who had asymptomatic carotid bruits.

Three hundred male patients underwent 374 peripheral vascular reconstructive procedures. Before surgery, they had GEE-OPG assessment of any incidental asymptomatic carotid bruits found by auscultation. A bruit was considered hemodynamically significant if the OPG test proved positive. Seventy-four patients (24.7%) had 118 carotid bruits. Twenty-five (22.3%) of the 112 bruits studied by OPG were hemodynamically significant. Three perioperative strokes occurred, yielding an incidence of 0.8%. The strokes occurred only in patients with hemodynamically significant bruits, yielding an incidence of perioperative strokes of 16% in such patients. Strokes occurred 24 to 48 hours after surgery. All 3 patients who sustained perioperative strokes had undergone reconstructive surgery for aortoiliac occlusive disease. All 3 patients had had bilateral carotid bruits, and in 2, the dense cerebral infarcts were ipsilateral to the hemodynamically significant carotid bruits.

A perioperative stroke incidence of 16% was found among patients who had positive OPG tests on their carotid bruits. A subgroup of patients with asymptomatic carotid bruits was identified as being significantly at risk for perioperative stroke.

▶ Patients scheduled for peripheral vascular reconstructive surgery for asymptomatic internal carotid artery disease should be examined thoroughly to rule out the presence of asymptomatic carotid artery bruits. The presence of such bruits may place the patient at risk for a perioperative stroke.—R.N. DeJong, M.D.

The Appropriateness of Carotid Endarterectomy

Winslow CM, Solomon DH, Chassin MR, Kosecoff J, Merrick NJ, Brook RH (Rand Corp, Santa Monica Calif; Univ of California, Los Angeles; Fink and Kosecoff, Inc, Santa Monica, Calif)
N Engl J Med 318:721–727, March 24, 1988   4–9

Carotid endarterectomy is commonly performed but controversial. To investigate the reasons for doing carotid endarterectomy, the appropriateness with which the procedure was performed was examined in 3 large geographic areas in the United States.

A list of 864 possible reasons for performing carotid endarterectomy was compiled from the literature. A panel of nationally known experts rated the appropriateness of each indication using a modified Delphi technique. These ratings were then applied to a random sample of 1,302

Medicare patients who had undergone the procedure in 1981. Thirty-five percent of these patients were judged to have carotid endarterectomy for appropriate reasons, 32% for equivocal reasons, and 32% for inappropriate reasons. Of those who had inappropriate surgery, 48% had less than 50% stenosis of the carotid artery that was operated on. Fifty-four percent of all procedures were done on patients without transient ischemic attacks in the carotid distribution. Of these procedures, 18% were considered appropriate, compared with 55% considered appropriate in patients with transient ischemic attacks in the carotid distribution. After the procedure, 9.8% of patients had a major complication—stroke with residual deficit at time of discharge or death within 30 days of surgery.

Carotid endarterectomy was substantially overused in the 3 geographic areas studied. Furthermore, when the complication rate is equal to or above the study's aggregate rate, carotid endarterectomy would not be warranted even in patients having appropriate indications because the risks would almost certainly outweigh the benefits.

▶ One wonders where the 3 geographic areas were. The authors don't come to the conclusion that the treatment is entirely useless, just that there are a great number done, many of which are probably unnecessary.—R.D. Currier, M.D.

Cardioembolic Stroke, Early Anticoagulation, and Brain Hemorrhage
Cerebral Embolism Study Group (Univ of Texas Health Science Ctr, San Antonio)
Arch Intern Med 147:636–640, April 1987   4–10

It is not known which cardioembolic patients are at risk for cerebral hemorrhage and therefore should not be given anticoagulation therapy. Nine patients were assessed and compared with historic cases to determine factors predisposing patients to hemorrhagic transformation.

Of the 9 patients with hemorrhage documented by computed tomography (CT), 8 were receiving anticoagulation therapy and 1, who had a small infarct, was not (Fig 4–2). The hemorrhage was confined to the basal ganglia in 2 patients and was cortical in 5 patients.

Retrospective analysis suggests that hemorrhage is not completely predictable in these patients. However, patients with large infarcts are at risk for this complication. Performing CT less than 12 hours after cardioembolic stroke may not allow detection of this transformation. Anticoagulation therapy may potentiate hemorrhage in patients liable to suffer this complication.

▶ The current efficiency of the heparin pumps and the false reassurance of the early negative CT scans have combined to produce this picture. We were better off when it took a day or so to obtain a CT scan and when our methods of giving heparin were not as efficient.

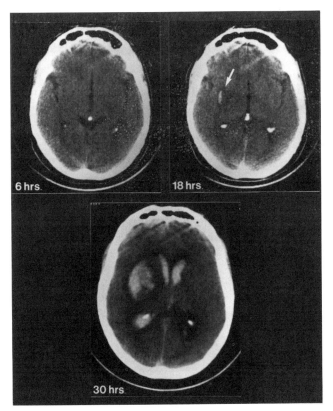

Fig 4–2.—Spontaneous hemorrhagic transformation of cardioembolic stroke in absence of antithrombotic therapy. Patient had a small infarct, and initial CT scan obtained 6 hours after stroke onset did not show hemorrhage. A second CT study obtained 18 hours after stroke onset showed a hemorrhagic infarct. There was clinical worsening, and a third CT study obtained 30 hours after stroke showed intracerebral and intraventricular hemorrhage. (Courtesy of Cerebral Embolism Study Group: *Arch Intern Med* 147:636–640, April 1987.)

Why don't we wait 3 or 4 days after the embolic stroke, repeat the CT scan, and then, if we think that the patient should be heparinized for the prevention of further emboli, do it? For that matter, why not forget the heparin and start with warfarin?—R.D. Currier, M.D.

Platelet Activating Factor Receptor Blockade Enhances Recovery After Multifocal Brain Ischemia
Kochanek PM, Dutka AJ, Kumaroo KK, Hallenbeck JM (Naval Med Research Inst, Bethesda, Md; Children's Hosp Natl Med Ctr, Washington, DC)
Life Sci 41:2639–2644, Dec 14, 1987   4–11

Studies suggest that platelets accumulate in regions of low blood flow after multifocal cerebral ischemia and that platelet aggregates are produced after stroke. Inhibition of platelet activation is a reasonable approach to preventing and treating cerebral vascular disease. The efficacy of a specific platelet activating factor receptor blocking agent, kadsurenone, in improving the outcome of multifocal brain ischemia induced by air embolism in dogs was investigated.

Four anesthetized dogs were treated with kadsurenone before 60 minutes of multifocal ischemia induced by air embolism. Neuronal recovery, blood flow, and autologous ^{111}In-labeled platelet accumulation were measured for 4 hours after ischemia. Four anesthetized dogs underwent identical ischemia and served as controls. Kadsurenone, 3 mg/kg, given 5 minutes before ischemia and continuously in 1 mg/kg doses every hour throughout ischemia and recovery significantly enhanced recovery of cortical somatosensory evoked response amplitude when compared with controls. Platelet accumulation was estimated as ^{111}In activity in the injured hemisphere minus that in the uninjured hemisphere. Dogs treated with kadsurenone did not exhibit significantly altered ^{111}In-labeled platelet accumulation when compared with controls.

Kadsurenone given prophylactically improved outcome after multifocal cerebral ischemia induced by air embolism. Improved evoked response amplitude was not accompanied by a change in platelet accumulation.

▶ I don't know how far this is from clinical use, even experimental clinical use, but it seems like a logical thing to prevent platelet accumulation and we look forward to hearing more.

Recent comments on stroke include the conclusions of a study by Colditz et al. (*N Engl J Med* 318:937–941, 1988), on the risk of cigarette smoking in women. Strokes definitely correlate with smoking in women, and the number of cigarettes increases the number of strokes. So women are not exempt. The Italian stroke study group has studied hemodilution after stroke and finds that it is of no benefit (*Lancet* 1:318–320, Feb 13, 1988).

Soria, Fine, and Paroski have very nicely summarized lacunes in the *New York State Journal of Medicine* (87:650–655, December 1987). It was copied and given to our residents. You might wish to do the same.— R.D. Currier, M.D.

Determinants of Long-Term Mortality After Stroke
Viitanen M, Eriksson S, Asplund K, Wester PO, Winblad B (Univ of Umeå, Umeå, Sweden)
Acta Med Scand 221:349–356, 1987   4–12

The effect of clinical parameters on survival after stroke in 409 patients with well-defined cerebrovascular disease (CVD) was examined prospectively. The mean age of the patients was 72.2 years (range, 30–95 years). The patients were compared with an age-matched healthy population.

Compared with patients aged younger than 70 years, the relative risk of dying during the first 3 months after stroke was 2.2 times higher for patients in their 70s and 4 times higher for older patients; this difference

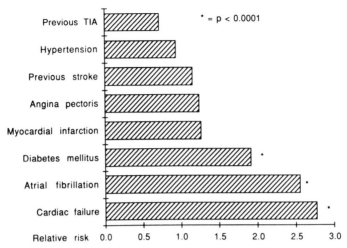

Fig 4–3.—Relative risk of dying for patients with cerebrovascular disease in relation to disease present before cerebrovascular disease. (Courtesy of Viitanen M, Eriksson S, Asplund K, et al: *Acta Med Scand* 221:349–356, 1987.)

disappeared after the first year. A history of cardiac failure, atrial fibrillation, and diabetes mellitus affected survival after stroke (Fig 4–3). Nearly all comatose patients died in the first week. Multivariate analysis indicated that impaired consciousness was the most important risk factor, followed by age, a history of cardiac failure or diabetes mellitus, male sex, and the diagnosis of intracerebral hemorrhage.

These results demonstrate that age and impairment of consciousness are the most important risk factors for death resulting from stroke. A history of heart failure, diabetes mellitus, or intracerebral hemorrhage is also associated with increased risk.

The Prognostic Value of Stress Hyperglycaemia and Previously Unrecognized Diabetes in Acute Stroke
Gray CS, Taylor R, French JM, Alberti KGMM, Venables GS, James OFW, Shaw DA, Cartlidge NEF, Bates D, (Royal Victoria Infirmary, Newcastle upon Tyne, England)
Diabetic Med 4:237–240, May–June 1987   4–13

The increased risk of stroke in patients with diabetes is well documented. Recent evidence suggests that hyperglycemia in the acute phase is associated with enhanced morbidity and mortality in stroke, although whether this reflects stress hyperglycemia or the clinical course of acute stroke in diabetic patients is not known. Considerable variation has been reported in the prevalence of recognized and unrecognized diabetes in patients with stroke. A study was done to investigate the prevalence of diabetes and hyperglycemia in acute stroke patients and to differentiate between diabetes and stress hyperglycemia as risk factors in mortality from acute stroke.

Eighty-six patients admitted in a 10-month period with a clinical diagnosis of stroke were studied. Blood glucose and HbA₁ were estimated within 72 hours of onset of acute stroke. The prevalence of previously diagnosed diabetes mellitus was 8%; whereas 28% were assumed to have unrecognized hyperglycemia preceding the acute event, as identified by a stable HbA_1 raised more than 2 standard deviations above the mean reference value. Only patients with normal blood glucose on admission had complete functional recovery of the limbs within 4 weeks of the stroke. None of the patients who had raised blood glucose on admission had full functional recovery within 4 weeks. Cumulative mortality at 4 weeks was significantly higher in patients with elevated blood glucose values, regardless of their HbA_1 values.

These findings confirm both the high prevalence of undetected hyperglycemia in patients with stroke—28%—and the adverse prognostic implications of hyperglycemia on admission. Admission blood glucose concentration is of greatest importance in predicting early mortality and morbidity.

▶ This is a curious conclusion. Complete recovery from the stroke was confined to those patients with a normal admission blood glucose. Stroke is, of course, more common in diabetics, and many patients with stroke have undiagnosed diabetes, but why does the presence of diabetes make recovery incomplete? Is it because the small vessel disease decreases collateral perfusion? Or do the individual cells recover less well in the presence of a higher sugar content?

In January 1988 the *Archives of Internal Medicine* (148:36–39, 1988) published a report from The National Cholesterol Education Program Panel on Detection, Evaluation and Treatment of High Blood Cholesterol in Adults. This is encyclopedic in content and a nice reference in case you get into arguments with your confreres about diets, treatment, and definitions of hypercholesterolemia.—R.D. Currier, M.D.

Mycotic Aneurysm, Subarachnoid Hemorrhage, and Indications for Cerebral Angiography in Infective Endocarditis
Salgado AV, Furlan AJ, Keys TF (Cleveland Clinic Found)
Stroke 18:1057–1060, November–December 1987   4–14

Ruptured mycotic aneurysms are responsible for about 5% of the neurologic complications of infective endocarditis. It is not known whether there are any neurologic or clinical predictors associated with an increased risk of mycotic aneurysm in infective endocarditis. The long-term risk of intracranial hemorrhage from unsuspected mycotic aneurysm in patients treated for infective endocarditis and the indications for cerebral angiography in these patients are also not established. A study was done to investigate these issues.

Comparative Data on Infective Endocarditis Patients
With and Without Mycotic Aneurysm

	With MA		Without MA	
	No.	Percent	No.	Percent
Number	68		147	
Age (mean)	31.4 yrs		52.0 yrs	
Sex				
Women		54.4		22.4
Men		45.6		77.6
Underlying cardiac disease				
Not mentioned		25		0
Rheumatic heart disease		25		21
Congenital heart disease		17.5		38
None known		23.5		41
Other		9.0		0
History of IV drug abuse		8.8		2.0
Type of valve at time of IE				
Native		98.5		68.6
Prosthetic		1.5		31.2
Valve involved				
Mitral only		52*		29.2
Aortic only		33.3*		55.1
Most frequent microorganism isolated				
Streptococcus viridans		33.8		30.6
Group D *Streptococcus*		10.3		23.8
Other *Streptococcus*		11.8		2.7
Staphylococcus aureus		17.6		19.9
Staphylococcus coagu-lase-negative		1.5		10.8
Others†		5.9		8.4
Not mentioned		14.7		0
Negative blood cultures		4.4		4.0
Incidence and nature of neurologic complications during IE				
SAH/ICH		57.4		0
Focal deficit		23.5		19.0
Headache		13.2		6.8
Bacterial meningitis		2.9		1.3
Seizures		1.5		0.7
Change in mental status		1.5		10.9
Cerebrospinal fluid pleocytosis				
	(17/39)	43.6	(7/12)	58.3

MA, mycotic aneurysm, IE, infective endocarditis, SAH, subarachnoid hemorrhage, ICH, intracerebral hemorrhage.
*In 48 patients for whom information was available.
†Gram-negative bacilli, diphtheroids, yeast, and lactobacillus.
(Courtesy of Salgado AV, Furlan AJ, Keys TF: *Stroke* 18:1057–1060, November–December 1987.)

The clinical course of 68 patients with infective endocarditis and mycotic aneurysm and 147 patients with infective endocarditis but no mycotic aneurysm was compared (table). Fifty-seven percent of the patients with mycotic aneurysm had subarachnoid hemorrhage without warning. Forty-three percent had a neurologic prodrome 2 days to 18 months before the aneurysm was discovered. A focal deficit consistent with embolism, found in 23%, was the most common prodrome. However, no significant differences were observed in the frequency of neurologic symptoms between the patients with and those without mycotic aneurysm. Patients were followed up for an average of 40 months. There were no occurrences of subarachnoid hemorrhage or mycotic aneurysm among 121 patients discharged after a full course of antibiotic therapy.

In this series, the risk of rupture of an unsuspected mycotic aneurysm after a full course of antibiotics was low. When a prodrome preceded a mycotic aneurysm, it was most often a focal deficit consistent with embolism. Angiography was recommended for all patients with infective endocarditis who experience a focal deficit with good recovery.

▶ Before the advent of antibiotics, infective endocarditis was not treatable and its mortality rate was extremely high. Today, most patients recover, but mycotic aneurysms develop in many; these may rupture and cause intracranial hemorrhages. The authors of this report recommend that patients with a history of infective endocarditis who experience a focal neurologic deficit, even with recovery, should have cerebral angiography to see whether they have a mycotic aneurysm.—R.N. DeJong, M.D.

Cocaine-Related Intracranial Hemorrhage: Report of Nine Cases and Review

Mangiardi JR, Daras M, Geller ME, Weitzner I, Tuchman AJ (New York Med College, Bronx, NY)

Acta Neurol Scand 77:177–180, March 1988   4–15

The use of free-base cocaine and combined intravenous cocaine and heroin is increasing. These uses of cocaine may have played a role in the development of intracranial hemorrhage in 9 patients seen at 1 center in the past 6 months. Findings in these 9 patients and in 5 described in the literature were reviewed.

The patients were 3 women and 6 men, aged 22–41 years. All had used intravenous drugs, including cocaine, heroine, or both, over a long period of time. A history of "crack" use was reported by 5 patients. All patients had urine that tested positive for cocaine in the initial toxicology screening in the emergency room. The diagnosis of subarachnoid hemorrhage was established in 5 patients by computed tomographic (CT) scan, lumbar puncture, or both. In the remaining 4 patients, CT scan revealed an intracerebral hematoma in 2 (Fig 4–4) and intraventricular hemorrhage in 2. Arteriography done in 6 cases revealed an aneurysm in 1 and an arteriovenous malformation in 2. Two patients had consistently in

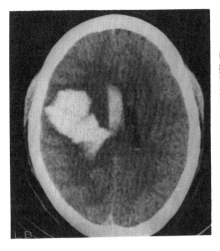

Fig 4–4.—Large intracerebral hematoma involving the right frontoparietal and basal ganglia with midline shift and rupture into the lateral ventricles. (Courtesy of Mangiardi JR, Daras M, Geller ME, et al: *Acta Neurol Scand* 77:177–180, March 1988.)

creased arterial pressure. Only 2 patients survived, 1 of whom left the hospital with a significant left hemiplegia and hemianopsia. Three patients died during the first week of hospitalization. Of the other 4, 1 died from recurrent bleeding, 1 from severe subacute bacterial endocarditis, and 2 from pneumonia and sepsis.

In these nine cases of intracranial hemorrhages related to cocaine use, a relationship between severe cocaine-induced hypertension and the development of subarachnoid or intracerebral hemorrhage was noted. This relationship was apparently associated with sudden transient increases of blood pressure resulting from cocaine use.

▶ Transient increases in blood pressure related to cocaine use may cause intracerebral and subarachnoid hemorrhage. Increasing numbers of cases of this complication are being reported following use of "crack" (free-base cocaine), a new, very potent form of cocaine that has recently been used in epidemic proportions in many major inner-city centers.—R.N. DeJong, M.D.

Do Cerebral Arteriovenous Malformations Increase in Size?
Mendelow AD, Erfurth A, Grossart K, MacPherson P (Inst of Neurological Sciences, Glasgow, Scotland)
J Neurol Neurosurg Psychiatry 50:980–987, 1987   4–16

Arteriovenous malformations of the brain are well-recognized causes of subarachnoid and intracerebral hemorrhage. To determine whether cerebral arteriovenous malformations increase in size, the angiograms of patients with an arteriovenous malformation who had a second angiogram after an interval of time were reviewed.

From 1965 to 1985, 326 patients seen at one institution were found to have an arteriovenous malformation on arteriography. Nine patients had a second angiogram 4–25 years later. Of these, 5 had increases in the size of the malformation. A sixth patient was identified anecdotally. The minimum incidence rate was estimated to be 0.6 per 100,000 per year. The 6 patients were aged 8 months to 24 years. Three were female, and 2 were male.

Girl, 14 years, had paresthesia, weakness, and clumsiness in one hand. She recovered spontaneously but returned 3 years later with a fixed deficit. Angiography revealed a large arteriovenous malformation that was not operable. She had several episodes of dysphagia, became epileptic, and sustained a subarachnoid hemorrhage 10 years after initial angiography. Repeat angiography at this time demonstrated the increased size of the malformation.

The frequency of spontaneous enlargement among 6 patients with cerebral arteriovenous malformations that occurred in a period of 4–20 years was estimated to be 0.2% to 2.8% per annum. This rate of enlargement should be considered when treatment options are reviewed and should be added to the risk of hemorrhage.

▶ This subject has been argued in rounds with the neurosurgeons for years. Most thought that the malformations enlarged, but little proof was available, and now we finally have it.—R.D. Currier, M.D.

5 Child Neurology

A Catch in the Reye
Orlowski JP, Gillis J, Kilham HA (The Children's Hosp, Camperdown, New South Wales, Australia; Cleveland Clinic Found)
Pediatrics 80:638–642, November 1987   5–1

The cause of Reye's syndrome remains a mystery. Between 1973 and 1982, 23 cases of Reye's syndrome were diagnosed at the Children's Hospital, Camperdown, Australia. In a retrospective chart review of these cases, 20 cases met the United States Public Health Service Centers for Disease Control criteria for Reye's syndrome. Only 1 child had ingested aspirin or salicylate-containing products; 6 had ingested paracetamol (acetaminophen). Pathologic confirmation of the diagnosis of Reye's syndrome was confirmed in 90% of cases, compared with less than 20% in U.S. studies. The incidence of Reye's syndrome in New South Wales, Australia, was estimated to be 9 cases per 1 million children, compared with 10 to 20 cases per 1 million children in the U.S. and 3 to 7 cases per 1 million children in Great Britain. The mortality rate of the cases of Reye's syndrome in Australia was 45% compared to a 32% case-fatality rate in the United States. In Australia, aspirin usage in children had been virtually nil for the past 25 years, for both over-the-counter and prescription forms. Paracetamol (acetaminophen) was the most frequently used pediatric analgesic and antipyretic for at least 25 years.

These findings show no association between the development of Reye's syndrome and ingestion of aspirin or salicylates in Australia. Despite this, it is interesting to note that the incidence of Reye's syndrome is declining in Australia, since no cases have been reported at the Children's Hospital since 1983.

▶ We have invited Owen B. Evans, M.D., Associate Professor of Pediatrics and Neurology and Director of Pediatric Neurology and Child Development at the University of Mississippi School of Medicine, to comment on the following 2 abstracts—R.D. Currier, M.D.

▶ The authors report what many clinicians have suspected: Reye's syndrome is becoming rare. Attributing the declining incidence to the effort to reduce aspirin exposure in children was perhaps too easy. In Australia, where aspirin exposure in children has always been low, there has also been a declining incidence. The cause for this decline, as the cause for the disease itself, remains unknown. In that Reye's syndrome is often associated with influenza viral infections, especially type B, it is notable that none of the patients reported here had a preceding influenza viral infection.— O.B. Evans, M.D.

Multiple Sclerosis in Childhood: Clinical Profile in 125 Patients

Duquette P, Murray TJ, Pleines J, Ebers GC, Sadovnick D, Weldon P, Warren S, Paty DW, Upton A, Hader W, Nelson R, Auty A, Neufeld B, Meltzer C (Multiple Sclerosis Clinics, Montreal, Halifax, London, Hamilton, Ottawa, Canada, et al)

J Pediatr 111:359–363, September 1987   5–2

The onset of multiple sclerosis (MS) usually occurs in early adulthood. However, age at clinical onset varies markedly. The implications of the age of onset on clinical presentation and course are not clear. A population-based retrospective study of 125 patients with onset before age 16 years was done.

Nine Canadian MS clinics completed questionnaires on various aspects of their MS populations. Of 4,632 patients with MS, 125 (2.7%) had initial manifestations before age 16 years. Average age of onset was 13 years. The earliest age at onset was 5 years in a boy and 7 years in a girl (Fig 5–1). Eight patients had onset before age 11 years. Among the group with onset in childhood, 75.2% were female and 24.8% were male, yielding a sex ratio of 3:1; among the entire MS population, the female/male ratio was 2.1:1.

Initial clinical manifestations in the childhood group were pure sensory in 26.4%, optic neuritis in 14%, diplopia in 11%, pure motor in 11%, gait problems in 8%, blurred vision in 6%, cerebellar ataxia in 5%, sensory and motor in 5%, optic neuritis with simultaneous involvement of an additional structure of the CNS in 3%, transverse myelitis in 3%, ves-

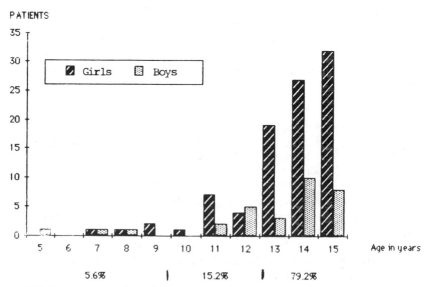

Fig 5–1.—Age at onset of MS in patients with onset before 16 years. (Courtesy of Duquette P, Murray TJ, Pleines J, et al: (*J Pediatr* 111:359–363, September 1987.)

tibular syndrome in 1.6%, and sphincter problems in 0.8%. Data on degree of recovery from the first episode were available for 102 patients. Sixty-eight percent had complete recovery, and 24% had partial recovery. Eight percent had no recovery. Of the patients, 80% had definitive MS, 12% had probable MS, and 8% had possible MS. Further, 56% had a relapsing-remitting course, 22% had an initially progressive course, and 22% had a mixed course. Duration of disease was 15 years. Kurtze scores after 10 years of disease were available for 51 patients: 60% had a score of <3, 24% had a score ranging from 3 to 6.5, and 16% had scores ≥7. Of 118 patients, 21% had a positive family history. Thirteen of 32 patients had increased IgG levels in cerebrospinal fluid; 19 had normal levels. Of 39 patients, 32 had 2 or more oligoclonal bands on electrophoresis.

This study of MS onset in childhood demonstrated that childhood MS is more frequent in girls, that it has a relapsing-remitting course, that initial bouts usually involve afferent structures of the CNS, that recovery from these is often complete, and that the pace of the disease is slow.

▶ This study is the largest study of MS in childhood. Unfortunately, only 8 of the 125 children were younger than age 11 years. Most were actually adolescents or young adults. The key features are that the disease is more common in girls and more frequently affects sensory and visual symptoms initially. The children are likely to remit completely. In addition, 82% of the patients had abnormal CSF studies. It would appear from this study that MS in children in general does not differ significantly from that in adults. A significant factor is its actual infrequency in children; only 2.6% of the total MS patient cohort (4,632 patients) were children.— O.B. Evans, M.D.

Prognosis in Severe Guillain-Barré Syndrome
Cole GF, Matthew DJ (Hosp for Sick Children, London)
Arch Dis Child 62:288–291, March 1987   5–3

Guillain-Barré syndrome is an inflammatory demyelinating disease of the peripheral nerves with a generally benign course. However, 7% of adult patients die and others are left with disability. Adult patients who require ventilation are considered to have the worst prognosis. Data on 11 children with Guillain-Barré syndrome seen at the authors' hospital over a 7-year period were reviewed with reference to their ventilation requirements to determine whether ventilation is related to prognosis in children.

Eight children required ventilation; 2 children died. Seven of the 9 survivors had a complete recovery and 2 children were left with very minimal disability.

It appears that, in contrast to adult patients, children with

Guillain-Barré syndrome who require ventilation do not have an unfavorable prognosis. In general, the outcome of severe Guillain-Barré syndrome appears to be better in children than in adults. Provided the child survives the acute phase, the prognosis for a functional recovery is excellent.

▶ It appears that the need for early mechanical ventilation is not necessarily a bad prognostic sign for neurologic recovery in children with the Guillain-Barré syndrome.— R.N. DeJong, M.D.

Plasmapheresis for Myasthenic Crisis in a Young Child

Snead OC III, Kohaut EC, Oh SJ, Bradley RJ (Univ of Alabama, Birmingham)
J Pediatr 110:740–742, May 1987   5–4

Two reports of exchange transfusion for neonatal myasthenia gravis (MG) have been described, but plasmapheresis for myasthenic crisis has been reported in only 1 older child. A child, aged 14 months, was seen whose symptoms began at less than 1 year of age and rapidly progressed to a life-threatening myasthenic crisis, which was successfully treated with plasmapheresis.

Infant, female, developed normally until age 8 months, when increased fatigability developed. Bilateral ptosis developed at 11 months and MG was diagnosed on the basis of a positive edrophonium test. Pyridostigmine treatment was initiated, but the child became progressively weaker and was brought to the hospital with profound, diffuse weakness and acute respiratory failure at age 14 months. There was no family history of MG.

A test dose of edrophonium, 0.15 mg/kg of body weight, produced transient improvement in strength and spontaneous ventilatory effort with decreased ptosis and full extraocular movements, but the heart rate decreased to 65 beats per minute and atropine was required. The dose of pyridostigmine was increased to a maximum of 1 mg/kg of body weight over the next 6 days, but severe muscarinic side effects developed, which were only partially alleviated with glycopyrrolate. On hospital day 4, prednisone therapy was begun at 2 mg/kg of body weight per day, and on day 5, subclavian and femoral vein catheters were surgically implanted. On day 6, a two-volume membrane plasmapheresis was begun, and it was carried out every other day for 16 days. The patient gradually improved, and the ventilator was removed 2 days after the last plasmapheresis.

The patient's acetylcholine receptor antibody titers decreased from 17.8 to 1.5 nmol/L, concomitant with her improvement (Fig 5–2). The patient was discharged after hospital day 28 with a titer of 3 nmol/L. Before plasmapheresis, there was a profound decremental response to repetitive stimulation of the peroneal nerve, with a 72% decrement at a stimulation rate of 10/sec. Immediately after plasmapheresis, there was dramatic improvement to only a 9% decrement. Nine months after the initial episode, the patient required plasma-

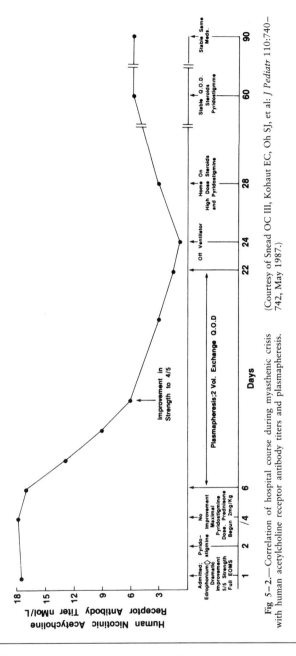

Fig 5–2.—Correlation of hospital course during myasthenic crisis with human acetylcholine receptor antibody titers and plasmapheresis. (Courtesy of Snead OC III, Kohaut EC, Oh SJ, et al: *J Pediatr* 110:740–742, May 1987.)

pheresis after she again went into myasthenic crisis; at age 25 months thymectomy was performed.

Plasmapheresis allowed postponement of thymectomy until the child was older, which may have been life-saving.

Neurologic Uncertainty in Newborn Intensive Care

Coulter DL (Boston Univ; Boston City Hosp)

N Engl J Med 316:840–844, April 2, 1987

5–5

difficult treatment decisions. These decisions are often difficult because of medical uncertainty, which develops when the diagnosis and prognosis are unclear; and moral uncertainty, which develops when the expected benefit of treatment is unclear. In general, the medical diagnosis and prognosis must be determined first, and resolution of medical uncertainty may then clarify the moral and ethical issues.

Three types of neurologic disease in newborn infants include brain death, a persistent vegetative state, and survival with disabilities, which often cause uncertainty and can be distinguished by their eventual outcomes. To resolve uncertainty, it is necessary to identify the criteria for brain death. These criteria can be recognized when the cause of the neurologic condition is known; when there is no clinical evidence of any cerebral or brain-stem functions; and when contrast arteriography shows no evidence of intracranial blood flow. If brain death is not present, it is important to assess the cause and extent of brain damage, which can be accomplished by obtaining appropriate laboratory tests and pediatric neurologic consultation. The third and most difficult step in resolving neurologic uncertainty is to wait; the more time that passes, the clearer the prognosis becomes.

The importance of distinguishing among the 3 categories is self-evident. Infants in a vegetative state should be treated with a conservative and cautious approach because of the prognostic uncertainty. However, infants with a neurologic disorder who are not in a vegetative state and who are likely to survive with or without a disability should receive all appropriate medical treatment.

▶ The prognosis for infants with a neurologic disease in a newborn intensive care unit is uncertain. If such infants are not in a vegetative state and are likely to survive with or without disability, Coulter recommends that they be given all appropriate medical treatment, because the actual outcome may be much better than anyone might expect.—R.N. DeJong, M.D.

Carbamazepine-Exacerbated Epilepsy in Children and Adolescents

Horn CS, Ater SB, Hurst DL (Fitzsimons Army Med Ctr, Aurora, Colo; Univ of Colorado, Denver; Texas Tech Univ Health Sciences Ctr, Lubbock)

Pediatr Neurol 2:340–345, November–December 1986

5–6

The records of 26 children and adolescents whose seizures reportedly worsened while receiving carbamazepine (CBZ) were studied retrospectively. Twenty-two patients had increases in seizure frequency, 8 had increases in duration of individual seizures, and 11 had onset of new seizure types. Twelve patients had 2 changes and 1 patient had all 3 of these changes in seizure activity.

The most commonly affected seizure type was absence. Eleven patients had increased frequency of their absence seizures while receiving CBZ. There were tonic-clonic seizures in 7 patients, myoclonic in 3, atonic in 2, and 2 were unclassifiable. Eleven other patients developed new-onset absence seizures while receiving CBZ, including 3 patients who developed absence status. Electroencephalography showed new generalized spike-and-wave discharges in 11 patients. Four epileptic syndromes worsened with CBZ therapy; there was childhood absence in 6 patients, frontal-lobe in 6, severe myoclonic epilepsy of infancy in 2, and Lennox-Gastaut syndrome in 2. Additionally, 3 patients had Lennox-Gastaut syndrome and 3 had new onset of childhood absence epilepsy.

These data agree with those of previous studies on problems with CBZ-exacerbated epilepsy. They support evidence of a primary adverse effect of CBZ on generalized seizure types, as opposed to a coincidental worsening with CBZ as part of the natural evolution of a patient's particular seizure disorder. An abrupt exacerbation of generalized/mixed seizures with the introduction of CBZ in therapeutic doses has been observed. A stepwise increase in seizure frequency can occur as CBZ doses and levels are increased, as seen in at least 10 patients in this study. Withdrawal of CBZ can result in improved seizure control. Five of these patients had stable seizure rates for months to years while receiving CBZ; they became seizure-free after CBZ withdrawal without the addition of other antiepileptic drugs.

Caution is needed when prescribing CBZ for a child or adolescent with absence or mixed seizures. Patients who develop uncontrolled, generalized seizures should be examined for CBZ-exacerbated epilepsy. A marked improvement in epilepsy control may result from CBZ being discontinued in these patients.

Psychologic and Behavioral Effects of Antiepileptic Drugs in Children: A Double-Blind Comparison Between Phenobarbital and Valproic Acid
Vining EPG, Mellitz ED, Dorsen MM, Cataldo MF, Quaskey SA, Spielberg SP, Freeman JM (Johns Hopkins Med Insts, Baltimore)
Pediatrics 80:165–174, August 1987   5–7

Physicians treating children with epilepsy must prevent seizures while minimizing side effects. Methods of assessing subtle side effects that can interfere with school and social performance are needed. A double-blind, counterbalanced, crossover study of 21 epileptic children who were given phenobarbital and valproic acid for 6 months each was performed to compare cognitive and behavioral function.

There was no difference in seizure control between the 2 regimens. Children receiving phenobarbital performed significantly worse on 4 tests of neuropsychological function and were rated significantly worse by parents on 3 behavioral items. These children were also considered significantly more hyperactive.

Although children receiving antiepileptic drugs may appear to be tolerating medication, subtle changes in higher cortical function and behavior may be occurring. More sensitive methods of monitoring these children are required. Future studies are required to determine what side effects are associated with each drug, which patients are prone to these side effects, and whether these effects are reversible.

▶ The authors show rather convincingly that antiepileptic drug therapy affects behavior and cognition in children. Most of the data that have been accumulated thus far have been from adults, particularly healthy adult volunteers. This particular study looks at children by using the child as his own control in a well-designed double-blind crossover trial. A key feature is the documentation of the adverse cognitive and behavioral effects of phenobarbital. Although phenobarbital is an excellent anticonvulsant drug as well as being inexpensive, the adverse side effects, including cognitive impairment and behavior problems, should restrict its widespread use in children.— O.B. Evans, M.D.

Neurological Findings in the Fetal Alcohol Syndrome
Marcus JC (Downstate Med Ctr, Brooklyn, NY)
Neuropediatrics 18:158–160, 1987   5–8

The damaging effects of alcohol on the fetus have been recognized for hundreds of years. The constellation of central nervous system abnormalities, marked growth failure, dysmorphic facies, and a lesser incidence of cardiac and skeletal abnormalities was labeled fetal alcohol syndrome (FAS) 10 years ago. Formal neurologic deficits not related to higher cortical functions, however, have received little attention. Five children with FAS noted to have neurologic abnormalities were described.

The patients were 3 boys and 2 girls, aged 2¼ to 10 years. All had facial features typical of FAS and growth failure. Neurologic features common to all were kinetic tremor and axial ataxia (table). Three children also had dysdiadochokinesis. Only 2 had reduced intelligence. Three children had signs of attention deficit disorder, and 4 had speech problems. Motor deficits were not found to be a feature. The single cases of complex partial epilepsy and febrile convulsions were not considered remarkable. Clinical findings suggested diffuse cortical and cerebellar dam-

	Neurologic Findings				
	Kinetic Tremor	Dysdiadocho-kinesis	Axial Ataxia	Dysarthria	I.Q.
1.	+	+	+	+	50
2.	+	+	+	+	100
3.	+	+	+	−	55
4.	+	−	+	−	95
5.	+	−	+	+	85

(Courtesy of Marcus JC: *Neuropediatrics* 18:158–160, 1987.)

age. The mothers of all the children drank heavily during pregnancy, including beverages such as beer, wine, and vodka. Three children were born prematurely, and 1 was delivered by cesarean section. Birth weights ranged from 1.65 to 3.15 kg.

Five children with FAS and abnormal neurologic findings were described. Such findings were primarily cerebellar. Attention deficit disorder was found in 3, mental retardation in 2, and epilepsy in 1.

▶ The fetal alcohol syndrome has been recognized for many years. Babies delivered by mothers who drink heavily during pregnancy have cerebellar findings and attention deficit disorders and may have mental retardation and epilepsy. These symptoms indicate the presence of diffuse cortical and cerebellar damage. Every effort must be made to prevent the development of this syndrome. There is no effective treatment.— R.N. DeJong, M.D.

Minor Anomalies in Offspring of Epileptic Mothers
Gaily E, Granström M-L, Hiilesmaa V, Bardy A (Helsinki Univ, Pitäjänmäki Epilepsy Research Ctr, Helsinki)
J Pediatr 112:520–529, April 1988   5–9

Controlled studies have suggested an excess of minor anomalies in the offspring of women with epilepsy. One hundred twenty-one children of epileptic mothers and 105 control children were examined prospectively at age 5½ years for the presence of 80 minor physical anomalies. In the study group, 106 children were exposed to antiepileptic drugs during pregnancy and 82 were exposed to phenytoin. Forty-four mothers had generalized seizures during pregnancy. The parents of both study and control children also were assessed.

There was a significant excess of anomalies characteristic of hydantoin syndrome in the children of epileptic mothers and also in epileptic mothers themselves. Only hypertelorism and digital hypoplasia were associated with phenytoin exposure. None of the phenytoin-exposed children had all of the important features of hydantoin syndrome, including typical acrofacial findings, intellectual deficiency, growth retardation, and microcephaly. There was no excess of other minor anomalies in any group.

Children of epileptic mothers in this series did not have life-threatening major anomalies. The typical minor anomalies associated with phenytoin exposure were not accompanied by serious developmental abnormalities. There would seem to be limited teratogenic risk from well-monitored antiepileptic drug therapy during pregnancy. The estimated risk of serious developmental disturbance in phenytoin-exposed children is 1%–2%.

▶ Armin F. Haerer, M.D., Professor of Neurology, Department of Neurology, University of Mississippi Medical Center, Jackson, comments on this study.— R.D. Currier, M.D.

▶ It is reassuring to note that someone has finally succeeded in destroying the myth of the "hydantoin syndrome." Many of us felt we couldn't distinguish the pictures of children with this supposed syndrome from those with the "fetal alcohol syndrome" and others. Anomalies in offspring of epileptics seem to have multiple etiologies, including epilepsy and drugs.—A.F. Haerer, M.D.

Guidelines for the Determination of Brain Death in Children
Task Force for the Determination of Brain Death in Children
Neurology 37:1077–1078, June 1987   5–10

The unique issues in determining brain death in children are all medical ones, and are directly related to the more difficult task of confirming it in young children. The following criteria are useful 7 days after a neurologic insult in term newborns aged older than 38 weeks.

The critical initial assessment is the clinical history and examination. Determining the proximate cause of coma to ensure the absence of remediable or reversible conditions is the most important factor. Especially important are detection of toxic and metabolic disorders, sedative-hypnotic drugs, paralytic agents, hypothermia, hypotension, and surgically remediable conditions. Coma and apnea must coexist, and complete loss of consciousness, vocalization, and volitional activity must be exhibited. There must be absence of brain-stem function; the patient must not be significantly hypothermic or hypotensive for age. Excluding spinal cord events such as reflex withdrawal or spinal myoclonus, flaccid tone and absence of spontaneous or induced movements should exist. The examination should remain consistent with brain death throughout the observation and testing period.

Regarding observation periods, the Task Force recommends 2 examinations and electroencephalograms (EEGs) separated by at least 48 hours for children aged 7 days to 2 months, and 2 examinations and EEGs separated by at least 24 hours for children aged 2 months to 1 year. If a concomitant radionuclide angiographic (CRAG) study shows no visualization of cerebral arteries, a repeated examination and EEG are not necessary. Laboratory testing is not required when an irreversible cause exists, and an observation period of at least 12 hours is recommended in children aged older than 1 year. When the assessment of extent and reversibility of brain damage is particularly difficult, such as in cases of hypoxic-ischemic encephalopathy, and when the first examination is performed soon after the acute event, a period of at least 24 hours is recommended. This period may be reduced if the CRAG does not visualize cerebral arteries and if the EEG demonstrates electrocerebral silence.

If EEG is performed, it should be done over a 30-minute period; a CRAG demonstrating arrest of carotid circulation at the base of the skull and the absence of intracranial arterial circulation can be considered confirmatory of brain death.

Brain Death in Children: Part II

Ashwal S, Schneider S (Loma Linda Univ, Loma Linda, Calif)
Pediatr Neurol 3:69–77, 1987   5–11

Assessment of brain death in children is increasingly reliant on various neurodiagnostic studies. When using EEG recording to confirm brain death in infants and children, technical problems in intensive care units must be taken into account, as well as the relatively rapid cardiac and respiratory rates and the lower amplitude of cortical potentials in premature and newborn infants. The effects of hypothermia and CNS depressant drugs on EEG amplitudes are uncertain. Radionuclide angiography is a sensitive means of demonstrating absence of cerebral blood flow (CBF) in children, as in adults. Doppler and real-time cranial ultrasound methods also are used to determine the absence of CBF in newborn and young infants.

Clinical evaluation of pediatric patients in cases of suspected brain death involves the assessment of state of consciousness and the brain-stem reflexes after stabilization of the environment and under conditions of normal blood pressure without volume depletion. Blood and urine studies are done as appropriate to rule out toxic and metabolic disorders. Laboratory studies are required for confirmation in patients younger than 2 months of age. If the initial EEG is isoelectric in a child younger than 1 year old, a CBF study may be obtained using radionuclide angiography. Such a study is also indicated if the initial EEG shows activity. If CBF is present, brain death is not diagnosed. Loss of neuroendocrine and neurovascular control in the brain-dead patient must be treated if organ donation is considered.

▶ Rae Hanson, M.D., Assistant Professor of Pediatrics and Neurology at the University of Mississippi Medical Center, Jackson, comments on this study.— R.D. Currier, M.D.

▶ Ashwal and Schneider have written a concise and up-to-the-minute review of the topic of brain death in children. Their discussion of the adult criteria and their application to children, as well as the issues of normal CNS development in premature infants, fairly represents our understanding of these matters at the present time. Recommendations are given for evaluation of brain death in children that clinicians can easily apply to their patients. This article should be read by all physicians who deal with issues of cerebral death in pediatric patients.

Ahmann et al. (*J Pediatr* 110:723–728, 1987) studied brain-dead children using pulsed Doppler ultrasound, finding a characteristic waveform in most. The Task Force for the Determination of Brain Death in Children reported its findings in the June issues of *Neurology* and *Annals of Neurology*. The criteria change with each age group.— R. Hanson, M.D.

6 Epilepsy

Syncope
Linzer M (Montefiore Med Ctr; North Central Bronx Hosp; Mt Sinai Med Ctr, New York; Duke Univ)
South Med J 80:545–552, May 1987   6–1

Syncope, a transient loss of consciousness, is a frequent diagnostic problem that is not definitively characterized in up to half of cases. The differential diagnosis of syncope is broad (table, p. 68). The role of neurologic events in producing syncope remains unclear. Several new drugs can cause postural syncope. Situational syncope is a prominent disorder in the elderly, in whom syncope in general is frequent. A related issue is that falls are an important form of trauma in elderly persons. So-called bedtime syncope is a disorder seen in healthy young adults ambulating at night, with associated periods of asystole.

Routine electroencephalographic recording has a very low yield in patients with syncope. Nuclide brain scans are most useful in patients with abnormal neurologic findings. Holter monitoring is indicated where no cause of syncope is apparent, and possibly in persons with suspected neurologic factors. Programmed electrical stimulation may be useful in patients with recurrent syncope and organic heart disease. Carotid sinus massage deserves further attention in evaluating unexplained syncope.

Most patients with syncope do very well, but those with cardiac syncope have increased mortality. Models predicting both short-term and long-term outcome are needed, as are valid diagnostic criteria. Pre- and post-test probabilities of a specific diagnosis, such as cardiac syncope, should also be a topic of future research.

▶ The isolated syncopal episode is often benign and self-limited, but it may represent serious neurologic or cardiac disease. This paper reviews our current advances in understanding syncope and determining prognosis.— R.N. DeJong, M.D.

Classification of the Epilepsies: Influence on Management
Dreifuss FE (Univ of Virginia, Charlottesville)
Rev Neurol (Paris) 143:375–380, 1987   6–2

A classification of epileptic syndromes is needed not just for purposes of communication, but for appropriate use of treatment and/or its judicious withholding, and for determining prognosis in an individual patient. The Commission on Classification and Terminology of the Interna-

---

Differential Diagnosis of Syncope

I. Vasovagal

II. Cardiac
   A. Stokes-Adams, sick sinus syndrome, supraventricular and ventricular tachycardias, heart block, drugs (eg, quinidine), "bedtime syncope"
   B. Aortic stenosis, hypertrophic cardiomyopathy, mitral valve prolapse
   C. Carotid sinus hypersensitivity, pulmonary hypertension (including pulmonary embolism), myocardial ischemia, atrial myxoma, pericardial tamponade

III. Neurologic
   A. Transient ischemic attacks (rare)
   B. Unwitnessed seizure

IV. Other Causes
   A. Postural
      1. Volume depletion
      2. Autonomic insufficiency
      3. Drug-induced (eg, prazosin, nitrates)
   B. Situational
      1. Micturition
      2. Posttussive
      3. Postdefecation
      4. Postdeglutition
      5. Postprandial
   C. Psychiatric
      1. Hysteria
      2. Hyperventilation
   D. Metabolic
      1. Hypoglycemia
      2. Hypoxemia
      3. Systemic mastocytosis
   E. Miscellaneous
      1. Takayasu's disease
      2. Glossopharyngeal neuralgia
      3. Subclavian steal syndrome

V. Syncope of Unknown Origin

(Courtesy of Linzer M: *South Med J* 80:545–552, May 1987.)

---

tional League Against Epilepsy proposed a classification for the epilepsies.

The main categories of seizures include generalized seizures and partial seizures. Generalized seizures include absence, myoclonic, tonic, atonic, and tonic-clonic. There are 2 main subdivisions under partial seizures: simple partial seizures, in which consciousness is preserved, and complex partial seizures, in which consciousness is impaired. Simple partial seizures are subclassified according to the area of cortex predominantly involved; it is understood that they may progress to complex partial seizures or to secondarily generalized tonic-clonic seizures. Complex partial seizures involve limbic structures. Consciousness is impaired. These seizures may progress to secondarily generalized tonic-clonic seizures.

Syndromes are also classified. Localization-related epilepsies and syndromes include idiopathic and symptomatic types. Generalized epilepsies and syndromes are either idiopathic, such as benign neonatal familial convulsions, benign neonatal convulsions, benign myoclonic epilepsy in infancy, childhood absence epilepsy, juvenile absence epilepsy, juvenile myoclonic epilepsy, and epilepsy with grand mal seizures on waking; idiopathic and/or symptomatic, such as West syndrome, Lennox-Gastaut syndrome, epilepsy with myoclonic-astatic seizures, and epilepsy with myoclonic absences; or symptomatic, of nonspecific or specific etiology. Epilepsies and syndromes undetermined, whether focal or generalized, include those with both generalized and focal seizures, such as neonatal seizures, severe myoclonic epilepsy in infancy, epilepsy with continuous spike-waves during slow-wave sleep, acquired epileptic aphasia, and those without generalized or focal features. Special syndromes include situation-related seizures, isolated apparently unprovoked epileptic events, epilepsies characterized by specific modes of seizure precipitation, and chronic progressive epilepsia partialis continua of childhood.

This proposed classification can facilitate treatment for epileptic patients. Therapy should be as specific as possible, considering the seizure, the medication most specifically useful for that type of seizure, and determination of the syndrome to which the seizure belongs. This, in turn, allows formulation of a prognosis.

▶ This classification of epileptic syndromes aids in ascertaining treatment and prognosis of individual cases.— R.N. DeJong, M.D.

CT Findings in Late-Onset Epilepsy
de la Sayette V, Cosgrove R, Melanson D, Ethier R (Montreal Neurological Hosp)
Can J Neurol Sci 14:286–289, August 1987   6–3

Epilepsy beginning in late adult life may be caused by a variety of disorders such as cerebrovascular disease, brain tumors, degenerative and inflammatory cerebral processes, or metabolic disturbances. It is uncommon, and limited data are available on its clinical characteristics and causes. Establishing an etiologic diagnosis and excluding an expanding intracerebral lesion as the cause of seizures are important. Computed tomography is commonly used to investigate epilepsy in elderly patients. The clinical and CT findings of 387 patients older than 50 years with new-onset seizures were reviewed to establish clinical and radiologic correlations in late-onset epilepsy and to study the role of CT scanning in this condition.

The radiologic files from 1978 to 1984 at 1 institution were reviewed. Seizures were found to be generalized in 212 patients, focal in 160, and indeterminate in 15. The CT scanning demonstrated cerebral atrophy in 113 patients, ischemic lesions in 75, cerebral neoplasms in 20, and no abnormality in 177. Only 3 patients with generalized seizures were found to have tumors; all 3 had focal neurologic deficits at the time of CT diagnosis. Seventeen neoplasms were found among patients with a focal seizure disorder.

This review showed that most patients with late-onset epilepsy had a normal CT scan. Cerebral atrophy was the most common abnormality detected. Cerebral vascular disease appeared to be the most commonly identified cause of late-onset epilepsy in this series; cerebral neoplasms were uncommon.

▶ The first thought of most physicians when confronted with late-onset epilepsy (after the age of 50) is "brain tumor." This carefully carried out study, however, shows that cerebral neoplasms are uncommon in these patients and that cerebrovascular disease is the most common cause of seizures.—R.N. DeJong, M.D.

Outcome From Coma After Cardiopulmonary Resuscitation: Relation to Seizures and Myoclonus

Krumholz A, Stern BJ, Weiss HD (Sinai Hosp of Baltimore, Johns Hopkins Univ)
Neurology 38:401–405, March 1988   6–4

Seizures and myoclonus often follow cardiopulmonary resuscitation (CPR). However, the relationship of these disorders to outcome is not well established. The effect of seizures and myoclonus after CPR on the outcome of all comatose adult survivors of CPR in an 8-year period was investigated.

From 1977–1985, 114 consecutive adults who survived CPR for more than 24 hours and were referred to the neurology service in coma were prospectively studied. Patients with prior contributing neurologic disor-

Neurologic Recovery of Patients Comatose After CPR

	No.	Conscious at discharge	Conscious at any time
I. All patients	114	21 (18%)	25 (22%)
II. No seizures or myoclonus	64	15 (23%)	17 (27%)
III. Seizures or myoclonus	50	6 (12%)	8 (16%)
IV. Status (seizures and/or myoclonus)	36	1 (3%)†	2 (6%)†
A. Status epilepticus other than MSE	10	1 (10%)	2 (20%)
B. Myoclonic status epilepticus (MSE)	19	0†	0†
C. Status myoclonus other than MSE	7	0	0

*Significantly different from patients without this condition, $P < .05$.
†Significantly different from patients without this condition, $P < .01$.
‡Significantly different from patients without this condition, $P < .001$.
(Courtesy of Krumholz A, Stern BJ, Weiss HD: *Neurology* 38:401–405, March 1988.)

ders were excluded from the study. Of the 114 patients, 50 suffered either seizures or myoclonus. Seizures occurred in 41 patients, or 36%, and myoclonus occurred in 40 patients, or 35%. Status epilepticus or status myoclonus occurred in 36 patients, or 32%. Nineteen, or 17%, had myoclonus status epilepticus. Seizures and myoclonus per se were not found to be significantly related to outcome. However, status epilepticus, status myoclonus, and especially myoclonic status epilepticus were predictive of poor outcome as judged by survival and recovery of consciousness (table).

Seizures and myoclonus after CPR per se are not associated with poorer prognosis. However, severe and prolonged paroxysmal disorders, such as status and particularly myoclonic status epilepticus, are related to significantly higher mortality and morbidity.

▶ Either seizures or myoclonus occurred in nearly 50% of all adult survivors of cardiopulmonary resuscitation. These were not significantly related to outcome, but status epilepticus and status myoclonus, and particularly myoclonic status epilepticus, were predictive of poor outcome as judged by survival and recovery of consciousness.— R.N. DeJong, M.D.

Complex Partial Status Epilepticus Presenting as Fever of Unknown Origin
Semel JD (Highland Park Hosp, Lake Forest Hosp, Rush-Presbyterian-St Luke's Med Ctr, Chicago)
Arch Intern Med 147:1571–1572, September 1987   6–5

Patients with fever of unknown origin present a diagnostic challenge to clinicians. In a woman with periodic episodes of fever, the eventual diagnosis was complex partial status epilepticus.

Woman, 61, was assessed for intermittent fever; each episode lasted 24–72 hours. The patient had memory loss associated with the fever. One of the patient's children had epilepsy. Initial evaluations, as well as evaluations following other febrile episodes, revealed no abnormality. Nine months after the initial evaluation, the patient was readmitted to the hospital after being observed to undergo cycles of nonresponsiveness, speech arrest, staring, lip smacking, and hand movements before fever onset. Complex partial epilepsy was diagnosed, and carbamazepine therapy was initiated. Eleven months later, the patient discontinued the medication and seizures with fever again occurred. An electroencephalogram showed bilateral, independent, temporal-lobe epileptogenic foci. Carbamazepine therapy was reinstated, and the patient remained seizure free after 1 year.

Fever may be associated with seizures in adults as a result of epilepsy; thus, epilepsy should be considered in the diagnosis of intermittent fever. Observation, electroencephalography, or a trial of anticonvulsant medication may help to confirm the diagnosis.

Withdrawal of Anticonvulsant Drugs in Patients Free of Seizures for Two Years: A Prospective Study

Callaghan N, Garrett A, Goggin T (Cork Regional Hosp, Univ College, Cork, Ireland; Parke-Davis, McDonnell-Douglas Systems, London)
N Engl J Med 318:942–946, April 14, 1988   6–6

Because anticonvulsant drugs are known to have long-term toxic effects, their prolonged use in the treatment of epilepsy should be avoided. An attempt was made to identify risk factors associated with relapse of epilepsy after withdrawal of monotherapy with either phenytoin, sodium valproate, or carbamazepine.

The study population included 40 male and 52 female patients with epilepsy (mean age, 24 years), who had remained free of seizures during 2 years of single-drug therapy prior to this study, and who had had epilepsy for a mean duration of 2 years before drug treatment was first initiated. Of these 92 patients, 72 had responded to the first drug prescribed, 15 to the second drug prescribed, and 5 to the third drug prescribed. Drug treatment was withdrawn gradually over a 6–12 month period.

During a mean follow-up of 26 months after drug withdrawal, 31 (33.7%) patients relapsed and 61 patients remained free of seizures. The average remission in patients who relapsed lasted 8 months. Drug treatment was reinstated in those who relapsed.

Statistical analysis of the data showed that complex partial seizures with secondary generalization were associated with the highest risk of relapse. Generalized seizures carried a 65% lower risk of relapse, whereas complex or simple partial seizures without secondary generalization carried a 97% lower risk of relapse. Electroencephalographic Class 4 epilepsy, defined as abnormal before treatment and unchanged before drug withdrawal, was associated with the highest risk of relapse (73.7%). Of the 3 drugs used for treatment, sodium valproate was associated with the highest relapse rate.

Clinicians should consider withdrawal of anticonvulsant medication in patients who have been free of seizures for at least 2 years.

▶ As expected, complex partial seizures with secondary generalization were the ones least likely to remain absent after medications were stopped. It does appear that the EEG is of use in predicting the return of seizures.—R.D. Currier, M.D.

The First Seizure in Adult Life: Value of Clinical Features, Electroencephalography, and Computerised Tomographic Scanning in Prediction of Seizure Recurrence

Hopkins A, Garman A, Clarke C (St Bartholomew's Hosp, London)
Lancet 1:721–726, April 2, 1988   6–7

Up to 5.9% of the population will experience at least 1 nonfebrile seizure at some stage of life. Such patients may ask whether they will have subsequent seizures, what factors are related to recurrence, whether there is some definite cause for the first seizure, and what investigations are appropriate. A study was done to address these questions.

All patients older than age 16 years referred with a first seizure were followed up. Of the 408 patients studied, almost 40% were aged 20–29 years. Initial seizures were tonic-clonic with no evidence of partial onset in 85.3% and with clinical evidence of partial onset in 12.2%. Initial seizures were partial complex or simple in the remaining 2.2%. The actuarial risk of seizure recurrence was highest in the early weeks. For patients seen within the first week, the risk of recurrence was 52% by the end of 3 years. The time of day of the initial seizure, age younger than 50 years, and a family history of seizures of any type tended to be associated with recurrence. Such risk factors appeared to be additive, so the risk of recurrence at 1 year for a person with all 3 risk factors was about 3 times that of a person with no risk factors. Sex, type of seizure, and EEG features were not predictive. Computerized tomography demonstrated tumors in 3% of the subjects, who were particularly likely to have recurrent seizures.

This study demonstrated a high rate of recurrence after an initial seizure in adulthood—at least 52% by 3 years. Age, sex, family history, or seizure type were not statistically significant variables by univariate analysis.

▶ The thing that is curious about this study is the failure of the electroencephalogram to be of predictive value. The follow-up length was 4 years, so perhaps an argument could be made that the EEG might be valuable if follow-up were longer.

On the other hand, a report by Callaghan, Garrett, and Goggin (*N Engl J Med* 318:942–946, 1988), shows that the EEG is of value in predicting the success of withdrawal from medications in patients free of seizures for 2 years. So perhaps we shouldn't pull the plug on the EEG machine yet.—R.D. Currier, M.D.

Early Treatment and Prognosis of Epilepsy
Reynolds EH (Maudsley Hosp, Kings College Hosp, London)
Epilepsia 28:97–106, March–April 1987   6–8

A more optimistic perspective on the prognosis for control of epilepsy has emerged in recent years. Community and hospital-based studies indicate that about 75% of newly diagnosed epileptics achieve long-term remission with currently available medication.

The author presents data on 106 adolescent and adult patients with newly diagnosed and previously untreated epilepsy who were seen at Kings College Hospital over a 10-year period. All patients had experienced at least 2 tonic-clonic or partial seizures in the year before treatment. Treatment was with either phenytoin (61 patients) or carbamazepine (45 patients), initially in a small dose; the dosage was increased if seizures recurred. If 2 or more seizures were experienced, after the dosage had been raised to optimum blood level range, a second drug was added. At 2-year follow-up, 73% of patients were in 1-year remission, and at 8-year follow-up, 92% had achieved 1-year remission (Fig 6–1).

Most individuals who develop chronic epilepsy can be identified within the first 2 years of treatment. Prompt treatment during this period is crucial. If treatment fails to arrest the evolution of chronic epilepsy, it is usually due to the presence of brain lesions and neuropsychiatric handicaps. There is some evidence that chronic epilepsy is a process tending toward escalation unless halted by treatment.

In some cases, benign epilepsy remits spontaneously; it is not known whether prompt drug treatment might improve the prognosis for natural remission. Usually, a person who experiences a single afebrile tonic-clonic seizure not attributable to alcohol or drug abuse or to acute metabolic disturbance will later become epileptic. Research is needed to establish recommended treatment modalities in such cases. Further studies of the comparative efficacy of currently available drugs are needed. It presently appears that the major drugs are equally effective when prescribed appropriately by a practitioner experienced in long-term management of epilepsy. Other considerations in the initiation of an early treatment program include identification of avoidable precipitating factors, ensuring an understanding attitude in the patient's family, and emphasizing the importance of good compliance.

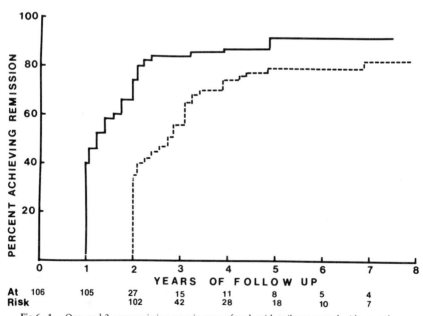

Fig 6–1.—One- and 2-year remission rates in new referrals with epilepsy treated with monotherapy. Actuarial percentage of patients completely free of seizures for 1 year *(solid line)* and 2 years *(broken line)*. (From Reynolds EH: *Epilepsia* 28:97–106, March–April 1987. Courtesy of Elwes RDC, Johnson AL, Shorvon SD, et al: *N Engl J Med* 311:944–947, 1984.)

► Early treatment is crucial in determining the subsequent course of epilepsy. The longer seizures continue, the less likely they are to be controlled. Recent studies have shown that there are no significant differences in the efficacy of the major antiepileptic drugs, and the choice of drug is determined by its costs and associated side effects, especially cognitive and behavioral effects.—R.N. DeJong, M.D.

If a Well-Stabilized Epileptic Patient Has a Subtherapeutic Antiepileptic Drug Level, Should the Dose Be Increased?: A Randomized Prospective Study

Woo E, Chan YM, Yu YL, Chan YW, Huang CY (Univ of Hong Kong; Queen Mary Hosp, Hong Kong)
Epilepsia 29:129–139, 1988   6–9

A prospective 2-year study was conducted to determine the proper management of stabilized epileptic patients with subtherapeutic anticonvulsant drug levels. The 80 patients in the study had been free of seizures for 3 months to 2 years. All had a documented seizure disorder of the primary generalized tonic-clonic type without focal clinical or electroencephalographic features, and all were taking a single antiepileptic drug. Either the dose was unchanged from its subtherapeutic level, or it was increased until serum levels of phenytoin or phenobarbital were in the therapeutic range.

Seizures were comparable in the 2 groups during a mean follow-up of 2 years, but patients taking increased drug doses had more neurotoxic side effects. Systemic toxicity was comparable in the 2 groups. Markedly significant differences in serum drug levels persisted, whether phenytoin or phenobarbital was taken.

It is not necessary to increase the dose of anticonvulsant drug in patients with subtherapeutic serum levels if they are relatively well stabilized. This approach minimizes the need for dose adjustments as well as the need for expensive drug monitoring. Monitoring remains valuable when physiologic changes or concurrent disease can lead to altered drug disposition. It also is helpful in identifying noncompliance with treatment.

► The answer is "no," a conclusion that is not really surprising.—R.D. Currier, M.D.

Corpus Callosotomy for Epilepsy: I. Seizure Effects

Spencer SS, Spencer DD, Williamson PD, Sass K, Novelly RA, Mattson RH (Yale Univ; VA Med Ctr, West Haven, Conn)
Neurology 38:19–24, January 1988   6–10

Corpus callosum section can be used to control generalized seizures. Results have been promising but difficult to compare. The experience with corpus callosum section in 22 patients followed up for more than 2 years was reviewed.

From 1979 to 1983, patients were considered for the procedure if control of secondarily generalized or partial seizures was not obtained medically for at least 4 years; if seizures were of sufficient frequency or character to interfere significantly with daily living; and if no single resectable epileptic focus could be identified. The 22 patients treated were 5 females and 17 males, aged 5–39 years. Nine had partial callosal sectioning and 13 had total sectioning. At 2 or more years after corpus callosum section, 41% of the patients were found to have a class 1 outcome—elimination of secondarily generalized and complex partial seizures; 32% had a class 2 outcome—elimination of secondarily generalized seizures; and 27% had a class 3 outcome—no appreciable change. Total section was found to be twice as effective in eliminating secondarily generalized seizures as partial section; success rates were 77% and 35%, respectively. Significant associations were observed between focal computed tomographic lesions and class 1 outcome and between IQ of less than 45 and class 2 or 3 outcome.

Total corpus callosum section can prevent secondarily generalized seizures in at least 75% of patients. The findings were consistent with those previously reported. Total callosotomy was twice as effective as partial section in controlling secondarily generalized seizures.

▶ Conditions in the majority of patients were improved by this procedure, and the longer the section, the greater the chances of success. The neurologic and neuropsychologic outcomes are reported in a following article in the same issue of *Neurology* (38:24–28, 1988).

These workers are leading the way in a rather tough area, and one hopes their attempts to treat these difficult patients will continue.— R.D. Currier, M.D.

Valproic Acid Hepatic Fatalities: A Retrospective Review
Dreifuss FE, Santilli N, Langer DH, Sweeney KP, Moline KA, Menander KB
(Univ of Virginia, Charlottesville; Abbott Laboratories; Univ of Health Sciences/
Chicago Med School, North Chicago, Ill)
Neurology 37:379–385, March 1987   6–11

Since its introduction to the American market in 1978, valproic acid (VPA) has been proved effective as an anticonvulsant in seizure therapy. However, there have been reports of fatal hepatotoxicity in patients undergoing treatment with VPA. The authors reviewed and analyzed data on cases of fatal hepatotoxicity to clarify the overall incidence rate of fatal hepatotoxicity and to identify factors that might indicate individual predisposition to hepatic failure.

The manufacturer of valproate received reports of 37 hepatic fatalities, coincident with VPA therapy during a 7-year period. Of nearly 400,000 patients who were treated with valproate during this time, there were 23 male and 14 female fatalities. Patients ranged in age from 5 months to 71

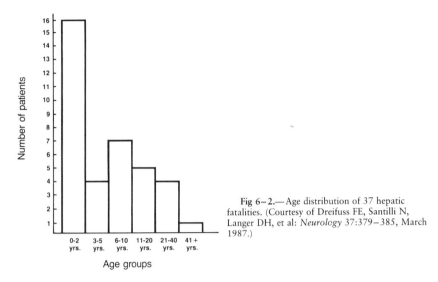

Fig 6–2.—Age distribution of 37 hepatic fatalities. (Courtesy of Dreifuss FE, Santilli N, Langer DH, et al: *Neurology* 37:379–385, March 1987.)

years (Fig 6–2). In all but 1 instance, seizures were accompanied by other disorders including mental retardation, congenital abnormalities, and various neurologic diseases. More than 86% of the fatalities occurred in patients undergoing polytherapy involving 1 to 4 additional anticonvulsant drugs, with phenytoin and phenobarbital being the most common. The dosage of VPA in relation to body weight was known in only 24 cases, and it ranged from a low of 13 mg/kg of body weight per day to a high (in 4 cases) of 120 mg/kg of body weight per day, which is twice the recommended maximum dosage. Patients at greatest risk were children aged younger than 2 years whose seizures were accompanied by other serious medical problems and who were undergoing polytherapy. The infant fatality rate with VPA monotherapy was substantially lower. Most of the polytherapy patients in this age group had already failed treatment with other anticonvulsants. The risk declined with age, and no hepatic fatalities occurred in patients aged older than 10 years receiving valproate as monotherapy.

The benefits of VPA therapy must be carefully weighed against the fatal hepatotoxicity risk in children aged younger than 2 years. In older patients, the risk of fatality is very low, particularly with valproate monotherapy; thus, it is best to use VPA as the only anticonvulsant drug whenever possible. Regular clinical monitoring for prodromal symptoms of hepatic toxicity is extremely important.

▶ This is a review of all patients in the United States who died of hepatotoxicity associated with the use of valproic acid between 1978 and 1984. The primary risk is in children under the age of 2 years receiving valproate as part of polytherapy.— R.N. DeJong, M.D.

7 Extrapyramidal Disorders

Clinical Assessment of 31 Patients With Wilson's Disease: Correlations With Structural Changes on Magnetic Resonance Imaging
Starosta-Rubinstein S, Young AB, Kluin K, Hill G, Aisen AM, Gabrielsen T, Brewer GJ (Univ of Michigan, Ann Arbor)
Arch Neurol 44:365–370, April 1987   7–1

Wilson's disease (WD) is a genetic disorder of copper metabolism that is frequently misdiagnosed in its early stages as a psychiatric disorder, a different neurologic disease, or liver disease. Excessive amounts of copper accumulate in the central nervous system, liver, cornea, kidney, and other organs, producing psychiatric, neurologic, hepatic, hematologic, renal, articular, or ocular abnormalities. The authors describe their experience with 31 patients with WD in whom brain lesions detected by magnetic resonance imaging (MRI) were correlated with clinical manifestations of WD.

Seventeen men and 14 women were studied. The mean patient age was 28 ± 6 years, and the mean age at onset of symptoms was 21 ± 5 years. All but 10% of patients had been treated with penicillamine; of these, the conditions of 31% had initially deteriorated despite treatment, and 50% never recovered to pretherapy baseline. The most prevalent neurologic findings included dysarthria (97%), dystonia (65%), dysdiadochokinesia (58%), rigidity (52%), gait and postural abnormalities (42%), and tremor (32%). Twenty-two patients underwent MRI. Scans were abnormal in 18 of 19 symptomatic patients, and scans were normal in the 3 asymptomatic patients. Lesions were most frequently found in the caudate, putamen, subcortical white matter, midbrain, and pons. Generalized atrophy of the brain was commonly detected. In a few cases, lesions were found in the thalamus, cerebellar vermis, globus pallidus, midbrain tegmentum, red nucleus, and dentate nucleus. Putamen lesions correlated with dystonia and bradykinesia. Putamen and caudate lesions corresponded with dysarthria. However, because of multiplicity of lesions and comparisons, no causal relationships can be assumed.

Because of the rarity of WD, it is suggested that cooperative studies be initiated for further investigation, and that patients be referred to specialized treatment centers. The current initial recommended penicillamine doses may be too high. Perhaps a more gradual introduction of penicillamine, combined with a low-copper diet, could reduce the side effects of current therapy.

▶ In this detailed clinical study of 31 patients with Wilson's disease, 22 had MRI. Of the neurologic findings, dystonia and bradykinesis were correlated with putamen lesions, and dysarthria was correlated with both putamen and caudate lesions. Attempts to avoid the complications of penicillamine therapy need further study.— R.N. DeJong, M.D.

Progressive Supranuclear Palsy and a Multi-Infarct State
Dubinsky RM, Jankovic J (Baylor College of Medicine, Houston)
Neurology 37:570–576, April 1987   7–2

Progressive supranuclear palsy (PSP) is defined by the combination of dementia, parkinsonism, and supranuclear ophthalmoparesis. Because all of these features may also be caused by strokes, the frequency of cerebrovascular disease in PSP was investigated.

Fifty-eight consecutive patients with PSP were assessed in the Movement Disorder Clinic at Baylor College of Medicine. Nineteen of 58 (32.8%) had computed tomography (CT), magnetic resonance imaging (MRI), or autopsy evidence of a multi-infarct state (Fig 7–1). The clinical findings in the infarct syndrome were similar to idiopathic PSP. There were 5 multi-infarct PSP patients who had had a stroke, 4 who had focal dystonia, 2 who had hemiparesis, and 1 who had an intention tremor of recent onset. In contrast, only 5.9% of 426 Parkinson's disease patients had evidence of strokes. There was 1 case of PSP studied pathologically that was attributed to cerebral amyloid angiopathy.

Although the multi-infarct PSP is clinically similar to PSP, the former can be differentiated by prior strokes, presence of focal dystonia, hemiparesis, and intention tremor. The neuroimaging studies (CT, MRI) reveal a much higher incidence of multi-infarct in PSP than in Parkinson's disease, but autopsies will be needed to differentiate the multi-infarct PSP from the idiopathic PSP.

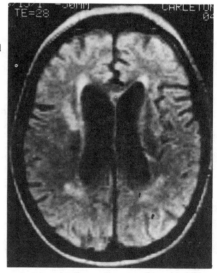

Fig 7–1.— Magnetic resonance imaging showing right internal capsule, right occipital, and bilateral periventricular with infarcts. (Pulsing sequence, TR = 2.0 seconds, TE = 28 msec) (Courtesy of Dubinsky RM, Jankovic J: *Neurology* 37:570–576, April 1987.)

▶ Idiopathic progressive supranuclear palsy and the progressive supranuclear palsy caused by a multi-infarct state may be differentiated by a history of prior strokes and the presence of focal dystonia, hemiparesis, and intention tremor in the latter. Neuroimaging studies (computed tomography and magnetic resonance imaging) also aid in the differential diagnosis.—R.N. DeJong, M.D.

Spasticity
Young RR, Wiegner AW (Harvard Univ; Massachusetts General Hosp, Boston)
Clin Orthop 219:50–62, June 1987   7–3

Spasticity represents a velocity-dependent hyperactive state of the stretch reflexes; it is therefore only 1 aspect of the syndrome produced by an upper motoneuron lesion. Imbalance in the strength of antagonistic muscle groups can contribute to joint contracture, but spasticity is not responsible for most of the functional disability of patients having upper motoneuron lesions. Paresis, lack of dexterity, and fatigability also are important. Spasticity appears to be related to increased excitation at the segmental spinal level. Reciprocal inhibition utilizing Ia interneurons is an important mechanism affected in the development of spasticity. The chief source of functional disability is disconnection of more rostral motor centers from those at the segmental spinal level.

Surgical treatment of spasticity is designed to produce discrete lesions in the stretch reflex arc to reduce hyperactivity. Recovery from negative symptoms is not aided. Selective dorsal rhizotomy can be used to destroy fibers mediating pain and flexor reflexes. Medical treatment has been relatively ineffective, since most neurotransmitters involved in the motor system are unknown.

Dantrolene is used to produce a dose-dependent reduction in calcium release from the sarcoplasmic reticulum, thereby uncoupling muscular contraction from electrical excitation. Other antispastic agents work within the central nervous system and produce significant drowsiness as a side effect. Clinical neurophysiologic testing can show which antispastic drug will be most effective in a given patient. Combined surgical and medical treatment is often necessary.

▶ Robert R. Young, Director of the Laboratory of Clinical Neurophysiology at the Massachusetts General Hospital, Harvard Medical School, is an authority on abnormalities of muscle tone. This article, which discusses spasticity and attempts to treat it, is an extremely important one.—R.N. DeJong, M.D.

Young Onset Parkinson's Disease
Quinn N, Critchley P, Marsden CD (Inst of Psychiatry, King's College Hosp Med School, London)
Movement Disord 2:73–91, 1987   7–4

Parkinson's disease rarely begins before age 40 years. Sixty patients with Parkinson's disease, 56 of whom were classified as having young-onset Parkinson's disease and 4 as having juvenile parkinsonism, were studied. The latter patients had an onset before age 21 years.

One fifth of patients with young-onset Parkinson's disease had a relative with probable parkinsonism, and 5 had a relative with essential tremor. About half the index patients had an akinetic-rigid syndrome; the rest had the triad of akinesia, rigidity, and resting tremor. Eight patients had dystonic features. Intellectual function was normal in most patients. Of 45 patients undergoing treatment with levodopa for 2 years or longer, 80% had an excellent response, and the rest had substantial benefit from treatment. Fluctuations were the rule on long-term levodopa therapy. All patients with juvenile parkinsonism had an affected relative. All 3 patients given levodopa had an excellent initial response, but 1 deteriorated after a short time. All 3 patients had treatment-related complications.

This study fails to confirm a very high familial incidence of parkinsonism or essential tremor in the relatives of patients with young-onset Parkinson's disease. It might be of interest to seek environmental causes of Parkinson's disease in young-onset patients. Patients with genetically determined juvenile parkinsonism probably have an illness other than Parkinson's disease, but pathologic data are lacking.

▶ These workers divide parkinsonism into 3 groups—juvenile, young onset, and the older onset (after age 40) idiopathic type. The younger the onset, they say, the more likely the disease is to be familial and the more benign in terms of later dementia. This could be a useful classification.—R.D. Currier, M.D.

Pathophysiology and Biochemical Mechanisms Involved in MPTP-Induced Parkinsonism
Poirier J (Clinical Research Inst of Montreal)
J Am Geriatr Soc 35:660–668, July 1987   7–5

The recent discovery of a new dopaminergic neurotoxin, 1-methyl-4-phenyl-1,2,3,6-tetrahydropyridine (MPTP), has led to an understanding of some of the possible mechanisms involved in the neurodegenerative process of idiopathic Parkinson's disease (IPD). Systemic administration of MPTP in human beings can induce a syndrome similar to IPD; although L-dopa has been shown to reverse those symptoms, after a certain period of time, the MPTP-treated patients presented the same treatment complications usually observed in the idiopathic form of the disease.

Animal models have shown that MPTP can no longer be considered as a single target toxin, since it significantly affects some of the peripheral organs. It decreased catecholamines in mouse hearts and in the adrenal glands of frogs, increased adrenal levels of dopamine and noradrenaline in monkeys, and produced duodenal ulcers in rats. In the liver, MPTP is transformed into a toxic metabolite, MPP+.

It is evident that MPTP neurotoxicity is caused by a combination of short- and long-term effects, which eventually lead to cell death. The transformation of MPTP into MPP+ passes through the formation of MPTP+, which in turn is transformed into MPP+. The exact location of this transformation is still not known. Once formed, MPP+ accumulates in different areas of the brain for a few hours, then is rapidly removed, except in the substantia nigra, where it continues to accumulate for more than 72 hours.

Neurodegeneration induced by MPTP in the central nervous system is more specific than that observed in IPD, but no Lewy bodies have been found in MPTP-treated monkey brains. The MPTP models have, however, served to clarify the role of the dopaminergic neurons with respect to the onset and evolution of the parkinsonian symptoms. Whereas MPTP, a neutral molecule, can cross the blood-brain barrier of rodents and primates, MPP+ cannot; however, MPP+ is avidly accumulated by the catecholaminergic neurons whereas MPTP is not. These 2 compounds present complementary features that determine their neurotoxicity. There are still some major differences in terms of neurochemistry, pathology, and evolution of the syndromes, despite clinical similarities between MPTP-induced parkinsonism and IPD in human beings.

Deprenyl Versus Placebo in Parkinson Disease: A Double-Blind Study
Lieberman AN, Gopinathan G, Neophytides A, Foo SH (New York Univ; New York Infirmary-Beekman Downtown Med Ctr, New York)
NY State J Med 87:646–649, December 1987   7–6

Deprenyl, alone or with levodopa, may delay or prevent the progression of Parkinson's disease. Animal studies have shown that deprenyl blocks the oxidation of 4-methyl-4-phenyl 1,2,3,6 tetrahydropyridine (MPTP) to its toxic metabolite 1-methyl-4-phenyl-pyridine (MPP+) and prevents the development of MPTP-induced parkinsonism. If the cause of idiopathic Parkinson's disease is related to the formation of an MPP+-like substance, deprenyl may delay the disease progression. Deprenyl is currently available only on an experimental basis in the United States. A study was done to evaluate the drug's safety and efficacy in patients with Parkinson's disease.

Thirty-three patients were admitted to the randomized, double-blind study. None was responding satisfactorily to levodopa. Seventeen patients received 10 mg of deprenyl per day in addition to levodopa, and 16 received placebo with levodopa. A modified Columbia University Scale was used to assess the patients. Patients also kept 24-hour diaries to help evaluate daily fluctuations. Age, duration of Parkinson's disease, duration of levodopa therapy, and the presence of "wearing off" phenomena were comparable in the 2 treatment groups. After 8 weeks, patients receiving deprenyl had a significant 22% decrease in symptoms, a 17.4% decrease in signs, and a 21% decrease in levodopa use. No significant changes were noted in the number of hours "on." Adverse effects were minimal and similar to those produced by levodopa.

This study demonstrated a significant improvement in patients with

Parkinson's disease after receiving deprenyl. Deprenyl was concluded to be an effective and safe antiparkinson agent.

▶ If MPTP has anything to do with idiopathic parkinsonism, the use of deprenyl raises hope that the progression of the disease itself may be slowed, since the drug prevents the oxidation of MPTP to MPP+, the toxic component. This drug is not available in the United States.— R.D. Currier, M.D.

Embryonic Substantia Nigra Grafts Innervate Embryonic Striatal Co-Grafts in Preference to Mature Host Striatum
de Beaurepaire R, Freed WJ (Saint Elizabeth's Hosp, Washington, DC)
Exp Neurol 95:448–454, February 1987   7–7

Embryonic substantia nigra (SN) grafts can partially reinnervate denervated striatum. The efficacy of these grafts could be limited, because the adult striatum is not the ideal target tissue for growing dopaminergic axons. The ability of SN grafts to innervate adult striatum or embryonic striatal grafts was investigated in 12 adult Sprague-Dawley rats.

When embryonic striatum and embryonic SN were implanted together, adjacent to denervated adult striatum, only the embryonic striatum was reinnervated at 5 months. When embryonic SN was transplanted alone, reinnervation of the host striatum could be observed.

It appears that immature striatum is a better target tissue for SN graft reinnervation than is adult striatum. The difference may result from specific trophic factors.

▶ This is another experiment with transplantation of grafts to the basal ganglia in order to reinnervate the dopamine-denervated corpus striatum. This and the adrenal medulla grafts done in Mexico City illustrate new awareness of basic neurologic research.— R.N. DeJong, M.D.

Transplantation in Parkinson's Disease: Two Cases of Adrenal Medullary Grafts to the Putamen
Lindvall O, Backlund E-O, Farde L, Sedvall G, Freedman R, Hoffer B, Nobin A, Seiger Å, Olson L (Univ of Lund, Sweden; Haukeland Hosp, Bergen, Norway; Karolinska Hosp, Stockholm; Univ of Colorado, Denver)
Ann Neurol 22:457–468, October 1987   7–8

Grafts of fetal mesencephalic dopamine neurons from several species, including man, reinnervate the denervated rat striatum and compensate for motor deficits induced by lesioning the nigrostriatal dopamine pathway. Adrenal chromaffin cells have countered the motor symptoms of 6-hydroxy-dopamine-induced parkinsonism.

Autologous adrenal medullary tissue was transplanted to the putamen, unilaterally, in 2 patients having severe Parkinson's disease. Rigidity and hypokinesia were the chief symptoms. There was little tremor, and the patients were not demented. They had some response to L-dopa and bromocriptine, but severe side effects were a problem. One patient had improved motor performance for 2 days, and longer periods of normal function for about 2 months. The other patient had minor improvement in balance and gait for 2 months. Electrophysiologic studies suggested increased catecholaminergic activity in the basal ganglia after transplantation in both patients. No adverse effects were evident.

Transplantation of catecholamine-rich cellular implants of adrenal medullary tissue in the basal ganglia transiently improved these 2 patients with severe Parkinson's disease. In rats, addition of nerve growth factor to the graft area promotes nerve fiber formation and lengthens the time of clinical benefit.

▶ These Swedish workers report improvement lasting perhaps 2 months in 2 patients who were transplanted with adrenal graft into the putamen. A note by Robert Joynt (*Ann Neurol* 22:455–456, October 1987) in the same issue of the *Annals* and one in *Science* last April by Roger Lewin (236:149, April 10, 1987) both advised caution in analysis of transplantation results. I prefer the view expressed by Van Manen and Speelman in a letter to the *Lancet* (1:175–176, January 23, 1988) in which they note that the approach through the frontal premotor cortical area combined with some destruction of the caudate nucleus (or putamen?) had been done with some success in the treatment of parkinsonism years ago without the introduction of extraneous tissue. The transplantation of adrenal may be unnecessary.—R.D. Currier, M.D.

8 Headache

Headache and Subacute Sinusitis in Children and Adolescents
Faleck H, Rothner AD, Erenberg G, Cruse RP (Cleveland Clinic Found)
Headache 28:96–98, March 1988   8–1

Chronic, nonprogressive, daily headaches without ominous CNS symptoms or abnormal neurologic signs are usually attributed to stress or tension. Sinus pathology is rarely considered in the differential diagnosis of chronic headache in the absence of associated respiratory symptoms. Fifteen children and adolescents presenting with daily headaches who were subsequently found to have sinus pathology on radiographs were described.

The charts of 150 children and adolescents presenting with chronic headaches in 1984 and 1985 were reviewed. Fifteen had sinus pathology diagnosed radiologically, although none had prominent respiratory symptoms. The patients were 7 girls and 8 boys, aged 4–19 years. In 11 patients, headaches occurred daily. Head pain location was variable. Description of the pain was also variable and included pounding, aching, and sharp with equal frequency. Although 8 patients reported a history of respiratory problems or allergy, only 1 was truly atopic. Eleven patients were examined with sector computed tomographic scans of the sinuses, and 4 underwent standard sinus radiography. Multiple sinus involvement or pansinusitis was found in 13 patients and maxillary sinusitis was found in 2. All patients improved with a course of antibiotics and decongestants.

Sinus pathology was diagnosed radiographically in 15 of 150 children and adolescents presenting with chronic headaches in a 2-year period. None of the 15 patients had prominent respiratory symptoms, and all improved with therapy directed toward the sinus condition. Including sinusitis in the differential diagnosis of chronic headache in children is important.

▶ A large percentage of patients with recurring headaches will state that they have "sinus headaches." When I was in medical school 50 years ago, I was taught that sinus disease is never the cause of chronic headache, and I have always believed it. These physicians from the Cleveland Clinic found that 10% of children and adolescents with recurrent headache did have sinus involvement without prominent respiratory symptoms and that the headaches improved with treatment of the sinus disease. In the same issue of the journal *Headache,* an editorial by John Edmeads states that this article "could begin the rehabilitation of that disreputable concept, sinus headaches" (*Headache* 28:96–98, 1988). At the very least, the Cleveland Clinic group have shaken up our complacency a little, and that can only be helpful.—R.N. DeJong, M.D.

Red Wine as a Cause of Migraine

Littlewood JT, Gibb C, Glover V, Sandler M, Davies PTG, Rose FC (Queen Charlotte's Hosp, Charing Cross Hosp, London)
Lancet 1:558–559, March 12, 1988   8–2

About 25% of patients with migraine believe that their attacks can be provoked by food or drink. Alcoholic beverages, especially red wine, are implicated most often. However, whether such attacks are induced by alcohol or some other compound is disputed. An experiment was done to compare the ability of red wine with that of vodka to induce migraine in patients who believe they are specifically sensitive to red wine.

Nineteen patients who believed their migraine could be provoked by red wine but not vodka or gin were studied. Five patients with migraine who did not believe themselves sensitive to red wine and 8 healthy controls also participated. The first group was given either red wine or a vodka and diluent mixture of equivalent alcohol content. The drinks were consumed cold out of dark bottles to disguise flavor and color. The red wine, which had a negligible tyramine content, provoked a typical migraine attack in 9 of 11 patients in the first group, whereas none of the 8 challenged with vodka had an attack. Neither red wine nor vodka provoked migraine attacks in the other migrainous or healthy persons.

Red wine induced migrainous headaches in patients who believed they were susceptible to it. Vodka did not induce an attack. The major chemical difference between red and white wines is in their content of phenolic flavonoids; thus, these are plausible migraine-inducing agents. Such flavonoids include the catechins and anthocyanins that give red wine its color.

▶ On looking at this article all I can say is hurrah, hurrah. Finally we are beginning to analyze the chemistry of the foods that are thought to cause migraine. The authors note that it may not be tyramine after all. My aching head cheers on these investigators.—R.D. Currier, M.D.

Exteroceptive Suppression of Temporalis Muscle Activity in Chronic Headache

Schoenen J, Jamart B, Gerard P, Lenarduzzi P, Delwaide PJ (Univ of Liège, Liège, Belgium)
Neurology 37:1834–1836, December 1987   8–3

The pathogenesis of tension headache is largely unknown, although pain may develop from sustained contraction of head and neck muscles. If abnormal temporalis muscle activity is a factor, impaired physiologic control of corresponding motoneurons would be expected. The authors compared exteroceptive suppression of the temporalis electromyogram in 20 patients having common migraine, 25 with tension headache, and 22 healthy persons matched with the patients for age and sex. In study patients, tension headaches had occurred nearly daily for at least 6 months.

Early and late exteroceptive suppression periods were elicited by electrical stimulation of the labial commissure during teeth-clenching. The duration of late suppression for single shocks was reduced in tension headache patients. At a stimulation rate of 2 Hz, late suppression was abolished in 40% of this group and in none of the migraine patients. Neither the early silent period nor the latency of the late silent period differed among the 3 study groups.

Exteroceptive suppression in the temporalis muscle is mediated by inhibitory brain-stem interneurons, under the control of limbic structures. There may be deficient activation or excessive inhibition of these interneurons in tension headache. Future studies should seek correlations among electrophysiologic, psychological, and pain threshold data.

▶ These authors have shown what apparently is a clear physiologic difference between patients with tension headaches and normal individuals. However, they have not shown that these results are not secondary to the headache and its subsequent muscle contractions, rather than a factor preceding or leading to the headache itself.

A recent letter from the Netherlands (Van Gijn, J.: *J Neurol Neurosurg Psychiatry* 50:1700–1701, 1987) points out the benefit to headache by 20 minutes of running—all headaches responded but 1. Otto Appenzeller has been heard to say the same thing—he's never had a migraine that did not respond to a 5-mile run. The thought of running with a migraine is personally nauseating—they must be tough fellows.—R.D. Currier, M.D.

Delayed Hyperemia Following Hypoperfusion in Classic Migraine: Single Photon Emission Computed Tomographic Demonstration
Andersen AR, Friberg L, Olsen TS, Olesen J (Univ of Copenhagen; Bispebjerg Hosp, Copenhagen)
Arch Neurol 45:154–159, February 1988   8–4

The role of vascular pathogenesis in classic migraine attacks has received increased attention. It has been difficult to study regional cerebral blood flow (rCBF) because of the short duration of the aura and the spontaneity of the attacks. Patients with migraine were followed up by repeated rCBF measurements into the later phases of a spontaneous classic attack to detect whether regionally delayed hyperemia is interposed between the observed hypoperfusion and later normalization of rCBF. If so, it would suggest that rCBF previously was reduced to or below the ischemic level during the aura phase.

Seven patients were studied. The rCBF was measured during classic migraine attacks. Single-photon emission computed tomography (CT) was done soon after hospitalization and 3–8 hours, 20–24 hours, and 1 week after the onset of symptoms. Initially decreased rCBF persisting up to 3 hours was seen in the hemisphere appropriate to the focal neurologic deficit. Hyperfusion was observed later in the same region in these patients. At 24 hours, rCBF was normal in 4 patients and hyperemia continued in 2; 1 patient was not restudied. The area of interest showed a mean decrease of 19% ± 7% in side-to-side asymmetry when compared with the contralateral area. In 3–8 hours, this reversed to a mean increase of 19% ± 4%. No asymmetry was seen after 1 week. The late hyperemic asymmetry often continued beyond the duration of the headache.

The tardive regional hyperfusion observed resulted from previous focal arteriolar vasoconstriction. This vascular sequence of events further highlights the diagnostic merit of studying rCBF in patients with migraine by noninvasive single-photon emission computed tomography.

▶ This pretty well nails down the fact that cerebral blood flow is decreased in the area of cerebral involvement during the migraine attack and increases after recovery. The question still to be resolved might be, What is the circulation like before the attack?—R.D. Currier, M.D.

Migraine Prophylaxis: A Comparison of Propranolol and Amitriptyline
Ziegler DK, Hurwitz A, Hassanein RS, Kodanaz HA, Preskorn SH, Mason J (Univ of Kansas)
Arch Neurol 44:486–489, May 1987   8–5

Propranolol hydrochloride and amitriptyline hydrochloride are commonly prescribed drugs that have been shown to be effective in the prophylaxis of migraine. These drugs were compared in 30 migraine patients in a double-blind, placebo-controlled, crossover study. The psychological effects of the drugs were monitored by the Zung and Hamilton depression tests and the Spielberger state test for anxiety.

Both drugs were significantly superior to placebo. Neither was significantly better than the other. No correlation was found between therapeutic effectiveness and change in mental state as measured by the Zung and Hamilton tests and the Spielberger test.

Both propranolol and amitriptyline were effective against migraine. However, there was no correlation between this effect and depression or anxiety reduction. The results do not support the hypothesis that these drugs provide prophylaxis from migraine through psychological effects in a population without psychological disturbance.

▶ This is an interesting article, but it brings us no farther in the treatment and prophylaxis of migraine. Both drugs help to a degree, but we do not understand why they help. But every venture into the prevention and amelioration of this frequently incapacitating illness is progress.—R.N. DeJong, M.D.

Hindbrain Hernia Headache
Nightingale S, Williams B (Midland Ctr for Neurosurgery and Neurology, West Midlands, England)
Lancet 1:731–734, March 28, 1987   8–6

Only a small percentage of patients with recurrent headaches have a structural abnormality. For most patients with headache, an accurate history of the duration, frequency, and character of the symptoms together with a neurologic examination is sufficient to make a diagnosis. A study was conducted of data from 6 patients with episodic, severe, and disabling headaches in whom the symptoms were caused by hindbrain herniation into the foramen magnum with resulting craniospinal pressure dissociation.

Woman, 28, described a 15-month history of pounding occipital head pain provoked by coughing, laughing, straining at stool, any heavy exertion, or standing suddenly. The headache would begin a few seconds after the precipitating maneuver and then gradually die away in less than a minute. Sometimes the pain could be relieved by stooping with the neck flexed anteriorly or by lying down. The headaches were not associated with neurologic symptoms. Air encephalography revealed descent of the cerebellar tonsils into the foramen magnum. Combined lumbar and ventricular pressure recording during and after the Valsalva maneuver demonstrated that the timing and severity of headache was related to pressure dissociation across the craniospinal junction. The patient underwent a surgical decompression of the foramen magnum and no longer experiences these headaches.

Five other patients were seen who experienced disabling headaches that were also caused by hindbrain herniation into the foramen magnum. This syndrome may be recognized by eliciting the typical history. In all 11 patients, myelography revealed hindbrain herniation or Arnold-Chiari deformity. Surgical decompression of the foramen magnum led to complete resolution of the headaches.

▶ Headaches have been with us since history began, but new headache syndromes continue to appear. This is an interesting type of headache, and it is well delineated. As we look for cases, I am sure they will appear.—R.N. De-Jong, M.D.

Treatment of Migraine With Intramuscular Chlorpromazine
McEwen JI, O'Connor HM, Dinsdale HB (Queen's Univ, Kingston, Ont)
Ann Emerg Med 16:758–763, July 1987   8–7

A prospective, randomized, double-blind, placebo-controlled clinical trial was designed to assess the efficacy and safety of intramuscular parenteral CPZ in the treatment of 39 patients with acute migraine attacks. Excluded were those younger than 18 or older than 60 years of age, pregnant, with new neurologic signs, using phenothiazines, or in whom the use of phenothiazines was contraindicated. Patients were given either CPZ (1 mg/kg) or a saline placebo and were observed for 1 hour.

Of the 19 patients receiving CPZ, 9 (47.4%) had enough relief from their headache to carry on with daily activities. Only 4 (23.5%) of the 17 patients in the control group experienced such relief. This difference was not statistically significant; however, CPZ was significantly more effective than placebo in providing some relief from headache and in relieving nausea. Significant adverse effects included drowsiness and an asymptomatic drop in blood pressure of 10 mm Hg, systolic.

Although CPZ is a safe medication that provides some relief from migraine headaches, it appears to be less efficacious than previously reported.

▶ It is sad to hear that our original optimism about CPZ in the relief of migraine in the emergency room was misplaced. This brings this particular treatment down to the same level as the rest of the emergency room treatments, which, after all, are fairly effective.

J.N. Blau in the *Lancet* is looking for a new name for tension headaches (1:222, July 25, 1987). I certainly would agree to the need. Neither muscle tension nor psychogenic tension are the chief cause of ordinary headache, in my opinion, and the present nomenclature is misleading to medical students and insurance carriers. The International Headache Society Ad Hoc Committee on the classification of headache has suggested the term "tension-type" headaches and is asking for comment on a proposed new headache classification. Dr. Jes Olesen of Copenhagen is chairman of the committee and Dr. Seymour Solomon of the Headache Unit, Montefiore Medical Center, 111 East 210th Street, Bronx, N.Y. 10467, can be contacted with any suggestions.

Scarani, Beghi, and Tognoni of Milan (*Headache* 27:345–350, 1987) have studied the records of 500 patients with primary headache seen by multiple physicians. They found that the type, number, and character of drug treatments were irrational and plead for more accurate drug studies of a standardized nature to give rational data on which sensible treatment can be based. The problem is not confined to Italy.

Heckerling et al. (*Ann Intern Med* 107:174–176, August 1987) found that headaches and dizziness correlate with carboxyhemoglobin levels higher than 10%. The level tends to correlate with cigarette smoking, gas kitchen stoves for heating, problems with some heating systems, and cohabitants with concurrent headache and dizziness. I have always thought that cigarettes were contraindicated in people with headaches but never really knew why.—R.D. Currier, M.D.

Headache Caused by Serious Illness: Evaluation in an Emergency Setting
Shesser R (George Washington Univ, Washington, DC)
Postgrad Med 81:117–125, Feb 15, 1987   8–8

One of the most challenging problems facing the physician in an emergency department is evaluation of severe headache. Although these patients generally look ill and uncomfortable, they rarely have life-threatening illness. However, it is important to differentiate benign headaches of vascular origin or those caused by muscle tension, sinusitis, or nonmeningitis infections from headaches caused by subarachnoid hemorrhage and meningitis.

All patients suspected of subarachnoid hemorrhage should undergo a careful physical examination with neurologic emphasis. A specialist should be consulted if the findings suggest a local lesion, and the patient should be hospitalized. Particular attention should be given to the neck, subconjunctival and preretinal areas, and ocular fundi. Electrocardiographic and cardiac rhythm abnormalities may occur in patients with acute intracranial problems such as subarachnoid hemorrhage. The patient may also present with massive albuminuria or glycosuria. After simple studies are completed, the patient should undergo computed tomography and possibly lumbar puncture. The diagnosis of subarachnoid hemorrhage may be missed initially in 25% of patients. However, early diagnosis is important; prognosis is markedly improved in properly treated groups.

The patient with fever and headache presents another difficult diagnostic problem. Because many suppurative processes in the central nervous system cause fever and headache, physical examination again focuses on excluding neurologic disease. The absence of Kernig's or Brudzinski's sign should not dissuade the physician from performing lumbar puncture if the history and clinical findings suggest acute meningitis. It is important to distinguish viral meningitis from bacterial meningitis, and it is crucial to institute early treatment of bacterial meningitis. Lumbar puncture is always indicated if meningitis is suspected.

Severe headache is a common problem among patients in the emergency department. Because early therapy markedly reduces deaths from subarachnoid hemorrhage, the physician must use advanced technological and sometimes invasive tests to diagnose this condition. In patients with meningitis, the physician must assume there will be only 1 opportunity to make the correct diagnosis. Patients usually seek emergency care early in the course of meningitis when accurate detection on clinical grounds is difficult. A conservative approach and liberal use of all appropriate diagnostic techniques are recommended.

▶ Severe headache is a common problem among patients in an emergency facility. Prompt diagnosis and treatment may be life-saving.— R.N. DeJong, M.D.

Migrainous Stroke
Rothrock JF, Walicke P, Swenson MR, Lyden PD, Logan WR (Univ of California, San Diego; St John's Mercy Med Ctr, St Louis)
Arch Neurol 45:63–67, January 1988   8–9

Although migraine is common, migraine-associated stroke is rare. Twenty-two patients with acute migraine-associated stroke seen during a 7-year period were evaluated prospectively.

Ninety-one percent of the patients were female. Mean age at time of stroke was 35 years, with a range of 9–64 years. Mean age at onset of migraine was 16.5 years, with a range of 3–43 years. Eight patients had a history of complicated migraine, 5 of whom also had a history of migraine-associated stroke. Nine patients had a history of classic migraine, and 5 had common migraine only. Four patients also had chronic hypertension. Ninety-five percent of the patients experienced typical migraine acutely in association with stroke. Sixteen sustained permanent neurologic damage and 1 patient died. The incidences of major stroke risk factors and mitral valve prolapse were not higher among the 22 patients studied than for the general population of similar age. Computed tomography, magnetic resonance imaging, or radionucleotide scanning of the brain was done on all patients. Ischemic or hemorrhagic infarction was demonstrated in 12. Cerebral arteriography showed abnormalities related to the acute stroke in 5 of 12 patients studied overall and in 4 of 6 patients assessed within 72 hours of stroke onset. One patient became comatose shortly after arteriography was performed. The 21 surviving patients were followed up for a mean of 22 months; 1 suffered recurrent migrainous stroke.

Twenty-two patients with acute migraine-associated stroke were described. Although various processes alone or combined may contribute to migrainous stroke, extracranial and/or intracranial vasospasm apparently plays a major role in at least some of the cases.

▶ Extracranial or intracranial vasospasm is apparently the major etiologic factor in migrainous stroke. This type of stroke occurs in otherwise healthy persons, but is often serious and may cause permanent neurologic damage.—R.N. DeJong, M.D.

9 Acquired Immunodeficiency Syndrome

Subacute Encephalomyelitis of AIDS and Its Relation to HTLV-III Infection
de la Monte SM, Ho DD, Schooley RT, Hirsch MS, Richardson EP, Jr (Massachusetts Gen Hosp, Boston; Harvard Univ)
Neurology 37:562–569, April 1987   9–1

Patients with acquired immunodeficiency syndrome (AIDS) or AIDS-related complex (ARC) often have CNS disease. The nature and distribution of lesions of subacute encephalomyelitis in autopsies on 30 patients with AIDS or ARC were examined and correlated with the clinical course and the presence of the virus in neural tissue.

Distribution of CNS Lesions in Subacute
Encephalomyelitis of AIDS

Location	Frequency
Cerebral white matter	25/27 (93%)
Cerebral cortex	23/27 (85%)
Frontal	15/26 (58%)
Parietal	10/21 (48%)
Temporal	11/16 (69%)
Occipital	12/23 (52%)
Insula	6/14 (43%)
Basal ganglia	17/22 (77%)
Caudate	10/22 (45%)
Putamen	15/22 (68%)
Globus pallidus	9/20 (45%)
Thalamus	11/19 (58%)
Hypothalamus	3/6 (50%)
Hippocampus	14/22 (64%)
Amygdala	8/10 (80%)
Substantia innominata	1/9 (11%)
Midbrain	3/19 (16%)
Pons	6/22 (27%)
Medulla	5/24 (21%)
Cerebellum	4/20 (20%)
Spinal cord	5/18 (28%)

(Courtesy of de la Monte SM, Ho DD, Schooley RT, et al: *Neurology* 37:562–569, April 1987.)

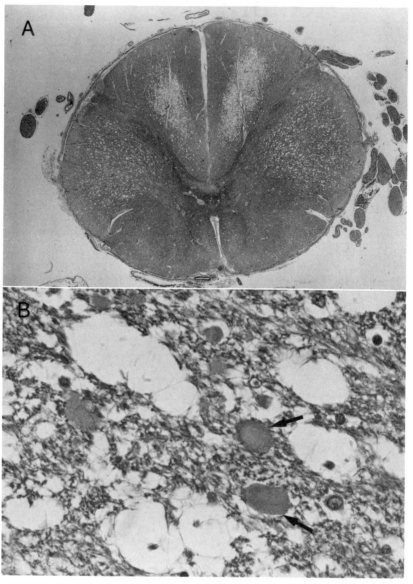

Fig 9–1.—Vacuolar myelopathy involving upper cervical spinal cord. **A,** vacuolation of posterior and lateral funiculi. **B,** vacuoles and axonal spheroids *(arrows)*. Note absence of inflammation and minimal gliosis. Luxol fast blue-hematoxylin-eosin; original magnification ×313. (Courtesy of de la Monte SM, Ho DD, Schooley RT, et al: *Neurology* 37:562–569, April 1987.)

In 90% of these patients, subacute encephalitis was seen. It was characterized by demyelination, gliosis, focal necrosis, microglial nodules, atypical oligodendrocyte nuclei, and cellular multinucleation. It occurred in 58% of frontal lobes, 69% of temporal lobes, 77% of basal ganglia,

80% of amygdala, and 64% of hippocampi (table). In 2 of 18 cases examined, the spinal cord had a vacuolar myelopathy (Fig 9–1). Patchy demyelinative peripheral neuropathy was seen in half of the specimens examined. Ten patients with moderate or severe subacute encephalitis had been demented, whereas 82% of those with mild subacute encephalitis had no recognized neurologic disorder. In 11 of 13 specimens, HTLV-III could be isolated from neural tissue or CSF. Ten of these patients had subacute encephalitis, and 1 had no CNS lesions.

In this series, moderate or severe subacute encephalitis accompanied dementia in 80% of cases. Mental deterioration was especially common when lesions were extensive and occurred in the frontal lobes. Cerebral white matter was the most frequently affected structure. Combined with peripheral nerve demyelination, this suggests that myelin-producing cells are vulnerable. It appears that HTLV-III is neurotropic and causes the subacute encephalitis associated with AIDS.

▶ Subacute encephalomyelitis is common in patients with acquired immunodeficiency syndrome and is most likely caused by central nervous system infection with neurotropic HTLV-III, now referred to as "human immunodeficiency virus" (HIV).—R.N. DeJong, M.D.

Neurological Complications in AIDS
Fischer PA and Enzensberger W (Frankfurt, West Germany)
J Neurol 234:269–279, 1987   9–2

Neurologic complications are a prominent part of acquired immunodeficiency syndrome (AIDS). There probably are neurotropic variants of the causative agent, human immunodeficiency virus. It is not clear whether infection of the nervous system by human immunodeficiency virus (HIV) automatically produces acute or chronic AIDS encephalitis, or whether the virus lies dormant in neural tissue for a long time, or perhaps indefinitely.

The most acute form of central nervous system (CNS) involvement by HIV infection is acute meningoencephalitis. An AIDS dementia complex, or chronic AIDS encephalopathy, is the most frequent neurologic complication seen in AIDS patients. At least half of all AIDS patients may be affected. Chronic deterioration of cognitive and behavioral functions begins insidiously. Apathy and a flat affect are usual. Also, severe dementia, mutism, paraplegia, and incontinence may be present. An atypical form of aseptic meningitis also is seen in AIDS patients, as is vacuolar myelopathy at autopsy. The peripheral and cranial nerves are involved in about 15% of patients.

Central nervous system toxoplasmosis may occur in AIDS, as may systemic cytomegalovirus infection involving the nervous system. Herpes virus encephalitis also may occur. Cryptococcal meningoencephalitis is seen in perhaps 10% of AIDS cases in this country. Central nervous system malignancies include primary lymphoma and systemic lymphoma involving the CNS. Cerebral involvement by Kaposi's sarcoma is rare.

The psychological and social consequences of AIDS require close attention. Patients with AIDS dementia complex will be limited intellectually and socially, and will no longer be able to live independently.

▶ As the authors state: "Mankind will be exposed to a fundamental revision of its social, sexual, psychological, economical, educational, and ethical principles in order to handle the implications and consequences of this new pandemic."—R.N. DeJong, M.D.

Early Penetration of the Blood-Brain-Barrier by HIV
Resnick L, Berger JR, Shapshak P, Tourtellotte WW (Univ of Miami; Univ of California, Los Angeles)
Neurology 38:9–14, January 1988   9–3

More than half of the patients with acquired immunodeficiency syndrome (AIDS) have progressive dementia. Neurologic complications may result from immune dysfunction, or from human immunodeficiency virus (HIV) infection of the nervous system. Human immunodeficiency virus isolation and antibody studies were performed on the cerebrospinal fluid (CSF) of 52 seropositive patients, 29 of whom had neurologic signs and symptoms. Twenty patients had a diagnosis of AIDS, 20 had AIDS-related complex, and 12 were seropositive patients from high-risk groups.

Ten patients had CSF cultures consistent with HIV infection. About one fifth of specimens from neurologically asymptomatic individuals and 17% of those from patients with symptoms were culture-positive. Only 1 patient with AIDS had a positive CSF culture. Human immunodeficiency virus was recovered from the blood in 6 of 8 AIDS patients and from 10 of 15 patients without AIDS. All the patients with CSF positive for virus had increased intra–blood-brain barrier total IgG synthesis. Six of the 10 patients had oligoclonal IgG bands in the CSF. Also, HIV-specific IgG synthesis was increased in three fourths of all patients, and 60% had CSF oligoclonal IgG bands.

Infectious HIV may be isolated from the CSF in patients with various stages of infection, including those without neurologic symptoms. The findings suggest that HIV involves the CNS early in the course of disease, and before AIDS-related neurologic abnormalities develop. Prospective studies are needed to define the spectrum of neurologic disease resulting from HIV infection, and to determine the actual incidence of subclinical CNS infection.

▶ Signs and symptoms of CNS dysfunction sometimes develop prior to onset of other manifestations of HIV infection. These studies demonstrate that HIV enters the CNS early in the course of viral infection, often prior to the development of HIV-associated neurologic abnormalities.—R.N. DeJong, M.D.

Neuropathological Findings in 31 Cases of Acquired Immunodeficiency Syndrome (AIDS)

Hénin D, Duyckaerts C, Chaunu MP, Vazeux R, Brousse N, Rozenbaum W, Hauw JJ (Hôpital de la Salpêtrière, Inst Pasteur, Paris; Hôpital Beaujon, Clichy, France)
Rev Neurol (Paris) 143:631–642, 1987   9–4

A 15-month prospective neuropathologic study was done to determine the prevalence of neurologic signs and symptoms in a cohort of 48 patients who died of acquired immunodeficiency syndrome (AIDS). Autopsy findings in 31 patients, 30 men and 1 woman, aged 22–58 years at the time of death, were described.

Twenty-eight men were homosexual, 1 patient had received several transfusions for treatment of a lymphoma, and 1 patient from Senegal had recently gone back home for a visit. The only woman in this cohort was originally from the Congo; she had received several blood transfusions. Eighteen patients manifested neurologic signs and symptoms several days to several months before death. In 2 patients, AIDS was first confirmed on the basis of neurologic findings at autopsy.

Autopsy of the brain revealed cerebral abnormalities in each patient, including malignant non-Hodgkin's lymphoma in 3, toxoplasmosis in 13, cytomegalovirus encephalitis in 4, cryptococcal meningitis in 3, and intracellular *Mycobacterium avium* infection in 1. Twenty-three patients had a single type of cerebral lesion, 6 had 2 types of lesions, and 2 had 3 types of lesions. Seventeen patients had subacute encephalitis caused by opportunistic infections, including 10 in whom characteristic lymphomonocytic focal infiltration and mild lymphomonocytic perivascular cuffs was demonstrated.

These results are in agreement with epidemiologic data from other studies as far as incidence of lymphoma, cryptococcosis, and mycobacterial infections. However, unlike other reported studies, no progressive multifocal leukoencephalopathy was observed. Only 1 patient had typical giant cells, and areas of mild demyelination were seen in only 1 case. The incidence of cerebral toxoplasmosis in this series was higher than that in other series. None of the patients had encephalitis caused by seroconversion secondary to primary human immunodeficiency virus (HIV) infection.

The findings of this neuropathologic study clearly demonstrate the neurotropic character of the HIV virus.

▶ This does not represent the largest pathologic study of AIDS but is of interest because every one of their 31 consecutive autopsies had abnormalities in the nervous system. Only 18 of the 31, however, had neurologic signs or symptoms before death. The recent supplement to the *Annals* on retroviruses includes a pathologic study by Petito (*Ann Neurol* 23(Suppl):S54–S57, 1988). She mentions that "over 90% have abnormalities in the nervous system."

When AIDS was first being described I was hoping that it would stay away from the nervous system, but that hope obviously is in vain. Indeed, the nervous system is involved close to 100% of the time, and some claim that it is the critical area, which may be true. The involvement, of course, is not just the secondary infections, but also the findings typical of AIDS encephalopathy: the glial nodules and multinucleated cells.

On the lighter side in *Nature* (329:61–65, Sept. 3, 1987), there is a report by Rothschild and Turnbull of a bear from the Pleistocene era (11,500 years ago) found in Indiana that tested positively with antisera for *Treponema*. The involvements were gummatous lesions of the bear's humerus and spine. The opportunity for humerus remarks is almost too great to pass over with this finding, but to be honest yaws, not syphilis, is the most likely explanation.—R.D. Currier, M.D.

10 Infections of the Nervous System

Alteration in the Natural History of Neurosyphilis by Concurrent Infection With the Human Immunodeficiency Virus
Johns DR, Tierney M, Felsenstein D (Massachusetts Gen Hosp, Boston)
N Engl J Med 316:1569–1572, June 18, 1987   10–1

Four patients with neurosyphilis were seen within 18 months. All were young homosexual men who were seropositive for human immunodeficiency virus (HIV). Two of the 4 patients had been treated with benzathine penicillin for syphilis. Meningovascular syphilis developed in 1 patient within 4 months of infection.

It appears that HIV may alter the natural course of syphilitic infection, presumably because of depression of the immune system. Lumbar puncture should be performed on all HIV-positive patients with syphilis. Neurosyphilis should probably be considered an infectious complication of acquired immunodeficiency syndrome and may be the first symptom to appear.

▶ In the same issue of the *New England Journal of Medicine* as this article there is a report by Berry et al. (316:1587–1589) recounting a failure of benzathine penicillin treatment of secondary syphilis in a patient with acquired immunodeficiency syndrome and an editorial (316:1600–1601) by Tramont, who concludes: "This means that anyone who has a compromised immune status for any reason and has contracted syphilis must be treated with higher doses of antibiotics for prolonged periods." He further admonishes that all HIV-infected patients be screened for syphilis and vice versa, and finally recasts Osler: "Know HIV infection in all its manifestations and relations and all other things clinical will be added unto you."—R.D. Currier, M.D.

Focal Encephalitis in a Young Woman 6 Years After the Onset of Lyme Disease: Tertiary Lyme Disease?
Broderick JP, Sandok BA, Mertz LE (Mayo Graduate School of Medicine, Rochester, Minn)
Mayo Clin Proc 62:313–316, April 1987   10–2

Lyme disease, which is caused by a tickborne spirochete, *Borrelia burgdorferi*, is a complex multisystem disorder. Early symptoms include fever, chills, malaise, headache, and a characteristic rash. There is also a neurologic triad including lymphocytic meningitis, cranial neuritis, and radiculoneuritis as well as rare involvement of the central nervous system

(CNS). The neurologic deficits usually resolve during a period of several months. A well-known late manifestation of Lyme disease is chronic arthritis. A patient was seen with Lyme disease and chronic involvement of the nervous system.

Girl, 13 years, experienced fever, chills, headache, stiff neck, sore throat, and malaise 1 to 2 weeks after being bitten by a tick. One week later, a macular rash developed, and 3½ weeks later, bilateral facial palsies appeared. Prednisone therapy was begun and the patient's symptoms resolved in the next few months. Six years after this illness, the patient experienced headaches and difficulty with language. At this time, she was alert, globally aphasic, and apraxic; she had little speech output and could follow only simple commands. It was then discovered that her serum contained antibodies against several specific *B. burgdorferi* antigens. Several other serologic tests confirmed the diagnosis of Lyme disease. The patient underwent a series of cerebrospinal fluid studies and treatment was begun with 20 million units of penicillin G daily. The patient's condition continued to deteriorate, and she was released to the care of her parents. Her clinical course was one of gradual and steady improvement. Approximately 3 months after onset of her headaches and language difficulties, she returned to normal.

It is likely that this patient had had classic untreated Lyme disease. It was hypothesized that her focal inflammatory encephalitis was a result of a persistent spirochetal infection of the CNS.

▶ Lyme disease is being diagnosed with increasing frequency, but we are familiar only with the acute and subacute manifestations. This patient showed evidence of a persistent spirochetal infection of the central nervous system. As with syphilis, we must also consider the possibility of a tertiary variety of *Borrelia burgdorferi* infection.— R.N. DeJong, M.D.

Chronic Meningitis Without Predisposing Illness: A Review of 83 Cases
Anderson NE, Willoughby EW (Auckland Hosp, Auckland, New Zealand)
Q J Med New Series 63:283–295, April 1987   10–3

Subacute or chronic meningitis is difficult to diagnose and to manage. A review was made of data on 83 previously healthy patients with chronic meningitis.

The most common cause of chronic meningitis was tuberculosis (40% of the patients), whereas cryptococcosis was the cause in 7% and malignancy in 8% (table). In 34% of the patients no cause was defined. Although tubercular meningitis and malignant meningitis generally fit the typical clinical picture of meningitis, meningitis resulting from other causes did not. Clinical features and changes in cell count and concentrations of protein and glucose in cerebrospinal fluid could not be used to distinguish the various types of meningitis, nor could cerebral and meningeal biopsy be used in this way.

Management of chronic meningitis is difficult. Treatment usually must

Causes of Chronic Meningitis*

	n	%
Tuberculous	33	40
Cryptococcal	6	7
Malignant	7	8
Eosinophilic	4	5
Syphilitic	2	2
Sarcoid	1	1
Leptospiral	1	1
Herpes zoster	1	1
Idiopathic	28	34
Responsive to anti-Tb drugs	14	17
Responsive to steroids	9	11
No sustained treatment	4	5
Unresponsive to treatment	1	1
Total	83	

*Anti-Tb, antituberculosis.
(Courtesy of Anderson NE, Willoughby EW: *Q J Med New Series* 63:283–295, April 1987.)

be initiated before the cause of the meningitis is identified. If the patient is seriously ill, it is recommended that treatment begin with isoniazid, rifampicin, and ethambutol immediately, as tuberculosis is the most common cause and results in high mortality if treatment is delayed. If the patient's condition continues to worsen, steroids should be added, but only if fungal meningitis has been excluded. If fungal disease is common in the region, amphotericin B should be tried before steroids. In patients who are reasonably healthy, treatment can be withheld until the causative organism has been identified. It should be noted that some patients with idiopathic chronic meningitis respond well to long-term treatment with steroids.

▶ As the authors point out, reviews of a series of patients with chronic meningitis are infrequent. Their comments are therefore valuable. The majority of patients had tuberculosis, but the study is influenced by the large Polynesian group coming into the Auckland Hospital with tuberculous meningitis. If the diagnosis of tuberculosis was not made and the patient's condition was deteriorating, they treated for it anyway, usually with good results. If that was unsuccessful, steroids were used next, often with good results. In their population there was a subgroup of patients with idiopathic chronic meningitis responsive to steroids. However, the authors do not recommend steroid therapy in areas of the world where fungal infections are common without a prior trial of amphotericin B.—R.D. Currier, M.D.

Treatment of Cryptococcal Meningitis With Combination Amphotericin B and Flucytosine for Four as Compared With Six Weeks

Dismukes WE, Cloud G, Gallis HA, Kerkering TM, Medoff G, Craven PC, Kaplowitz LG, Fisher JF, Gregg CR, Bowles CA, Shadorny S, Stamm AM, Diasio RB, Kaufman L, Soong S-J, Blackwelder WC, the National Institute of Allergy and Infectious Diseases Mycoses Study Group (Univ of Alabama, Birmingham; Virginia Commonwealth Univ, Richmond; Ctrs for Disease Control, Atlanta; Natl Inst of Health, Bethesda, Md)
N Engl J Med 317:334–341, Aug 6, 1987

10–4

Cryptococcal meningitis is the most common form of fungal meningitis in the United States and is an important cause of morbidity and mortality in immunocompromised patients. No therapeutic regimen has been uniformly effective or without serious toxicity. In 1979, it was reported that a regimen combining amphotericin B and flucytosine for 6 weeks was as effective as a low-dose regimen of amphotericin B alone for 10 weeks. The duration of this combination was shortened further, from 6 weeks to 4 weeks, to determine whether this would reduce toxicity without compromising efficacy, in a multicenter, prospective, randomized clinical trial.

The 194 patients enrolled in the study had cryptococcal meningitis. All patients received intravenous amphotericin B, 0.3 mg/kg/day, for 28 days, and oral flucytosine, 150 mg/kg/day, in equal doses every 6 hours, for 28 days. At the end of 4 weeks, patients were randomized to either a 4-week regimen calling for no additional treatment or a 6-week regimen that included 2 more weeks of therapy. Of the 91 patients who met pre-

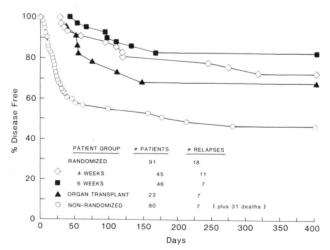

PATIENT GROUP	# PATIENTS	# RELAPSES	
RANDOMIZED	91	18	
◇ 4 WEEKS	45	11	
■ 6 WEEKS	46	7	
▲ ORGAN TRANSPLANT	23	7	
○ NON-RANDOMIZED	80	7	(plus 31 deaths)

Fig 10–1.—The probability of disease-free survival in randomized patients, patients with organ transplants, and patients not randomized. For the randomized and transplant groups, each symbol represents 1 patient relapse; for the group not randomized, each symbol represents either 1 relapse or 1 death. (Courtesy of Dismukes WE, Cloud G, Gallis HA, et al: *N Engl J Med* 317:334–341, August 1987.)

established criteria for randomization, cure or improvement was seen in 75% of those treated for 4 weeks and in 85% of those treated for 6 weeks. The estimated relapse rate for the group on the 4-week regimen was 27%, compared with 16% of the group on the 6-week regimen. The incidence of toxic effects for the shorter and longer regimens was 44% and 43%, respectively. Among 23 transplant recipients, 4 of 5 treated for 4 weeks relapsed (Fig 10–1). Thus the rest were treated for 6 weeks. Only 3 of the 18 treated for 6 weeks relapsed. Of the 80 patients who did not follow the initial protocol and therefore were not randomized, 38 died or relapsed. Three significant predictors of favorable response were identified by multifactorial analysis of treatment factors for all 194 patients: headache as a symptom, normal mental status, and a cerebrospinal fluid (CSF) white blood cell count of more than $20/mm^3$.

These findings concurred with other data suggesting that the 4-week regimen should be reserved for patients with meningitis without neurologic complications, underlying disease, or immunosuppressive therapy; with a pretreatment CSF white blood cell count of more than $20/mm^3$ and a serum cryptococcal antigen titer of less than 1:32; a negative CSF India ink preparation; and serum and CSF cryptococcal-antigen titers of less than 1:8 after 4 weeks of therapy.

▶ This looks helpful, but one really must have the criteria for use of the 4-week regimen written and at hand to be sure not to overstep the treatment bounds. A simultaneous note in the *American Journal of Medicine* by the same group (83:236–247, August 1987) gives a method for following flucytosine during therapy to prevent toxicity. They say that the "serum creatinine level should be monitored twice weekly and the creatinine clearance weekly during therapy in order to anticipate changes in serum flucytosine." In addition, it is recommended that the serum flucytosine level be determined once a week, 2 hours after an oral dose, and that the dose be adjusted to maintain a level of 50 to 100 μg/ml.—R.D. Currier, M.D.

Involvement of JC Virus-Infected Mononuclear Cells From the Bone Marrow and Spleen in the Pathogenesis of Progressive Multifocal Leukoencephalopathy

Houff SA, Major EO, Katz DA, Kufta CV, Sever JL, Pittaluga S, Roberts JR, Gitt J, Sain N, Lux W (Natl Inst of Neurological and Communicative Disorders and Stroke, Natl Cancer Inst, Bethesda, Md; VA Hosp, Washington, DC; George Washington Univ)

N Engl J Med 318:301–305, Feb 4, 1988   10–5

Progressive multifocal leukoencephalopathy (PML) is a subacute demyelinating disease resulting from infection of oligodendrocytes by JC virus and occurs almost exclusively in immunocompromised patients. The pathogenesis of PML remains obscure. Two patients with PML were examined for the presence of JC virus DNA and virion antigen.

The first patient was immunocompromised by acquired immunodeficiency syndrome. The second patient had no recognizable underlying disease that would impair immunity. Bone marrow biopsy and aspiration were performed, and in situ hybridization and immunocytochemistry were done. Scattered mononuclear cells containing JC virus DNA and virion antigens were found in the marrow specimens from both patients.

At autopsy, the first patient was found to have JC virus in mononuclear cells of the spleen and bone marrow. Electron microscopy of oligodendrocyte inclusions from an area of demyelination showed typical papovavirus-like virions in nuclei. Several mononuclear cells containing JC virus were found in the Virchow-Robin spaces, and JC virus-infected glial cells were often found in increased numbers in the perivascular parenchyma.

The JC virus can be present in mononuclear cells in the bone marrow during latency. Virus-infected lymphocytes may enter the perivascular space of the brain, which might result in glial cell infection.

▶ This is an important article reporting findings that provide insight into the pathogenesis of a rare neurologic disease. An editorial by E.P. Richardson, Jr., one of the neuropathologists who first recognized the disease 30 years ago, appears in the same issue of the journal (*N Engl J Med* 318:315–316, 1988). Unfortunately, the virus responsible was given the initials of the patient, J.C. This is confusing because these are also the initials, though reversed, of another important viral disease of the central nervous system, Creutzfeldt-Jakob disease.—R.N. DeJong, M.D.

Prions Causing Nervous System Degeneration
Prusiner SB, DeArmond SJ (Univ of California, San Francisco)
Lab Invest 56:349–363, April 1987   10–6

Slow infections appear to be caused by both viruses and so-called prions. Six diseases, 3 of animals and 3 affecting humans, are probably caused by prions (table). All known prion diseases are confined to the central nervous system. Prolonged incubation periods have been observed. The clinical course usually is rather stereotyped, progressing to

Prion Diseases*

Scrapie†	Sheep and goats
Transmissible mink encephalopathy	Mink
Chronic wasting disease	Mule deer, and elk
Kuru	Humans, Fore
CJD†	Humans
GSS	Humans

*Alternative terminologies include subacute transmissible spongiform encephalopathies and unconventional slow virus diseases.
†Prions cause scrapie and Creutzfeld-Jakob disease (CJD), and they are presumed to cause the other diseases listed.
(Courtesy of Prusiner SB, DeArmond SJ: *Lab Invest* 56:349–363, April 1987.)

death. The human prion diseases probably are variants of the same disorder. All likely require the appearance of an abnormal isoform of the prion protein, which is encoded by a single-copy gene in hamsters and mice. The human PrP gene appears to be a single copy.

There now is direct evidence of the presence of protease-resistant prion proteins in the brains of persons dying of Creutzfeldt-Jakob disease. Neurons contain the highest levels of PrP mRNA in the hamster brain; glial cells contain relatively little mRNA. The lack of an immune response to lethal slow infection remains to be elucidated. The degree of astrocytic gliosis often is out of proportion to that of nerve cell loss. Amyloid plaque formation is also a feature of prion disease. The prion protein probably accumulates selectively in nerve cells during the course of disease.

Scrapie prion proteins fulfill the criteria needed for classification as a form of cerebral amyloid. Interest in a possible causative role of amyloids in Alzheimer's disease has grown. It may be that many disorders will be found to be caused by prion-like macromolecules.. The genetic origin of prions and the slow amplification that characterizes their replication require further investigation.

▶ The concept of slow infections was introduced by Sigurdson in 1954. These are caused by either slow virus infections or prions. Prions are known to cause 6 diseases, 3 of animals and 3 of humans (see table). There are many excellent reviews of slow virus infections (Haase 1975, Jakob 1971, Gibbs et al, 1969). This article discusses diseases caused by prions.— R.N. DeJong, M.D.

The Epidemiology of Creutzfeldt-Jakob Disease: Conclusion of a 15-Year Investigation in France and Review of the World Literature
Brown P, Cathala F, Raubertas RF, Gajdusek DC, Castaigne P (Natl Inst of Neurological and Communicative Disorders and Stroke Bethesda, Md; Hôpital de la Salpêtrière, Paris, France)
Neurology 37:895–904, June 1987   10–7

A 10-year retrospective and 5-year prospective study of Creutzfeldt-Jakob disease (CJD) in France was concluded in 1982. Of 329 patients who died of CJD between January 1, 1968 and December 31, 1982, 56 were born outside of France. Six percent of patients had definite, and 3% had possible, familial disease. The annual mortality of CJD for the entire 15-year period was 0.42 per million in the whole of France, 0.75 per million in the Paris metropolitan area, and 1.21 per million in Paris itself; for the prospective period 1978–1981, the percentages were 0.56, 0.86, and 1.19 per million, respectively.

Age-specific mortality rates showed a broad peak between ages 55–74 years, and the age-specific mortality curve for foreign-born patients was similar to that of the native French population, but with rates about double the native population, particularly North Africans. Since the begin-

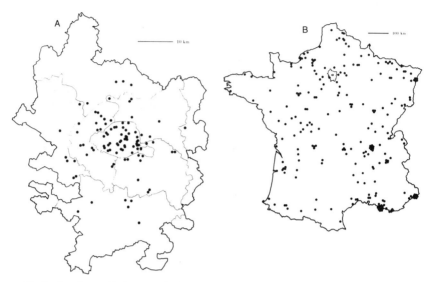

Fig 10–2.—Geographic location of adult residence of 329 patients with Creutzfeldt-Jakob disease dying in continental France during the period 1968–1982. Cases are shown in the Paris metropolitan area *(A)* and the rest of France *(B)*. (Courtesy of Brown P, Cathala F, Raubertas RF, et al: *Neurology* 37:895–904, June 1987.)

ning of prospective survey, there was no statistically significant upward or downward trend in the incidence of the disease in France. Major concentrations were seen in Paris, Lyon, Nice, and Marseilles, among other large metropolitan areas; numerous cases also occurred in a few smaller cities, and occasionally 2–3 cases in fairly close geographic proximity were noted in rural France (Fig 10–2). There was no correlation between densities or age distributions of regional populations.

There was a positive correlation of CJD related to population density, but in only 2 of the 239 cases was there contact between geographically close patient pairs, aside from the familial cases. The chance of contact with any other patient was unlikely for several patients. No association was found with exposure to animal sources of infection, nor could any meaningful conclusion be drawn among occupations. During the period between 1 and 5 years before the clinical onset of CJD, 8% of patients had surgery and 3% had trauma, and about twice as many patients had surgery or trauma at some earlier time. Even if contamination had occurred during every surgical procedure, iatrogenic transmission could not have been implicated in more than a small fraction of the case total.

The higher incidence of CJD in North African immigrants to France and Israel than in the native-born population suggests early life events could be important. Contaminated tissue from patients with CJD may be presumed to remain infectious outside the human host for long periods of time, since it is extraordinarily resistant to physical and chemical inactivation. If CJD is a naturally infectious disease, it must be minimally so, and takes from years to decades to incubate, with an as yet unidentified mode of transmission.

▶ This study describes 2 decades of epidemiologic research on Creutzfeldt-Jakob disease in France and other countries. It mentions, but I feel does not pay adequate attention to, the apparently dominantly inherited familial cases.—R.N. DeJong, M.D.

11 Multiple Sclerosis

Fatigue in Multiple Sclerosis
Krupp LB, Alvarez LA, LaRocca NG, Scheinberg LC (Albert Einstein College of Medicine, Bronx, NY)
Arch Neurol 45:435–437, April 1988   11–1

Fatigue is a common and often disabling symptom in multiple sclerosis (MS). Its relationship to disease activity, neurologic disability, and depression, however, is still poorly understood. Whether MS fatigue is similar to fatigue in healthy adults is also not known. To address these questions, patients with MS and normal healthy adults were interviewed about their fatigue.

Thirty-two patients with MS and 33 healthy persons were interviewed. The mean age in both groups was 39 years. Twenty-one healthy individuals and 23 patients with MS were women. Fatigue was significantly more frequent among the patients with MS than in the healthy group. Fatigue as measured by the visual analogue scale was also more severe among MS patients. Fatigue was considered the most troublesome symptom of MS by 28% of the MS patients. In 31% of MS patients, fatigue predated other symptoms of MS. The fatigue described by patients and healthy persons shared many features (table). In MS patients, fatigue was

Characteristics of Fatigue Common to Patients With Multiple Sclerosis (MS) and Normal Healthy Adults (NHA)

Qualitative Features	Answering Yes, %*		
	MS	NHA	χ^2
Fatigue is associated with			
Need to rest	75	78	0.02
Loss of patience	61	83	1.70
Decreased motivation	71	89	1.07
Fatigue is worsened by			
Exercise	71	61	0.11
Stress	71	83	0.33
Depression	54	71	0.54
Afternoon	80	94	0.58
Prolonged physical activity	88	70	1.02
Fatigue is improved by			
Resting	98	88	0.09
Sleeping	86	100	1.30
Positive experiences	65	72	0.02
Sex	45	64	0.29

*The *P* value was not significant for any feature.
(Courtesy of Krupp LB, Alvarez LA, LaRocca NG, et al: *Arch Neurol* 45:435–437, April 1988.)

unrelated to depression or global impairment, and there was no correlation between fatigue and neurologic disability.

Fatigue in MS appears to be a distinct clinical entity, often a disability, that can be distinguished from normal fatigue, affective disturbance, and neurologic impairment.

Correlation of Clinical and Immunologic States in Multiple Sclerosis

Mickey MR, Ellison GW, Fahey JL, Moody DJ, Myers LW (Univ of California, Los Angeles)

Arch Neurol 44:371–375, April 1987   11–2

Among patients with multiple sclerosis (MS), reduction of suppressor T lymphocytes has been reported in those with active disease. The response of this disease to cyclophosphamide has been attributed to a reduction in helper T cells. Fourteen MS patients whose disease was in the progression phase were given cyclophosphamide, with the dosage adjusted to maintain peripheral B lymphocytes and CD4 T cells at less than the fifty percentile for the normal population.

There was significant correlation between neurologic state and immunologic state. Clinical state improved after an increase in the percentage of CD8 cells and a decrease in the percentage of CD4 cells. There was no association of dosage and clinical effects.

This study indicates that a relative deficit in suppressor T cells is involved in the progression of MS. Control of this deficit may lead to control of MS.

▶ There is accumulating evidence from a number of studies, including this one, indicating that a relative deficiency of suppressive T cells is important in the production of clinical signs of multiple sclerosis and in the pathogenesis of the disease.—R.N. DeJong, M.D.

The Presence of Immunoreactive Myelin Basic Protein Peptide in Urine of Persons With Multiple Sclerosis

Whitaker JN (Birmingham, Ala)

Ann Neurol 22:648–655, November 1987   11–3

Myelin basic protein (MBP)-like material enters the cerebrospinal fluid (CSF) at the time of myelin damage to the central nervous system. An immunoassay was used to detect MBP-like material in urine in patients with multiple sclerosis (MS) and other neurologic disorders. In this study, a polyclonal antiserum detected nanogram amounts of MBP-like material in unconcentrated urine. The immunoreactive material crossreacted with human MBP peptides. It was dialyzable, and it was not an artifact of degradation of radioligand or salt effect. The octapeptide MBP 82–89, the smallest peptide containing the main epitope to which the antiserum was

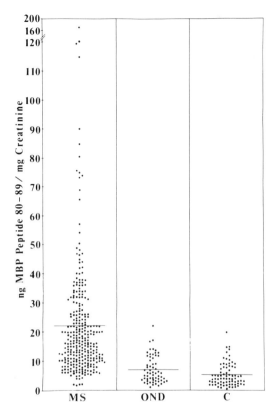

Fig 11–1.—Urinary myelin basic protein (MBP)-like material measured in unconcentrated urine in a double antibody radioimmunoassay against a standard of human MBP peptide 80–89 and expressed in relationship to urinary creatinine level in patients with multiple sclerosis (MS), other neurologic diseases (OND), and normal controls (C). (Courtesy of Whitaker JN: *Ann Neurol* 22:648–655, November 1987.)

directed, differed from the major epitope recognized by antisera detecting material in CSF.

Concentrations of urinary MBP-like material were significantly higher in 39 patients with MS than in either 48 with other neurologic disease or in 26 normal control subjects (Fig 11–1).

These results show that an MBP-like material is found in unconcentrated urine in higher amounts in patients with MS. Urine testing might provide a means of monitoring myelin damage in a clinically feasible manner. Precise identification of the chemical nature of this material might help analyze the in vivo catabolism of potentially autoantigenic MBP.

▶ John Whitaker has been looking for this particle in the urine for a long time and he has found it. It is hoped the work will continue to the point where we will have a urine test for myelin basic protein. Then young people with their first episode of demyelination could be tested.

Then all we would need is a decent and harmless treatment.— R.D. Currier, M.D.

The Role of NMR Imaging in the Assessment of Multiple Sclerosis and Isolated Neurological Lesions: A Quantitative Study

Ormerod IEC, Miller DH, McDonald WI, du Boulay EPGH, Rudge P, Kendall BE, Moseley IF, Johnson G, Tofts PS, Halliday AM, Bronstein AM, Scaravilli F, Harding AE, Barnes D, Zilkha KJ (Inst of Neurology and The National Hospitals, London)
Brain 110:1579–1616, December 1987
11–4

Nuclear magnetic resonance (NMR) imaging is highly sensitive in detecting lesions in patients with multiple sclerosis (MS). The form and distribution of NMR imaging abnormalities in 114 patients with clinically definite MS were compared with observations in other groups of individuals.

In addition to the patients with MS, NMR imaging was performed on 53 apparently healthy persons, 129 patients with isolated focal neurologic lesions with which MS often presents, and 105 patients with disorders that could be confused clinically or radiologically with MS. The latter group consisted of 55 patients with cerebral vascular disease, 24 with degenerative ataxic disorders, 8 with cerebellar tonsillar ectopia, 7 with sarcoidosis, and 11 with various other disorders. Periventricular abnormalities were seen in all but 2 MS patients, and discrete white matter was seen in all but 12. Periventricular changes in MS were characteristically irregular in outline. Periventricular abnormalities that were often milder and smooth in outline were noted in 37 patients with cerebral vascular disease, 9 of 24 with cerebellar degeneration, 5 of 7 with sarcoidosis, and 2 of 3 apparently healthy persons older than 60 years. Appearances in the 7 patients with dementia resembled those in advanced MS. Cerebellar and/or brain stem atrophy characteristic of the cerebellar degenerations, in the absence of white matter anomalies, aided in making the distinction from MS. More than half of the patients with symptoms attributable to isolated focal neurologic lesions had additional lesions. Multiple sclerosis could not be diagnosed in these patients at presentation, but repeat scans after 5–20 months in 25 patients with optic neuritis and in 10 with clinically isolated brain stem lesions showed new lesions in 20%. The patients with new lesions fulfilled the criteria for probable MS. In vivo measurements of T_1 and T_2 allowed the distinction of acute from chronic brain stem lesions. Quantitative differences in T_1 and T_2 were noted between the normal-appearing white matter in MS and normal brain. Postmortem brain studies showed that the NMR imaging abnormalities in MS corresponded with plaques.

Characteristic periventricular and discrete abnormalities in the white matter were seen on NMR images in 99% of patients with clinically definite MS, which corresponded to plaque distribution after death. An important source of the abnormal NMR signals in acute lesions appears to be edema and, in chronic lesions, gliosis.

▶ This is the first careful summary that I have come across concerning the differentiation of MS lesions from those of other causes (there must be others I missed). All but 2 of the patients with clinically definite multiple sclerosis had clear-cut lesions. The lesions were different from those resulting from cerebrovascular disease in being more irregular in outline and more pronounced.

The incidence of multiple sclerosis may be decreasing. The first note of this is by Cook, MacDonald, Tapp, Poskanzer, and Dowling, who have studied the incidence rate of multiple sclerosis in the Shetland Islands from 1938 through 1986 (*Acta Neurol Scand* 77:148–151, 1988). They feel that the decline began somewhere between 1951 and 1968 and appears to be significant. Is this the first hint that measles vaccination has been of use? What are the other changes in the Shetland Islands? When was the water fluorinated? When was the population vaccinated for measles? How complete was the vaccination? These authors do wonder about the failure to find a falling MS prevalence rate in the Shetland Islands despite the statistically significant decline in incidence rate and comment that it may be because patients are living longer.

If you are looking for a good summary on the immunotherapy of multiple sclerosis, we can recommend that of Weiner and Hafler (*Ann Neurol* 23:211–222, 1988).—R.D. Currier, M.D.

A Follow-Up Study of Very Low Field MRI Findings and Clinical Course in Multiple Sclerosis
Palo J, Ketonen L, Wikström J (Univ of Helsinki)
J Neurol Sci 84:177–187, 1988   11–5

Little is known of the evolution of plaques in the course of multiple sclerosis (MS). Seventy-three patients with definite MS underwent magnetic resonance imaging, 57 of whom were examined a second time after 6 months. Forty-one patients had a third examination and 25 had a fourth examination after up to 2 years. The mean patient age at initial assessment was 36 years. Studies used both inversion recovery and spin-echo sequencing.

Increased T_1 and T_2 relaxation times were most evident on spin-echo scans. Plaques were widely scattered in the periventricular regions and in cerebral and cerebellar white matter. Nearly 80% of the patients had abnormal results from initial scans. Plaques were most numerous in those with progressive disease and in more disabled patients. Two thirds of the patients with abnormal MRI scans had more than 3 lesions. New plaques appeared after 6 months in only 16% of the patients studied. Among patients studied a third time, more showed disappearance of plaques or a decrease in plaque size than had progression (Fig 11–2). New plaques sometimes appeared during clinical remissions, but the disappearance of old plaques correlated well with clinical improvement.

Initial MRI showed abnormal results in 78% of these patients with

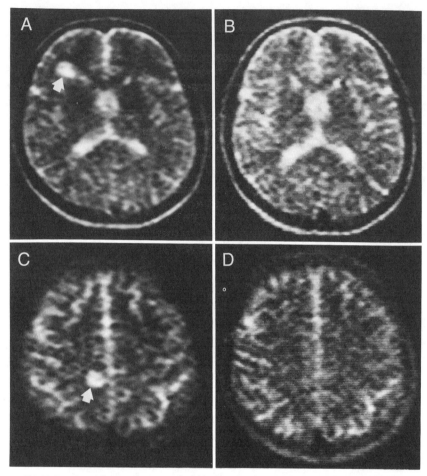

Fig 11–2.—A, axial spin-echo image through the ventricles of a 42-year-old woman with MS. A plaque with high signal intensity is adjacent to the right frontal horn *(arrow)*. **B,** the plaque has disappeared 6 months later. **C,** axial spin-echo image through the fovea semiovale of the same patient shows an MS plaque *(arrow)* on the right. **D,** no plaque can be seen in the same area 6 months later (TR 2000 msec, TE 150 msec). (Courtesy of Palo J, Ketonen L, Wikström J: *J Neurol Sci* 84:177–187, 1988.)

definite MS. Caution is necessary in predicting specific neurologic deficits from the MRI findings. However, MS no longer should be characterized as remitting or progressive solely on clinical grounds.

▶ Some of the questions relating to MS and MRI scanning are being answered. Evidently, plaques can come and go. As one might expect, they increase with increasing disability. However, there seems little doubt that in a "burned out" patient the plaques are also burned out.—R.D. Currier, M.D.

A Comparison Between Chemical Analysis and Magnetic Resonance Imaging With the Clinical Diagnosis of Multiple Sclerosis

Papadopoulos NM, McFarlin DE, Patronas NJ, McFarland HF, Costello R (Natl Inst of Health, Bethesda, Md)
Am J Clin Pathol 88:365–368, September 1987   11–6

The diagnosis of multiple sclerosis (MS) can be made clinically by taking a patient's medical history and conducting a neurologic examination. Additional criteria used to confirm the clinical diagnosis and aid in the differentiation of equivocal cases are magnetic resonance imaging (MRI) and electrophoretic and immunochemical analyses of serum and cerebrospinal fluid (CSF) proteins. The accuracy of these ancillary criteria in the diagnosis of MS was evaluated in 95 patients suspected of having MS on the basis of their medical history and neurologic examination. On the basis of clinical features, the patients were grouped as having clinically definite MS, not-definite MS, or no MS. Chemical analyses of paired serum and CSF samples were performed using simple zone electrophoresis and immunochemical quantitation tests to identify oligoclonal immunoglobulin (IG) bands and to estimate both the albumin quotient and the IgG index.

A high degree of positive correlation was achieved between clinically definite MS and chemical analysis in 73 of 73 patients. Chemical results were positive in 11 of 12 patients with not-definite MS and negative in all 10 patients without MS. The MRI scans had positive results in 48 of 51 patients with clinically definite MS and in 4 of 4 patients with not-definite MS. Five of 6 patients without MS had negative results for their MRI scans.

Combined electrophoretic and immunochemical determinations of serum and CSF proteins confirm the clinical diagnosis of MS, as well as aid in the differential diagnosis of not-definite MS. In atypical MS cases or cases with unequivocal clinical presentations, they can provide evidence to support the clinical impression of MS. Magnetic resonance imaging provides supplementary evidence for the accurate diagnosis of MS.

▶ A question comes to mind after reading this. What about the patient whom you suspect has multiple sclerosis both by history and neurologic examination but who has a negative MRI and spinal fluid? Will such patients in the long run have multiple sclerosis or something else and, if something else, what?—R.D. Currier, M.D.

Total Lymphoid Irradiation in Multiple Sclerosis: Blood Lymphocytes and Clinical Course
Cook SD, Devereux C, Troiano R, Zito G, Hafstein M, Lavenhar M, Hernandez E, Dowling PC (VA Med Ctr, East Orange, NJ; New Jersey Med School, Newark, Clara Maass Med Ctr, Belleville, NJ)
Ann Neurol 22:634–638, November 1987   11–7

Numerous attempts have been made to treat multiple sclerosis (MS) patients with immunosuppressive therapy, but no clear long-term benefits have been demonstrated in carefully controlled trials. A double-blind, randomized, prospective study was done to assess the efficacy of total lymphoid irradiation (TLI)—a potent immunosuppressive therapy—in treating patients with a chronic progressive course of MS.

The 45 patients studied were aged 20–60 years, had clinically definite MS for at least 3 years, and had progressive neurologic disability for at least 1 year, with scores of 4–8 on disability scale modified from the Kurtzke disability status scale. Most patients had received steroids or corticotropin (ACTH). Either TLI (1980 rad) or sham TLI was given for 29–64 days (mean 40 days) to 24 and 21 patients, respectively. The patients were followed for at least 6 months after completion of therapy. Patients with mean absolute lymphocyte counts of less than 900 in the first 3 posttreatment months did significantly better at all intervals than those with higher counts. At 24 months, 62% of patients with mean lymphocyte counts of less than 900 in the first 3 posttreatment months did not progress on functional scales, compared with 25% of those with higher counts. Patients with lymphocyte counts of less than 900 in the first year who received TLI showed less progression than patients with higher counts who received TLI; significances were reached at 6 and 12 months after treatment. Significant differences between those who received TLI and those who received sham TLI were also noted in the clinical course of patients with sustained lymphocytopenia in the first posttreatment year.

These findings suggest that a simple laboratory test, the absolute blood lymphocyte count, may serve as a valuable barometer for monitoring the amount of immunosuppressive therapy needed to prevent progression in patients with MS, and possibly other autoimmune diseases.

▶ Will this criterion for effectiveness—a total lymphocyte count of less than 900—be useful in following other methods of immune suppression? Total lymphoid irradiation certainly is simpler in the long run than other immune suppressive treatments. Some have reservations because of its irreversibility. We hope that these investigators will continue to inform us on the progress of this group.—R.D. Currier, M.D.

Cyclosporine Versus Azathioprine in the Long-Term Treatment of Multiple Sclerosis: Results of the German Multicenter Study

Kappos L, Patzold U, Dommasch D, Poser S, Haas J, Krauseneck P, Malin J-P, Fierz W, Graffenried BU, Gugerli US (Max Planck Society, Würzburg; Medizinische Hochschule Hannover, Hannover; Univ of Göttingen, West Germany; Univ of Zürich, Switzerland)
Ann Neurol 23:56–63, January 1988   11–8

Cyclosporine (CyA) is effective in preventing and suppressing autoimmune encephalomyelitis in animal models of multiple sclerosis (MS). The authors therefore compared CyA with azathioprine, which is standard immunosuppressive treatment for relapsing MS. Patients having clinically definite MS and increased autochthonous IgG production in the CNS

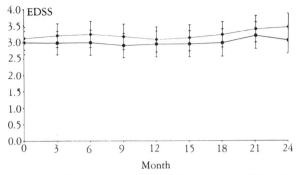

Fig 11–3.—Neurologic deficit vs. length of treatment. Mean scores with 95% confidence intervals in valid patients (*n* = 167). *Solid line with squares* = cyclosporine (*n* = 85); *dotted line with circles* = azathioprine (*n* = 82). EDSS = Expanded Disability Status Scale (Courtesy of Kappos L, Patzold U, Dommasch D, et al: *Ann Neurol* 23:56–63, January 1988.)

and/or oligoclonal bands in the cerebrospinal fluid participated in the trial. All had had active disease in the past 2 years, and were aged 18 to 50 years. The dose of orally given CyA was 5 mg/kg daily, and that of azathioprine was 2.5 mg/kg daily. The CyA dose was adjusted to maintain trough blood levels of 200–1,000 ng/ml, or 150–750 ng/ml later in the trial period.

Eighty-five CyA-treated patients and 82 treated with azathioprine completed 2 years of treatment. Clinical assessments showed no significant difference between the 2 groups (Fig 11–3), and rates of relapse were similar. Gastrointestinal side effects were frequent in both groups, and infections were equally frequent in the CyA and azathioprine groups.

Cyclosporine failed to exhibit the same benefit in this trial of MS patients as it has in transplantation. Deterioration was only minor with both CyA and azathioprine maintenance. Because of side effects, CyA alone is not the preferred choice for long-term immunosuppression of relapsing-remitting or relapsing-progressive MS. Less nephrotoxic compounds might prove more useful, or low-dose CyA could be combined with drugs having a complementary or additive action on the immune system.

▶ I had great hopes for cyclosporine. This is the first publication on its use in the treatment of multiple sclerosis. There is no difference between cyclosporine and azathioprine, which means at least to me that it probably will not turn out to be the answer unless it is a matter of dosage or method of administration. A third, placebo treated group would have told us whether either medication is better than nothing. Back to the drawing board.—R.D. Currier, M.D.

Treatment of Multiple Sclerosis With Gamma Interferon: Exacerbations Associated With Activation of the Immune System
Panitch HS, Hirsch RL, Schindler J, Johnson KP (Univ of Maryland and Biogen Research Corp, Cambridge, Mass)
Neurology 37:1097–1102, July 1987   11–9

There is evidence that viral infection or immune defects are involved in multiple sclerosis (MS). Therefore, clinical trials with interferons (IFNs) were undertaken. A pilot study of recombinant gamma IFN was performed in 18 MS patients in remission, to determine dosage and toxicity. Patients received 1 μg, 30 μg, or 1,000 μg of gamma IFN by infusion twice weekly for 4 weeks.

Serum levels of gamma IFN were proportional to the administered dose. No IFN was detected in cerebrospinal fluid. Of the 18 patients in this series, 7 had exacerbations during treatment. This rate was significantly higher than the rate of exacerbations prior to IFN treatment. Exacerbations occurred at all 3 treatment levels. The proportion of circulating monocytes with class II surface antigen, the proliferative response of peripheral blood leukocytes, and natural killer cell activity all increased during the treatment period.

Gamma IFN had pronounced effects on cellular immunity and increased the rate of disease exacerbation in MS patients. Therefore, gamma IFN is not a suitable treatment for MS. Perhaps therapy that inhibits the activity of gamma IFN should be investigated.

▶ The point seems to be that not only did gamma interferon not work in the treatment of multiple sclerosis, it actually seemed to have produced exacerbations. This is a not entirely unexpected support for the immunologic pathogenesis of multiple sclerosis. Improving or stimulating the function of the immune system seems to light up the disease.— R.D. Currier, M.D.

Controlled Pilot Trial of Monthly Intravenous Cyclophosphamide in Multiple Sclerosis
Killian JM, Bressler RB, Armstrong RM, Huston DP (Baylor College, Methodist Hosp, Houston)
Arch Neurol 45:27–30, January 1988   11–10

Cytotoxic immunosuppressive therapy has been used to treat multiple sclerosis (MS) for years in a variety of drugs and dosages with variable results. Some clinical benefit has been reported for monthly intravenous cyclophosphamide therapy. A randomized, double-blind, controlled trial was done to determine the efficacy of monthly intravenous bolus cyclophosphamide administration compared with placebo in patients with relapsing/remitting MS.

Eight patients received placebo and 6 received cyclophosphamide. Cyclophosphamide was given in an intravenous dose of 750 mg/m^2 and was repeated monthly for 12 months. A neurologic assessment, including determination of Kurtzke disability and ambulation indexes, was done at study entry, monthly intervals, and during exacerbations. The group receiving cyclophosphamide therapy had less frequent and less pronounced episodes than the group receiving placebos. When each group served as their own controls, the cyclophosphamide group had a significant reduction in episodes, whereas the placebo group did not. When the placebo group was given cyclophosphamide, they too experienced a significant decrease in episodes. The reduction in episodes was even more evident when all patients receiving cyclophosphamide were combined for analysis. Four of the 6 patients originally receiving cyclophosphamide therapy experienced monthly episodes of nausea and vomiting 8–12 hours after the intravenous treatment. Generally, adverse effects were considered minimal.

Intravenously given cyclophosphamide treatment may have a favorable effect on the frequency and duration of episodes experienced by patients with relapsing/remitting MS. Further studies are needed to determine this treatment's long-term effect on disability and disease progression.

► There has been much controversy regarding the use of long-term immuno-suppressive therapy in MS. This carefully carried-out study appears to show that monthly intravenously administered cyclophosphamide therapy brought about a significant decrease in the duration and frequency of relapsing-remitting episodes of MS in patients with the disease. What is this treatment's long-term effect on disability and disease progression?—R.N. DeJong, M.D.

A Pilot Trial of Cop 1 in Exacerbating–Remitting Multiple Sclerosis

Bornstein MB, Miller A, Slagle S, Weitzman M, Crystal H, Drexler E, Keilson M, Merriam A, Wassertheil-Smoller S, Spada S, Weiss W, Arnon R, Jacobsohn I, Teitelbaum D, Sela M (Albert Einstein College of Medicine, Bronx, NY, Weizmann Inst of Science, Rehovot, Israel)
N Engl J Med 317:408–414, Aug 13, 1987   11–11

Cop 1 is a random polymer simulating myelin basic protein, synthesized by polymerizing several L-amino acids. It suppresses experimental allergic encephalomyelitis, and is nontoxic in animals. A double-blind, placebo-controlled study of Cop 1 was undertaken in 50 patients having exacerbating-remitting multiple sclerosis. All patients had a definite diagnosis and were aged 20 to 35 years. At least 2 clear exacerbations had occurred in the past 2 years, but the Kurtzke Disability Status Scale score was not above 6. Study patients self-injected 20 mg of Cop 1 in saline daily over 2 years.

Fourteen of 25 patients in the Cop 1 group and 6 of 23 control patients had no exacerbations. The average numbers of exacerbations in 2 years were 0.6 and 2.7, respectively. The difference was greatest in patients who were less disabled at entry to the study. Less disabled patients also did better clinically during the 2-year study period. Only local side effects were significantly more frequent in the Cop 1 group (table).

Subcutaneous injections of Cop 1 appear to have substantial benefit in patients with definite multiple sclerosis, particularly those who are relatively less disabled when treatment is begun. The treatment is well toler-

Percentages of Patients Reporting
Side Effects

SYMPTOM	PLACEBO (N = 23)	COP 1 (N = 25)
Local		
Soreness*	35	92
Itching†	22	64
Swelling*	17	88
Redness	48	76
Other	35	36
Other		
Headache	39	32
Nausea	17	24
Vomiting	4	4
Dizziness	30	40
Constipation	30	40
Sweating	26	28
Rash	17	24
Palpitations	13	24
Cramps	9	12
Faintness	13	20
Joint pain	39	40
Gastrointestinal discomfort	22	12
Appetite loss	13	20
Drowsiness	26	20
Other	17	28

*$P < .001$ for the difference between placebo and Cop 1.
†$P < .01$ for the difference between placebo and Cop 1.
(Courtesy of Bornstein MB, Miller A, Slagle S, et al: *N Engl J Med* 317:408–414, Aug 13, 1987.)

ated. Further study of this agent in a full-scale multicenter trial is warranted.

▶ A random copolymer synthesized from L-analine, L-glutamic acid, L-lysine, and L-tyrosine simulates myelin basic protein. In a pilot trial on patients with multiple sclerosis, the results suggested that it might be of benefit in patients with mild cases of the exacerbating-remitting form of the disease. Confirmation by a more extensive clinical trial was advised. In an editorial in the same issue of the journal (*N Engl J Med* 317:442–444, 1987) Howard L. Weiner of Brigham and Women's Hospital, Boston, also advises further clinical studies, but points out several problems in the study, including whether effective therapy for the disease can be developed without knowing the exact cause. The Medical Advisory Board of the National Multiple Sclerosis Society also advises further clinical study. Cop 1 is not available for general use and remains an investigative agent. Future supplies of a uniform, standardized preparation are not yet assured, and it is not clear when this agent will again be available for clinical testing.— R.N. DeJong, M.D.

12 Myopathies and Myasthenia Gravis

Central Core Disease: Clinical Features in 13 Patients
Shuaib A, Paasuke RT, Brownell AW (Univ of Calgary)
Medicine 66:389–396, 1987   12–1

Central core disease (CCD) usually appears in infancy or childhood with hypotonia and proximal muscle weakness. The myopathy is generally nonprogressive; the deep tendon reflexes are often reduced or absent. A variety of skeletal defects may occur. The transmission of the myopathy has been shown to follow an autosomal dominant pattern. Findings in 13 patients with CCD were reviewed and compared with those in 62 patients reported in the literature.

Certain diagnoses of CCD can be made only by muscle biopsy. Cores lacking oxidative enzyme activity are present in most fibers. Central core disease was diagnosed in this series when the typical core lesions were seen in sections reacted for NADH dehydrogenase (Fig 12–1). Patients were grouped into 3 categories: those with muscle weakness who had not had in vitro contracture tests (IVCTs) to determine susceptibility to malignant hyperthermia; those with muscle weakness and susceptibility to

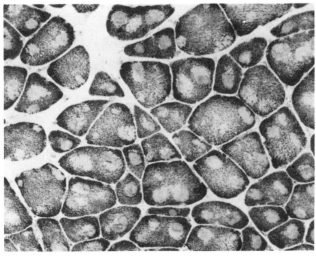

Fig 12–1.—Photomicrograph of NADH-dehydrogenase reacted sections showing the typical lesions of CCD (original magnification, ×125). (Courtesy of Shuaib A, Paasuke RT, Brownell KW: *Medicine* 66:389–396, 1987.)

malignant hyperthermia; and those with normal strength and susceptibility to malignant hyperthermia.

The 13 patients were from 6 different pedigrees. At diagnosis, patients ranged in age from 4 to 59 years; 7 were male. Five of the 13 patients had normal strength, 4 had generalized weakness, 2 had weakness in the upper and lower extremities, and 2 had weakness in the lower extremities only. The weakness did not significantly affect the daily activities of 7 patients; the eighth had been wheelchair-bound since age 4 years. In 6 patients the weakness was nonprogressive; in the remaining 2 its progression was gradual.

Muscle atrophy was observed in 5 patients, and varied from a mild generalized thinness in 4 to severe atrophy in 1. The 2 children in the series had hypotonia. Three patients had contractures, varying from mild and focal in 2 to severe and generalized in 1. Progressive vertebral column deformities were seen in 2 patients. Recurrent joint dislocation occurred in 2, muscle stiffness or soreness during exercise in 3, focal areflexia in 1, loose jointedness in 2, weakness after alcohol ingestion in 1, and weakness during muscular activity in the heat in 1. Six had elevated serum creatine kinase concentrations. One had recurrent cardiac arrhythmias. Three had mitral valve prolapse.

This study suggests that many patients with CCD do not show any myopathic features, that there is a high incidence of associated cardiac abnormalities, and that all patients with CCD should be considered at high risk for malignant hyperthermia unless IVCT results are normal.

▶ Central core disease, originally thought to be a congenital and nonprogressive myopathy, is now known to be a systemic disorder inherited in an autosomal nondominant pattern that has a high incidence of associated cardiac abnormalities and a high risk for malignant hyperthermia.—R.N. DeJong, M.D.

Chronic Enterovirus Infection in Patients With Postviral Fatigue Syndrome
Yousef GE, Bell EJ, Mann GF, Murugesan V, Smith DG, McCartney RA, Mowbray JF (St Mary's Hosp, London; Ruchill Hosp, Glasgow, Scotland)
Lancet 1:146–149, Jan 23, 1988   12–2

Preceding infection by Coxsackie B viruses has been related to chronic postviral fatigue syndrome (PVFS), or myalgic encephalomyelitis. Persistent enterovirus infection is demonstrable by detecting genomic sequences of Coxsackie B virus in muscle biopsy specimens from patients with dermatomyositis, polymyositis, and chronic myocarditis. Evidence of chronic enterovirus infection was found in patients with PVFS. The patients had excessive muscle fatigue on exertion, with myalgia, for at least 6 months, with or without preceding acute viral infection. All of the patients had dysphasia and difficulty in remembering and concentrating, and most had difficulty in accommodation. None, however, had apparent neurologic disease.

Viral isolation from concentrated fecal samples was attempted in 76 patients with PVFS and 30 matched control subjects. Positive cultures were obtained in 22% of patients and 7% of controls. Studies with an enterovirus group-specific monoclonal antibody directed against VP1 polypeptide demonstrated VP1 antigen in the serum of half of another 87 patients with PVFS. When IgM complexes were detectable, antigen was identified in 42 of 44 patients. When 17 of the initial patients were restudied, the same virus was again isolated from 29% of the group, and 76% had IgM responses to enteroviruses. About half were positive for VP1 antigen in serum.

Chronic enteroviral infection is present in many patients with PVFS. Detection of viral antigen in serum is a more sensitive test for enteroviral infection in PVFS than is viral isolation. Clinical improvement correlates with the disappearance of both VP1 antigen and IgM complexes from the circulation.

▶ This syndrome has gone under a variety of names. No single name has stuck. Years ago it was known as Iceland disease, Royal Free Bed Hospital disease, Jacksonville polio, etc. Postviral fatigue syndrome is as good as any. We have all seen patients with it and wondered whether their trouble was psychogenic or organic. The symptoms, as mentioned by the authors, are excessive muscle fatigue, myalgia, dysphagia, and difficulty with concentration and short-term memory. Fatigue is the chief complaint; it persisted for 6 months to 12 years in this group. The patients are all certain they have something, although after many months of being questioned they wonder themselves whether it is psychogenic.

It is hoped that these investigators will continue and that eventually there will be effective treatment.— R.D. Currier, M.D.

Seronegative Myasthenia Gravis
Soliven BC, Lange DJ, Penn AS, Younger D, Jaretzki A, III, Lovelace RE, Rowland LP (Columbia Univ)
Neurology 38:514–517, April 1988   12–3

Myasthenia gravis is ascribed to circulating antibodies to acetylcholine receptor (AChR), but antibody titers do not correlate consistently with the severity of symptoms. A review was made of data on 221 patients with myasthenia, 18.5% of whom had no detectable antibody to AChR. The series included 145 patients with generalized myasthenia and 30 with ocular myasthenia. Thirty-one patients were unavailable for follow-up.

Seventeen percent of patients with generalized myasthenia were seronegative. Antibody was absent in only 1 of 16 patients with ocular symptoms for less than 2 years. None of 8 patients with congenital myasthenia had antibody to AChR. No seronegative patient had thymoma, but 15% of seropositive patients did. About one fifth of both groups had myasthenic crisis. Seronegative patients had as good a response to thymectomy as did those who had antibody. More than 80% of both groups were asymptomatic after thymectomy. Four of 8 seronegative patients improved after a series of plasma exchanges.

It remains unclear why some patients with myasthenia gravis lack increased antibody against AChR. Absence of antibody does not necessarily indicate less-severe symptoms. Seronegativity does not contraindicate conventional treatments of myasthenia.

▶ S.H. Subramony, M.D., Associate Professor of Neurology, University of Mississippi School of Medicine, Jackson, writes the following comment.— R.D. Currier, M.D.

▶ The occurrence of a positive AChR antibody test in generalized myasthenia gravis in this study is similar to that reported in other series. Use of additional techniques of testing for antibody, for example, antibodies that block alpha bungarotoxin binding sites ("blocking antibodies") and those that cause loss of AChR from cultured muscle cells ("modulating antibodies") tends to increase the percentage of positive tests. Still, some patients with acquired generalized myasthenia gravis lack antibodies, perhaps because critical antigenic determinants on the AChR are lost during assay procedure or are lacking in the AChR used for assay, or because all AChR antibodies are bound to AChR with no circulating antibodies, or finally, because of the intriguing possibility that the antibodies are directed against end-plate determinants other than AChR itself. It is reassuring that the treatment modalities for seronegative myasthenia gravis are the same as for the seropositive disease, though the lack of thymic pathology in 3 out of 8 patients had led Mossman et al. (*Lancet* 1:116, 1986) to question the value of thymectomy in this group of patients.— S.H. Subramony, M.D.

Effects of Thymectomy in Myasthenia Gravis
Papatestas AE, Genkins G, Kornfeld P, Eisenkraft JB, Fagerstrom RP, Pozner J, Aufses AH, Jr (The Mount Sinai Med Ctr and School of Medicine, New York)
Ann Surg 206:79–88, July 1987   12–4

Thymectomy in myasthenia gravis has been observed to lead to remission of symptoms of the disease. But the role of thymectomy is not fully understood. Factors influencing the onset of remission in myasthenia gravis were assessed in 2,062 patients, of whom 962 had had thymectomy.

Follow-up data were obtained by patient examination or questionnaire. In 226 (11%) of the patients with myasthenia gravis, thymomas were observed. Eighty-one (6%) of the 1,254 patients with mild cases had thymomas; 145 (18%) of the 808 with severe symptoms had associated thymic tumors. Only one third of patients without thymomas had severe symptoms, whereas two thirds of those with associated thymomas did.

Seventy-two percent of patients who had thymectomy were operated

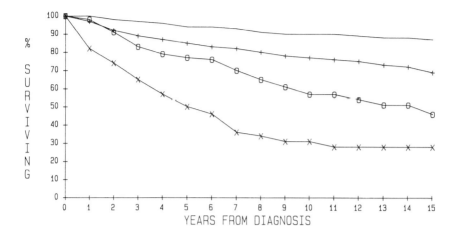

— SNT (n=788)   —+— NSNT (n=1048)   —⊖— ST (n=174)   —×— NST (n=52)

Fig 12–2.—Interval from diagnosis to death. *SNT*, thymectomy, no thymoma; *NSNT*, no thymectomy, no thymoma; *ST*, thymectomy thymoma; *NST*, no thymectomy, thymoma. (Courtesy of Papatestas AE, Genkins G, Kornfeld P, et al: *Ann Surg* 206:79–88, July 1987.)

on through the transcervical approach. The appearance of early remissions among all patients was significantly and independently affected by thymectomy, milder disease, and absence of coexisting thymomas. Sex and age did not influence the results.

Patients with thymomas who had surgery eventually had more remissions than patients with thymomas treated medically although they had considerable delay in remission onset. Short duration of disease before thymectomy in mild cases was also associated with earlier remissions. Mortality among all patients was significantly and independently affected by symptom severity, age, associated thymomas, and failure to remove the thymus. Patients without thymectomy and with thymomas had an earlier onset of extrathymic neoplasms. Morbidity after the transcervical approach was minimal (Fig 12–2).

Early thymectomy by the transcervical approach, when possible, was found to have significant clinical advantages over the transthoracic approach and should be advocated for all patients with myasthenia gravis, including those with ocular disease.

▶ This is a giant series that will remain unequalled for a long time.

The conclusions are that all myasthenics (including ocular) should have a thymectomy whether or not their disease is associated with thymoma, and that the transcervical approach is as good as the transthoracic and is associated with less operative morbidity. So, why are the surgeons here still reluctant to operate transcervically? There is probably something I don't understand.

But hold everything. Jaretzki et al. in a recently published report (*J Thorac*

Cardiovasc Surg 95:947–957, 1988) find that the wide-open surgical approach with a thorough search of the mediastinum and neck gives a 96% improvement rate in those without thymoma followed for 6 to 89 months—an unequalled result.

So, that's why. There was something I didn't understand.—R.D. Currier, M.D.

13 Amyotrophic Lateral Sclerosis

Guam Amyotrophic Lateral Sclerosis-Parkinsonism-Dementia Linked to a Plant Excitant Neurotoxin
Spencer PS, Nunn PB, Hugon J, Ludolph AC, Ross SM, Roy DN, Robertson RC
(Albert Einstein College of Medicine, Bronx, NY)
Science 237:517–522, July 31, 1987   13–1

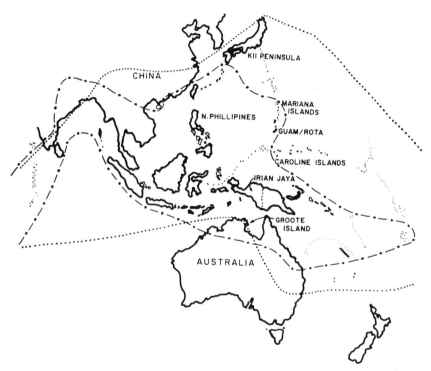

Fig 13–1.—Distribution of *Cycas* spp in relation to high-incidence foci of ALS in Guam and Rota, Kii Peninsula (Japan), and Irian Jaya (Indonesia). Area contained within *dotted lines* shows earlier distribution; that within *broken punctuated line* is taken from Read and Solt. Interest in possible foci of ALS has also centered on the North Philippines and Groote Island, Australia. No cases of ALS-PD have been reported in the Caroline Islands or in the islands east (Marshall and Gilbert Islands) or west (Palau Island) thereof, although *C. circinalis* was formerly used for food in Palau, Sonsorol (Palau Islands), Yap, Nukuoro (Caroline Islands), Majuro, and Arno (Marshall Islands). Other *Cycas* species were highly prized for food in Japan in the 18th century and, more recently, used in the Ryukyu Islands (South Japan) and Batanes Islands (North Philippines), and by the aborigines of northern Australia. (Courtesy of Spencer PS, Nunn PB, Hugon H, et al: *Science* 237:517–522, July 1987.)

The high incidence of amyotrophic lateral sclerosis (ALS), parkinsonism, and Alzheimer-type dementia has declined among the Chamorro population of the western Pacific islands of Guam and Rota. This fact, coupled with the lack of demonstrable viral and hereditable factors in this disease, suggests that an etiologic factor may be a gradually disappearing environmental agent associated with the culture. Seed of the neurotoxic plant *Cycas circinalis* L., a traditional source of food and medicine used less since the Americanization of the Chamorro people after World War II, is a candidate.

To test this agent, 13 1-year-old male cynomolgus monkeys in 6 groups received varying doses of synthetic β-N-methylamino-L-alamine (L-BMAA), identical to the natural free amino acid in *C. circinalis* seed. Neurologic deficits appeared 2 to 12 weeks later. Signs of motor-neuron dysfunction developed symmetrically or asymmetrically. After 1 month, animals in certain groups displayed stooped posture, unkempt coat, tremor and weakness of upper or all extremities, and reduced aggressive behavior. Clinical and electrophysiologic signs of motor deficit were observed, preceding concrete structural alterations in the corresponding areas of the CNS. Giant Betz cells undergoing chromatolysis were noted.

These results support the hypothesis that cycad exposure has an important role in the etiology of the Guam disease. Because human neurologic disorders comparable to ALS parkinsonism-dementia are reported to have a high incidence elsewhere in the distribution of Cycas spp (Fig 13–1), it is important to determine whether early exposure to slow toxins in certain plants has an etiologic role. The amino acid L-BMAA has a chemical and neuropharmacologic relationship to β-N-oxalylamino-L-alanine (L-BOAA), another unusual plant-derived nonprotein amino acid that induces corticomotoneuronal deficits in primates. L-BOAA has been implicated in the etiology of human lathyrism. This study demonstrated that L-BMAA and L-BOAA are linked to human motor system disease.

▶ This does seem like the answer after over 40 years of searching.

The significance of this in the etiology of worldwide idiopathic ALS is uncertain, just as the significance of 1,2,5,6-methylphenyl tetrahydropyridine in the chemical causation of parkinsonism is of uncertain relationship to idiopathic parkinsonism.

They both may be a clue, because they do provide an experimental tool and at the very least indicate there are multiple causes of both diseases.—R.D. Currier, M.D.

The Natural History of Motoneuron Loss in Amyotrophic Lateral Sclerosis
Munsat TL, Andres PL, Finison L, Conlon T, Thibodeau L (New England Med Ctr, Boston)
Neurology 38:409–413, March 1988   13–2

Current knowledge of the true course of amyotrophic lateral sclerosis (ALS) is anecdotal and unsubstantiated. A quantitative, reliable, sensitive, and valid measurement technique was used to analyze the rate and pat-

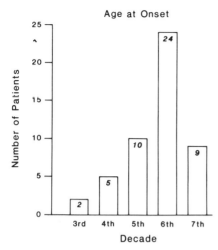

Fig 13–2.—Age of symptomatic onset by decade. (Courtesy of Munsat TL, Andres PL, Finison L, et al: *Neurology* 38:409–413, March 1988.)

tern of motor deterioration in 50 patients with ALS strictly defined for up to 67 months.

All patients with a firmly established diagnosis of uncomplicated ALS who had 8 or more monthly Tufts Quantitative Neuromuscular Examinations were selected. The patients were followed for 8–67 months, with a mean of 20 ± 13.4 months. The 24 women and 26 men had a mean age of onset of 53 years (Fig 13–2). The rate of motoneuron loss was linear and symmetric. Bulbar function deteriorated more slowly than respiratory, arm, or leg function. Loss of leg strength was slower than loss of arm strength. There was no correlation between age at onset or region of onset and rate of deterioration. Arm strength deteriorated more slowly in women than in men. Considerable variance in deterioration rates among individuals was observed, with lesser variance between different regions of neuraxis in the same patient.

In this study, the rate of motoneuron loss in patients with ALS was linear and symmetric. Bulbar deterioration was slower than respiratory, arm, or leg function deterioration, and loss of leg strength was slower than loss of arm strength. These findings should be useful in designing clinical trials and generating testable hypotheses of the etiology of ALS.

▶ The rate and pattern of motor neuron loss in patients with amyotrophic lateral sclerosis was linear and symmetrical. Bulbar function deteriorated more slowly than respiration or arm and leg function. It is hoped that these and subsequent careful analyses of the course of amyotrophic lateral sclerosis will be useful in developing new and treatable etiologic hypotheses.—R.N. DeJong, M.D.

Lowered Cerebral Glucose Utilization in Amyotrophic Lateral Sclerosis
Dalakas MC, Hatazawa J, Brooks RA, Di Chiro G (Natl Inst of Neurological and Communicative Disorders and Stroke, Bethesda, Md)
Ann Neurol 22:580–586, November 1987   13–3

There may be substantial discrepancy between the clinical signs of amyotrophic lateral sclerosis (ALS) and the extent of pathologic involvement, especially in the motor cortex. The regional cerebral metabolic rate for glucose (rCMRGlc) was determined in 12 patients with ALS, using positron emission tomography with [^{18}F] 2-fluoro-2-deoxy-D-glucose. Nineteen studies were carried out. Eight patients had clinical evidence of upper and lower motor neuron involvement, and 4 had progressive disease confined to the bulbar and spinal lower motor neurons.

Mean cortical rCMRGlc in patients with upper motor neuron signs was significantly lower than in age-matched controls. Hypometabolism extended through the cortex and basal ganglia, and its degree correlated with the duration of clinical abnormality. Three patients who were studied a second time had a further reduction in rCMRGlc, corresponding to clinical deterioration. Metabolic values were normal or nearly so in patients with disease confined to the lower motor neurons, and in 3 patients with lower motor neuron disease from old paralytic poliomyelitis. Patients with upper motor neuron involvement did not have undue atrophy.

Extensive neuronal hypometabolism is found in patients with ALS who have upper motor neuron disease. Some cortical neurons apparently exist in a state of neuronal nonfunction, rather than cell death. Determination of cortical rCMRGlc may prove useful in evaluating future experimental treatments for these patients.

▶ This article, one by Plaitakis and Caroscio (*Ann Neurol* 22:575–579, 1987) in the same issue, and that of Perry, Hansen, and Jones in *Neurology* (37:1845–1848, 1987) all point out metabolic problems of the same general type discovered by, in the first case, PET scanning, in the second case by analysis of fasting plasma and the result of oral glutamate loading, and in the third case by amino acid analysis of autopsied brains. Perry, Hansen, and Jones found a glutamate deficiency in the autopsied brains of ALS patients, whereas Plaitakis and Caroscio found an elevated plasma glutamate and aspartate level as compared to controls, thus tending to confirm their suspicion that glutamate acts as a neurotoxin. Dalakas et al. find a decreased glucose metabolic rate in the cerebral cortex of patients with ALS. Rather than their being at odds, I suspect that all 3 make sense, but explanation will require someone with greater biochemical knowledge than this editor.—R.D. Currier, M.D.

Controlled Acute Trial of a Thyrotrophin Releasing Hormone Analogue (RX77368) in Motor Neuron Disease
Guiloff RJ, Eckland DJA, Demaine C, Hoare RC, Macrae KD, Lightman SL (Westminster Hosp, London)
J Neurol Neurosurg Psychiatry 50:1359–1370, October 1987   13–4

Motor neuron disease is associated with spinal cord depletion of thytropin releasing hormone (TRH). The acute effects of L-pyroglutamyl-L-histidyl-L-3,3 dimethyl prolineamide (RX77368), a stabilized TRH analogue, were studied in 25 consecutive patients with motor neuron disease in a double-blind, randomized, crossover trial. After an initial pilot study, patients were randomized to receive RX77368 (300 µg/kg) intravenously (IV) over 2 hours or saline. Neurologic examination included detailed assessment of muscle force in 21 muscle groups.

Temporary improvements in bulbar symptoms, including speech, respiratory parameters, tongue movements, and swallowing, were noted. The most striking benefit of RX77368 was improvement in predominantly spastic dysarthria both in clarity and volume. In addition, an increase in fasciculations was noted as well as significant reductions in spasticity. Change in muscle force with RX77368 differed from placebo, but both increase and decrease in force were seen and did not result in detectable changes in function. Side effects were clinically significant in 50% of patients but cleared within 12 hours. Prolonged rise of thyroxine and an increase in plasma levels of prolactin, thyroid stimulating hormone (TSH), and growth hormone were seen and followed characteristic patterns.

Infusion of RX77368 is associated with temporary improvement in patients with motor neuron disease with bulbar syndrome.

▶ In this article and in a following article (Guiloff et al: *J Neurol Neurosurg Psychiatry* 50:1633–1640, 1987), the results of attempts at therapy of ALS with TRH are summarized.

The committee on health care issues of the ANA has released a report on TRH in the treatment of ALS (*Ann Neurol* 22:541–542, October 1987). They conclude that there is no evidence that TRH is clinically indicated or warrants a new controlled study or that it can be recommended in the management of patients with ALS. They further comment that "the TRH experience shows a need for double blind control studies of new therapeutic agents in ALS."

Mitsumoto, Hanson, and Chad have provided a nice review of ALS pathogenesis and therapeutic trials in the *Archives* (45:189–202, 1988). Swedish workers (Ronnevi et al: *Muscle Nerve* 10:734–743, 1987) have found something cytotoxic in the plasma of patients with ALS. Now *that* gets my interest. Do ALS patients have something circulating in their blood that is deadly to anterior horn cells?—R.D. Currier, M.D.

14 Neuropathies

Long-Stay Intensive Care as a Cause of Multiple Neuropathies
Barat M, Brochet B, Vital C, Mazaux JM, Arné L (Hôpital Tastet Girard, Bordeaux, France)
Rev Neurol (Paris) 143:823–831, 1987   14–1

There are only a few case reports in the literature concerning the development of polyneuropathy in the course of a prolonged stay in an intensive care unit. However, the prevalence of this syndrome has probably been underestimated, and its etiology has not yet been defined. Findings were reviewed in 4 patients with peripheral neuropathy. A diagnosis of polyneuropathy was made only after the patients were transferred to a neurologic rehabilitation center; this illustrates the difficulty in correctly diagnosing this complication.

Four men, aged 57–66 years, required mechanical ventilation because of multiple trauma after an automobile accident, severe asthma, acute respiratory distress, and coma. Each required prolonged treatment in the intensive care unit because of multiple complications associated with his primary admission. Neurologic evaluation consisted of retrospective examination of all medical data including duration and type of parenteral nutrition, intervening complications, potential iatrogenic neurotoxicity, serum protein levels, glucose metabolism, vitamin metabolism, and monoclonal antibodies. All 4 patients underwent electromyographic studies, and neuromuscular biopsy of the short peroneal muscle was performed in 2 for ultrastructure studies.

The precise onset of polyneuropathy was difficult to establish because of the patients' altered states of consciousness during their initial period in the intensive care unit, but it probably developed between day 10 and day 30. Electrophysiologic examination confirmed extensive polyneuropathy in all 4 patients and was suggestive of acute axonal lesions. Ultrastructure study of the biopsy specimens also suggested an acute axonal lesion in that there was a dramatic loss of myelinated fibers, and many myelinated fibers showed Bungner bands. Three patients recovered from their polyneuropathy within 3–4 months. One patient retained marked neuromuscular sequelae.

Thus, in patients with suspected peripheral neuropathy, early electrophysiologic and histologic study to search for axonal lesions would enable a much earlier diagnosis of polyneuropathy.

▶ Prolonged intensive care in itself may be a prominent cause for multiple peripheral neuropathy due to severe axonal degeneration and loss of myelinated fibers. Recovery occurs in most cases.— R.N. DeJong, M.D.

Acute Sensory Neuropathy-Neuronopathy From Pyridoxine Overdose

Albin RL, Albers JW, Greenberg HS, Townsend JB, Lynn RB, Burke JM, Jr,
Alessi AG (Univ of Michigan, Ann Arbor)
Neurology 37:1729–1732, November 1987   14–2

Pyridoxine, an essential, water-soluble vitamin (B_6), has several medical uses, including treatment for intoxication from the false morel mushroom, *Gyromitra esculenta*. However, the use of high doses of pyridoxine has been associated with risks. Two patients were described who experienced an acute profound, permanent sensory deficit after therapy with massive doses of parenteral pyridoxine.

A 27-year-old woman complained of nausea, diarrhea, and emesis after eating *G. esculenta*. She received about 132 gm of intravenous pyridoxine in a 3-day period. Symptoms persisted, and she began to experience blurred vision, slurred speech, dysphagia, and fatigue. During the next several days, her condition progressively deteriorated. Examination showed nystagmus in all directions of gaze, mild facial diparesis, mild tongue weakness, and symmetric proximal extremity weakness. Muscle stretch reflexes were absent, and plantar responses were flexor. Eight days after pyridoxine treatment, unequivocal objective sensory impairment became evident with diminished sensation in a stocking-glove distribution. Sensory disturbance progressed during the next few days, resulting in a profound loss of vibratory sense in all extremities and absent position sense at all joints except the neck. Severe appendicular ataxia was noted. Sural and ulnar sensory nerve action potentials (SNAPs) were absent, right median SNAP was reduced, and motor unit action potential (MUAP) recruitment showed an irregular pattern. Although she gradually began to improve, 1 year after onset she was still unable to walk and had not recovered her joint position sense.

The second patient, the 33-year-old husband of the first patient, had a similar initial illness after ingesting larger amounts of the mushrooms. His total intravenous pyridoxine dose was estimated at 183 gm given in 3 days. He complained of facial paresthesias and decreased facial sensation shortly after treatment. Within the next 2 days, he experienced diffuse numbness, dysarthria, slight upper extremity weakness, diminished muscle stretch reflexes, coarse nystagmus, decreased tongue strength, and moderate proximal lower extremity weakness. His subsequent course paralleled that of his wife. Despite intensive rehabilitation, 1 year after onset he was also unable to walk.

These 2 clinical pictures resemble that described in chronic pyridoxine neurotoxicity, except for rapid onset. They are also consonant with experimental models of acute pyridoxine intoxication, which is secondary to a sensory ganglion neuropathy. These patients also had transient autonomic dysfunction, mild weakness, nystagmus, lethargy, and respiratory depression, previously undocumented features that may be attributable to the preservative used in the parenteral pyridoxine preparation or to the exceptionally high doses of pyridoxine.

▶ This is a bizarre situation that produced a severe sensory neuropathy with a prolonged and possibly permanent residual deficit.

There is a similar report from Australia of a lady who took 1 gm of pyridoxine a day for 12 months. She recovered over a period of 4 months (*Med J Aust* 146:640–642, June 15, 1987).

Pyridoxine neuropathy has been gaining recognition since the original description by Schaumberg et al. in 1983; note the recent review of 103 possible cases by Dalton and Dalton et al. (*Acta Neurol Scand* 76:8–11, 1987) in which the intoxication resulted from the use of vitamin B$_6$ for the premenstrual syndrome. The average dose-time necessary to produce neuropathy was 117 mg/day for 2.9 years. The majority improved 3 months after the vitamin was stopped.

This is interesting. Physicians have been giving B$_6$ for premenstrual syndrome and nausea of pregnancy for decades. So why haven't we noticed this before? Were the doses in the average vitamin pill lower 30 years ago than now? There are physicians who still recommend pyridoxine and thiamine during the recovery phase of neuritis of unknown cause. The patient and the physician then may wonder why improvement is so slow.—R.D. Currier, M.D.

Neuropathy in the Miller Fisher Syndrome: Clinical and Electrophysiologic Findings

Fross RD, Daube JR (Mayo Clinic and Found, Rochester, Minn)
Neurology 37:1493–1498, September 1987   14–3

The Miller Fisher syndrome is a subacute disorder characterized by ophthalmoplegia, ataxia, and impaired or absent tendon reflexes. Minimal or no limb weakness is present. Peripheral nerve function was exam-

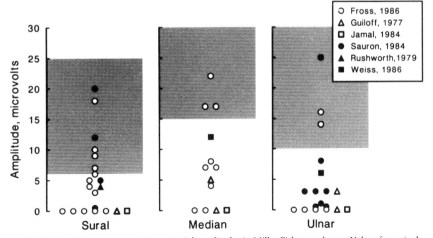

Fig 14–1.—Sensory nerve action potential amplitudes in Miller Fisher syndrome. Values from single limb and worst examinations are shown for each patient. Normal range is shaded. (Courtesy of Fross RD, Daube JR: *Neurology* 37:1493–1498, September 1987.)

ined in 10 patients, 6 women and 4 men with a mean age of 61 years. All had an antecedent acute febrile illness within 2 weeks before the onset of neurologic symptoms. Six patients had diplopia and 3 had gait difficulties. Most patients also had minor sensory complaints. The chief management was physical therapy, although 3 patients had short courses of high-dose steroid therapy. All patients but 1 recovered substantially or totally on follow-up for up to 3.5 years. One patient had persistent facial weakness at 3 months.

Half of the patients had mild abnormalities of nerve conduction in the extremities. Progressive loss of amplitude was documented in 2 cases. Motor conduction velocities were slowed by less than 20%. Sensory nerve action potential amplitudes were abnormal in all cases (Fig 14–1). Facial compound muscle action potential amplitudes were reduced in 5 of 7 patients. No marked electromyographic abnormalities were present.

It remains unclear what the immunologic target is in Miller Fisher syndrome, and how it differs from that in Guillain-Barré syndrome. The presence of peripheral nerve injury in the former state does not rule out the possibility of coexisting CNS damage.

▶ There has long been controversy whether the Miller Fisher syndrome is a peripheral neuropathy, related to the Guillain-Barré syndrome, or is of central origin. This editor has always favored the former. This study appears to favor peripheral nerve origin, although accepting that there may be coexisting central involvement.— R.N. DeJong, M.D.

Efficiency of Plasma Exchange in Guillain-Barré Syndrome: Role of Replacement Fluids

French Cooperative Group on Plasma Exchange in Guillain-Barré Syndrome
Ann Neurol 22:753–761, December 1987   14–4

Although deficits in Guillain-Barré syndrome (GBS) tend to resolve spontaneously, treatment is necessary to prevent complications, deaths, and residual disability. The presence of a humoral factor reproducing the electrophysiologic and histologic features of demyelination suggests that plasma exchange be tried. The short-term effects of plasma exchange were studied in a multicenter study of 220 patients; 109 were assigned to plasma exchange. Fifty-seven of those assigned to plasma exchange received diluted albumin as replacement fluid, whereas 52 received fresh frozen plasma. Four exchanges of 2 plasma volumes each were given on alternate days.

Patients treated by plasma exchange exhibited significant short-term clinical benefits (Fig 14–2). Fewer required ventilatory assistance, and the time to weaning from the ventilator declined. The times to onset of motor recovery and walking without aid also were shorter than in control patients. The course was similar in both actively treated groups, but patients given fresh frozen plasma had more complications from plasma exchange.

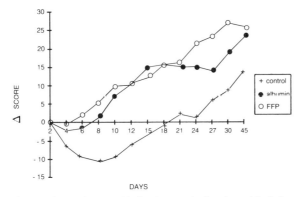

Fig 14–2.—Changes of mean Δ score with time in control, albumin, and fresh frozen plasma (FFP) groups. The Δ score is the algebraic difference between the score at each evaluation point and at randomization day. Between the control and plasma exchange groups, all the differences were significant from day 4 onward (Mann-Whitney test). No significant difference was observed between the albumin and the FFP groups. (Courtesy of the French Cooperative Group on Plasma Exchange in Guillain-Barré Syndrome: *Ann Neurol* 22:753–761, December 1987.)

Plasma exchange, begun early in the course of GBS, leads to clinical benefits. One patient in the present series died after contraindications to plasma exchange were overlooked. Diluted albumin is preferred to fresh frozen plasma as a replacement fluid.

▶ This work continues the tendency for studies of Guillain-Barré syndrome treated by plasma exchange to show that it really is effective during the acute phase. In addition, albumin is as good as fresh frozen plasma, which is helpful for those physicians and patients who are afraid of plasmapheresis because of the danger of AIDS.—R.D. Currier, M.D.

The Treatment of Guillain-Barré Syndrome by Modified Plasma Exchange—A Cost Effective Method for Developing Countries
De Silva HJ, Gamage R, Herath HKN, Karunanayake MGS, Peiris JB (Gen Hosp, Colombo, Sri Lanka)
Postgrad Med J 63:1079–1081, 1987   14–5

Plasma exchange for the treatment of Guillain-Barré syndrome is usually done with continuous flow cell separators, exchanging large amounts of plasma in a short time and replacing the removed plasma with 5% purified protein fraction or 5% normal serum albumin. This is a complex, expensive procedure. A simpler form of plasma exchange was developed that does not require cell separators or costly replacement fluids.

In 6 consecutive patients with progressive weakness of all 4 limbs, Guillain-Barré syndrome was diagnosed and treated with modified plasma exchange. A 17-gauge needle was inserted into an antecubital vein, and 0.5 L of blood was drawn into a collecting pack. After venesection, a 0.25-L unit of fresh frozen plasma (FFP) was infused. The blood pack was centrifuged in a Sorvall centrifuge, the supernatant plasma discarded, and the patients' blood cells reinfused. The cells and FFP were transfused through an intravenous cannula in a vein in the other arm. The procedure was done twice a day for 7–13 days in a row. Plasma exchange was begun within 20 days of illness onset in each case. Five patients had marked improvement in vital capacity, muscle power, facial weakness, and clinical grade. They were discharged, able to walk unassisted. None relapsed in 2–6 months of follow-up. The sixth patient's response to treatment was slower, and his vital capacity fell below 0.3 L. However, assisted ventilation was avoided. This patient was subsequently lost to follow-up.

Modified plasma exchange produced rapid improvement in 5 of 6 patients. This plasma exchange method was simpler and less expensive than the conventional method. The modified technique is recommended, particularly in developing countries with financial constraints and poor facilities.

▶ This seems a reasonable thing for those not blessed with plasma exchange machines. There is no doubt that this is not as effective as continuous exchange, but it appears to be of use.

While on the subject of treatment we must mention a recent editorial summary of the treatment of brain abscess in the *Lancet* 1:219–220, 1988). *Lancet* editorials are always unsigned, which is a shame because they are often superb, as is this one. The modern treatment of brain abscess has finally improved. The mortality rate, which had been 40% even after the introduction of antibiotics, is down to 10%. The authors credit 3 factors: the development of the CT scan, the introduction of more appropriate antibiotics, and the use of steroids to reduce the localized cerebral edema around the abscess capsule. I had just about given up hope that anything would be effective in this disorder, since the advent of antibiotics alone did not seem to have improved the mortality rate. The authors do remark that the operative handling—whether to remove the entire abscess or simply aspirate the pus—is still controversial.—R.D. Currier, M.D.

15 Treatment

A Controlled Trial of Nimodipine in Acute Ischemic Stroke

Gelmers HJ, Gorter K, de Weerdt CJ, Wiezer HJA (Streekziekenhuis, Almelo, St Antonius Ziekenhuis, Sneek, Scheper Ziekenhuis, Emmen, St Elisabeth Ziekenhuis, Venray, the Netherlands)

N Engl J Med 318:203–207, Jan 28, 1988   15–1

Elevated cellular calcium concentrations may be implicated in neuronal death after ischemia. A prospective, double-blind, randomized, placebo-controlled trial was carried out with 186 patients to determine whether treatment with a calcium–channel blocker would improve survival and neurologic outcome in acute ischemic stroke.

Nimodipine, 30 mg, was given every 6 hours, beginning within 24 hours of onset of symptoms of acute ischemic stroke. During the 4 weeks of treatment, death from all causes was significantly reduced among those receiving nimodipine compared with those receiving placebo. Mortality was 8.6% in the first group and 20.4% in the second. Improvement in survival was limited to men. During the 6-month follow-up period, an additional 8 patients died in each group.

Patients receiving nimodipine also had a significantly better neurologic outcome, as evaluated by the Mathew scale of neurologic deficit. Improvement in neurologic status was greatest in patients with a moderate to severe deficit at baseline. One episode of reversible azotemia may have been related to nimodipine treatment; there were no other important adverse effects.

Patients who sustain acute ischemic stroke may benefit from early treatment with nimodipine. However, the therapeutic effect noted appeared to be limited to men.

▶ We are not using calcium–channel blockers, but maybe we should. No doubt there will be continued discussion, since nothing seems clear-cut these days.—R.D. Currier, M.D.

Transluminal Angioplasty of the Vertebral and Basilar Artery

Higashida RT, Hieshima GB, Tsai FY, Halbach VV, Norman D, Newton TH (Univ of California, San Francisco)

AJNR 8:745–749, September–October 1987   15–2

Transluminal angioplasty is now being performed for atherosclerotic lesions of brachiocephalic vessels. A review was made of the results in 17 patients with vertebral artery stenosis and 1 with basilar artery stenosis who were treated by intravascular balloon dilatation. Presenting symp-

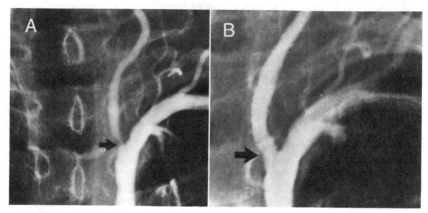

Fig 15–1.—A, high-grade stenosis of proximal left vertebral artery caused by atherosclerosis in a 60-year-old woman with symptoms of vertebral basilar insufficiency and transient ischemic attacks. **B,** angiogram 3 months after angioplasty shows complete return to normal luminal diameter of proximal vertebral artery *(arrow)*. (Courtesy of Higashida RT, Hieshima GB, Tsai FY, et al: *AJNR* 8:745–749, September–October 1987.)

toms included vertebral basilar insufficiency, transient ischemic attacks, and multiple strokes.

Successful transluminal angioplasty was performed in 16 patients with more than 70% narrowing of the dominant vertebral artery resulting from atherosclerosis (Fig 15–1). Continued patency was seen by angiography at 3-month and 1-year follow-up. Two patients had residual stenosis but were asymptomatic. The patient with basilar artery stenosis sustained a brain-stem infarct after angioplasty. One patient with vertebral artery stenosis had a transient ischemic attack after bilateral vertebral artery angioplasty. All patients who had successful dilatation were asymptomatic after 6 months to 2 years (mean, 15 months) of follow-up.

Vertebral artery angioplasty may be effective in the treatment of atherosclerotic lesions, with relatively low morbidity. Angioplasty of the basilar artery is more difficult and has a higher degree of risk because of the many branches supplying the brain stem. Long-term follow-up is required to validate this method.

The Optimal Intensity of Oral Anticoagulant Therapy
Hirsh J, Levine MN (McMaster Univ, Hamilton, Ont)
JAMA 258:2723–2726, Nov 20, 1987   15–3

About half a million patients in the United States receive oral anticoagulant therapy each year. It has long been the practice to use the 1-stage prothrombin time test to monitor warfarin therapy. However, the dose currently used to prolong the prothrombin time to 2 to 2.5 times control value is greater than that used to achieve the same effect in past years. This has gone largely unnoticed. It is a result of the test reagents being less responsive to a reduction in vitamin K-dependent clotting factors than the thromboplastins used in North America before the 1970s. The homemade reagents used then were more responsive to warfarin effect than present-day commercially prepared thromboplastins. The recommended therapeutic range did not change when commercial sources began to supply reagents for testing.

Randomized clinical trials are needed to compare different levels of anticoagulation for efficacy and safety. Available data suggest that both the older and the more intense regimens are effective in preventing venous thromboembolism, whereas the less intense regimen carries a much lower risk of bleeding complications. It would be desirable to use a common thromboplastin reagent worldwide, but this is not practical. An alternate solution is to standardize the reporting of prothrombin time results by relating them to a common standard. In addition, a less intense oral anticoagulant regimen is appropriate for both the prevention and treatment of venous thromboembolism, and the prevention of systemic embolism in patients with myocardial infarction, atrial fibrillation, and tissue heart valves.

▶ This was a shock because it seems all of us old-timers have been using the same control goal for anticoagulation with warfarin over the years and have been giving too much. The thromboplastins in the laboratory were changed in the 1970s, making the laboratory tests much less responsive. Now a goal of 1½ times the prothrombin time control value is correct, whereas we used to try for 2 to 2½ times. In a way this is irritating. Why didn't we know this? Why didn't our laboratory people tell us? Why didn't we ask? There is a defect in the system somewhere. One wonders how many patients have been over-anticoagulated.—R.D. Currier, M.D.

Parkinson's Disease in the Elderly: Current Management Strategies
Aminoff MJ (Univ of California, San Francisco)
Geriatrics 42:31–37, July 1987   15–4

Parkinson's disease becomes increasingly common with advancing age. The major symptoms of Parkinson's disease are tremor, rigidity, bradykinesia, and postural instability. The goal of therapy is to allow patients to lead a normal life for as long as possible.

A variety of drugs are used to treat Parkinson's disease. Anticholinergic drugs can be used. Orphenadrine and diphenhydramine are less likely to cause confusion as a side effect. Other side effects of anticholinergic drugs include constipation, urinary retention, visual blurring, and dryness of the mouth. Ethopropazine is the most effective drug for relief of tremor. When effective, amantadine helps relieve all symptoms of Parkinson's disease; side effects include confusion and ankle edema. Tricyclic compounds can be useful at all stages and in combination with other drugs, and can also help relieve accompanying depression. Dopaminergic therapy is the most effective treatment for Parkinson's disease. Early adverse reactions include anorexia, nausea, and postural hypotension. Mental side effects and dyskinesias become common as the duration of treatment increases.

One approach to managing these side effects is the drug holiday. Because levodopa appears to lose effectiveness with duration of treatment, most doctors prefer to introduce it as late as possible. Another problem with this therapy is the intermittent effectiveness or on-off phenomenon. One approach to managing this is the simultaneous administration of bromocriptine.

Typically, as a patient's disease worsens, anticholinergic drugs or amantadine is given. Once symptoms are troublesome, dopaminergic medication is introduced. Bromocriptine is added as the dosage of levodopa is increased. Physical therapy helps the patient to remain active. Educating patients and their families is emphasized.

Dietary Influences on the Antiparkinsonian Response to Levodopa
Juncos JL, Fabbrini G, Mouradian MM, Serrati C, Chase TN (Natl Insts of Health, Bethesda, Md)
Arch Neurol 44:1003–1005, October 1987   15–5

Dietary influences have been implicated in the pathogenesis of motor-response fluctuations that are common in patients with advanced Parkinson's disease. The absorption of levodopa can be reduced or retarded by concomitant food intake. Also, the transport of levodopa through the blood-brain barrier can be inhibited by large neutral amino acids (LNAA) derived from dietary proteins. To assess the acute effect of nutritional factors on the antiparkinsonian response to levodopa, the influence of various protein loads on plasma levodopa, LNAA levels, and motor performance was studied.

TABLE—Characteristics of Diets

	Protein Load	Diet A	Diet B*
Energy, kJ/kg (kcal/kg) body weight/meal	4.7 (19.7)	8.8 (37.0)	3.7 (15.5)
Protein, g/kg body weight/meal	0.40	0.26	0.13
Carbohydrate, g/kg body weight/meal	0.50	0.93	0.50
Fat, g/kg body weight/meal	0.13	0.45	0.13

*Large neutral amino acid composition (grams per 100 mg of protein as Ensure): leucine, 8.7; valine 5.0; tyrosine, 4.9; phenylalanine, 4.8; isoleucine, 4.5; methionine, 2.6; and tryptophan, 1.2,

(Courtesy of Juncos JL, Fabbrini G, Mouradian MM, et al: *Arch Neurol* 44:1003–1005, October 1987.)

Six patients with idiopathic Parkinson's disease, aged 59 ± 2.5 years, participated. Symptom duration ranged from 8 to 19 years; severity ranged from stage III to IV. All had received levodopa/carbidopa for 8 to 16 years and had motor performance fluctuations. In 1 study, 3 patients received serial plasma amino acid determinations and underwent neurologic assessment after the oral administration of a single protein-supplemented nutritional formula (table).

In a second study, 6 patients received 2 nominally isoenergetic diets— A and B—in a single-blind, balanced, crossover design. Results showed that the single oral administration of a high-protein formula significantly increased plama LNAA levels and prematurely terminated the antiparkinsonian response to levodopa/carbidopa. During oral or intravenous administration of levodopa, ingesting diets meeting the recommended daily allowance (RDA) for protein had no significant effect on plasma levodopa or LNAA levels or variance nor on parkinsonian scores or variance.

These findings suggest that although protein intake exceeding the RDA can diminish the antiparkinsonian response to orally administered levodopa/carbidopa in patients with advanced disease, diets adhering to the RDA protein guidelines have no clinically significant effect.

▶ The results of this study suggest that while excessive protein intake can diminish the antiparkinsonian response to orally administered levodopa/carbidopa in patients with advanced parkinsonism, diets adhering to the RDA for protein have no clinically appreciable effect. In an associated article, J.H. Pincus and K.M. Barry (*Arch Neurol* 44:1006–1009, 1987) state that a virtually protein-free diet until dinnertime followed by an unrestricted diet until bedtime permits near-normal daytime motor function.—R.N. DeJong, M.D.

Phenytoin Infusion in Severe Pre-Eclampsia
Slater RM, Wilcox FL, Smith WD, Donnai P, Patrick J, Richardson T, (Manchester Royal Infirmary, St Mary's Hosp, Manchester Med School, Manchester, England)
Lancet 1:1417–1420, June 20, 1987   15–6

Seizure prophylaxis is crucial in the treatment of eclampsia. However, there are problems with all therapies currently in use. Two eclamptic and 24 preeclamptic women were given intravenous phenytoin sodium to determine whether therapeutic blood levels could be reached without harm to either mother or baby.

The mean dose was 15.3 mg/kg. All patients had levels within the therapeutic range at 30 minutes and at 6 hours. No major side effects were reported. In 19 cases, the fetal heart rate remained within normal limits. Fifteen infants were admitted to the special care unit; all were premature and underweight. Thirteen infants born at term were cared for in the postnatal ward.

The ideal anticonvulsant to use in the treatment of eclampsia would work rapidly and predictably, with a wide safety margin, and be nondepressive and nontoxic for both mother and infant. None of the regimens currently used—diazepam, chlormethiazole, or magnesium sulfate—fulfill all these requirements. High-dose phenytoin can be administered to women at risk for preeclamptic seizures without complications and avoids the sedative effect of other anticonvulsants. Phenytoin should be compared with other regimens in large-scale trials.

▶ Here we have eclampsia treated successfully with phenytoin without the occasional serious side effects of magnesium sulfate. I have never understood why we used phenytoin for frequent seizures while our obstetric confreres 1 floor down used magnesium sulfate, with never a discussion of our therapeutic differences. I suppose each believes the other knows what he is doing. We have been giving intravenous phenytoin for 30 years and they have been giving magnesium sulfate for even longer. Perhaps the time has come for a comparative trial.

Speaking of in-hospital treatment of repeated seizures caused by metabolic dysfunction, Worthley and Thomas 2 years ago reported the successful treatment of seizures resulting from severe hyponatremia with 50 ml of 29.2% saline (250 mmol) intravenously (*Br Med J* 292:168–170, 1986). It evidently worked well, not only to restore the sodium and stop the seizures but also to reduce cerebral edema, all with a small volume of fluid.— R.D. Currier, M.D.

Double Blind Controlled Randomized Study on Azathioprine Efficacy in Multiple Sclerosis: Preliminary Results

Milanese C, La Mantia L, Salmaggi A, Campi A, Bortolami C, Tajoli L, Nespolo A, Corridori F (Inst Neurologico "C Besta," Milan, Italy)
Ital J Neurol Sci 9:53–57, 1988   15–7

Azathioprine treatment for multiple sclerosis (MS) was evaluated in a double-blind trial in patients with both progressive and remitting-relapsing disease. Study patients received azathioprine in tablet form in a daily dose of 2–2.5 mg/kg of body weight. All patients had definite MS; 19 patients had progressive disease and 19 had the remitting-relapsing form.

Twenty-three patients completed at least 1 year of treatment. The rate of progression in progressive cases was slower in actively treated patients than in placebo recipients, but the difference was not significant. In relapsing-remitting cases, relapses were less frequent in azathioprine-treated patients. Slowing of progression was evident only after 3 years of treatment. In 5 actively treated patients mild macrocytic anemia developed. One patient each had herpes zoster and late pancytopenia.

Azathioprine should be reserved for serious cases of MS because of its possible long-term side effects, including malignant disease. Prolonged treatment with azathioprine, 2 mg/kg of body weight daily, may slow the rate of progression after a period of 3 years.

▶ Here is a study showing azathioprine to be effective in multiple sclerosis with a long delay in discernible therapeutic result. I have a feeling this is correct. The worry about cancer and azathioprine is still there, although I don't believe anyone has confirmed the report of a 10% cancer rate in MS patients treated with azathioprine.— R.D. Currier, M.D.

Successful Chemotherapy for Recurrent Malignant Oligodendroglioma
Cairncross JG, Macdonald DR (Univ of Western Ontario, London, Ont)
Ann Neurol 23:360–364, April 1988   15–8

Chemotherapy is of only modest benefit in patients with malignant glioma who have recurrent disease after resection and irradiation. However, different histologic subtypes might respond differently to cytotoxic drugs. Eight consecutive patients with recurrent malignant oligodendroglioma received systemic chemotherapy, usually with a combination of procarbazine, lomustine, and vincristine. One patient each was treated with carmustine and diaziquone. The median interval from diagnosis to chemotherapy was 3 years. Six patients had repeated craniotomy for recurrent tumor. Half of the patients required steroid therapy.

One patient had a complete response; 7 had partial responses, but these often exceeded a 90% reduction in tumor size (Fig 15–2). In 2 partial responders, systemic metastases were completely controlled. Tumor

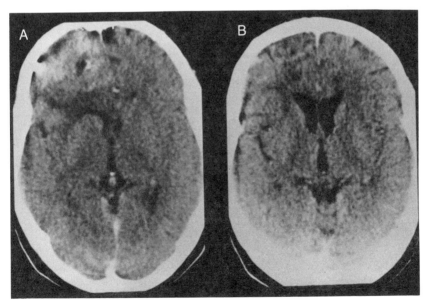

Fig 15–2.—**A,** computed tomographic scan in patient, before chemotherapy, demonstrating a contrast-enhancing right frontal tumor with compression of the ventricular system. **B,** computed tomographic scan 16 weeks later after 2 courses of procarbazine, lomustine, and vincristine, showing resolution of the enhancing mass. (Courtesy of Cairncross JG, Macdonald DR: *Ann Neurol* 23:360–364, April 1988.)

continues to be controlled in 4 patients. Treatment was well tolerated; there were no treatment-related hospitalizations or deaths.

At least half of these patients have responded to systemic chemotherapy for recurrent oligodendroglioma for longer than 1 year. Combination chemotherapy with nonoverlapping, non–cross-resistant drugs should be pursued. Another feasible approach is intensive adjuvant chemotherapy combined with focal radiotherapy.

▶ These patients previously had all been thoroughly treated with the usual surgery, radiation, and even chemotherapy. One might have expected their tumors to become more malignant, so I think the title of this paper is probably correct—success in this case being remission when one was not expected. It looks as though we are at the beginning of a new era of brain tumor treatment with combination chemotherapy. It is about time.—R.D. Currier, M.D.

16 Miscellaneous Topics

Contraindications to Lumbar Puncture as Defined by Computed Cranial Tomography
Gower DJ, Baker AL, Bell WO, Ball MR (Wake Forest Univ)
J Neurol Neurosurg Psychiatry 50:1071–1074, August 1987   16–1

Papilledema is not always an adequate predictor of complications of lumbar puncture, prompting many clinicians to use computed tomography (CT) for this purpose.

Man, 29, had severe headache and vomiting, followed by lethargy and neck stiffness. His temperature was 40C, and his white blood cell count was 28,000/mm³. Mild left hemiparesis was present. The cerebrospinal fluid contained 80 white blood cells/mm³ and had a protein concentration of 118 mg/dl. The patient suddenly became unresponsive, with fixed, dilated pupils and decerebrate posturing. Computed tomography showed a right thalamic mass lesion with midline

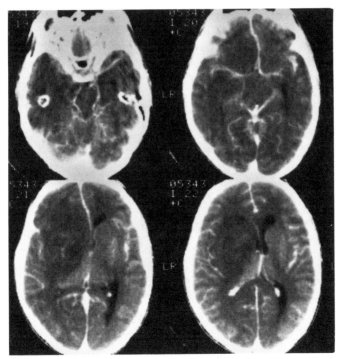

Fig 16–1.—Infused CT scan demonstrates midline shift and uncal herniation with displacement of the right posterior cerebral artery. (Courtesy of Gower DJ, Baker AL, Bell WO, et al: *J Neurol Neurosurg Psychiatry* 50:1071–1074, August 1987.)

shift (Fig 16–1). Despite mannitol, hyperventilation, and broad-spectrum antibiotic therapy, the patient was declared brain dead 24 hours after admission. Autopsy showed fungal cerebritis in the right thalamus; no source of fungal emboli was apparent.

In patients with unequal intracranial pressures, a shift of brain parenchyma can compress neural structures against a bony or dural prominence. Pressure may be inferred from the structural information in CT scans. Four criteria demonstrated on CT should be considered contraindications to lumbar puncture: (1) lateral shift of midline structures, (2) loss of the suprachiasmatic and basilar cisterns, (3) obliteration of the fourth ventricle, and (4) obliteration of the superior cerebellar and quadrigeminal plate cisterns with sparing of the ambient cisterns.

▶ This is a fine paper and no doubt will be the source of questions on various examinations in the future. The last of the 4 criteria is the tricky one. One must congratulate the authors on their perception.—R.D. Currier, M.D.

Spinal Cord Degeneration in Divers

Palmer AC, Calder IM, Hughes JT (School of Veterinary Medicine, Cambridge; London Hosp Med College, Med Division of Health and Safety Executive, London; Radcliffe Infirmary, Oxford, England)
Lancet 2:1365–1366, Dec 12, 1987   16–2

Examinations were made of spinal cords obtained from 11 divers, 8 of them professionals, who died in diving or nondiving accidents, to deter-

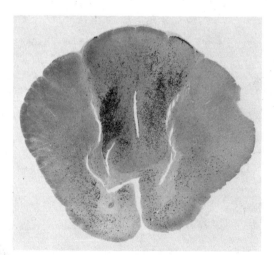

Fig 16–2.—Histologic features in degenerated spinal cord. Marchi-positive degeneration is seen in the afferent fibers of the posterior columns, in fibers of Lissauer's tract, and also scattered in the anterior and lateral columns. Marchi; original magnification, ×10. (Courtesy of Palmer AC, Calder IM, Hughes JT: *Lancet* 2:1365–1366, Dec 12, 1987.)

mine whether active divers can have unrecognized cord degeneration. Ten of the 11 men had been examined within 38 weeks before death.

Specimens from divers who died suddenly in diving accidents exhibited grossly distended empty blood vessels and, occasionally, perivascular hemorrhage. Perivascular proteinaceous globules, reflecting vasogenic edema, were noted in some of these cases. Chronic changes usually were minor. Vessels of the white matter were hyalinized in several cases, and corpora amylacea were a frequent finding. Three cords were stained by the Marchi method (Fig 16–2). Marchi-positive material always was extracellular; staining assumed a beaded appearance.

Tract degeneration may be found in the spinal cords of some professional divers. It is possible that these lesions contribute to some final diving accidents. A full neurologic examination might reveal the presence of tract degeneration before a dive.

▶ Although I was unaware of this as a cause of cord degeneration, it is an old problem. Spinal cord symptoms in divers were noted in the YEAR BOOK 80 years ago under the listing of "Caisson Myelitis," a report of 2 patients of Wassermeyer who had been underwater at 100 feet for many hours searching for a lost torpedo at Kiel (*Berliner Klin Woch, Feb 8, 1909).—R.D. Currier, M.D.*

Chronic Progressive Myelopathy: Its Relation to the Spinal Progressive Form of Multiple Sclerosis
Steiner I, Feir G, Soffer D, Pleet AB, Abramsky O (Hadassah Univ Hosp, Hebrew Univ, Jerusalem)
Acta Neurol Scand 77:152–157, 1988   16–3

A specific diagnosis may not be possible when chronic progressive myelopathy (CPM) is unaccompanied by signs of brain or peripheral nervous system dysfunction or systemic manifestations. Of 107 patients seen between 1979 and 1984 with a diagnosis of CPM, 76 had no apparent underlying cause of myelopathy.

Thirty-nine patients had a diagnosis of possible multiple sclerosis (MS). Most of these patients had motor dysfunction involving the legs, many of whom also had motor dysfunction in the hands. Only 11 patients had objective sensory impairment. Oligoclonal immunoglobulin was present in all patients. Twenty-two patients had spondylitic myelopathy, most of whom had a combined motor and sensory deficit. Nine patients had myelopathy resulting from other causes. In 37 patients, no definitive diagnosis was reached; these patients had been symptomatic for a mean of 4 years. About half of the patients had sensory symptoms in addition to motor dysfunction in the legs. The typical patient with myelopathy of unknown origin (MUO) was an early middle-aged man with a symmetrical mixed sensorimotor myelopathy that followed a relatively benign course.

It might be helpful to classify patients with CPM of unknown cause in 2 groups, on the basis of the presence or absence of oligoclonal immunoglobulin in the cerebrospinal fluid. However, it is not possible to definitively diagnose multiple sclerosis at this stage. Patients with oligoclonal Ig do have more active disease and follow a less benign course than do others.

▶ Here is a nice study of that devilish disease, progressive myelopathy, which tests negatively for multiple sclerosis. Some patients will remain in the group with myelopathy of unknown origin even when studied thoroughly with IgG and MRI. However, we still await information on such a group followed for a number of years with IgG and MRI analysis. Will there be any left in the MUO group if, say, an entire group is followed carefully for 20 years?—R.D. Currier, M.D.

Late Denervation in Patients With Antecedent Paralytic Poliomyelitis

Cashman NR, Maselli R, Wollmann RL, Roos R, Simon R, and Antel JP (McGill Univ, Montreal; Univ of Chicago)
N Engl J Med 317:7–12, July 2, 1987
16–4

A "postpoliomyelitis syndrome" has been observed, including weakness, fatigue, and pain, many years or decades after acute paralytic poliomyelitis. A study of the syndrome was undertaken in 18 patients with a past history of poliomyelitis. Thirteen of them described new weakness for 1 to 20 years. The new symptoms first appeared a mean of 36 years after acute poliomyelitis. Five other patients had no new weakness at the same stage.

Nine patients with weakening also had new atrophy, and 10 patients

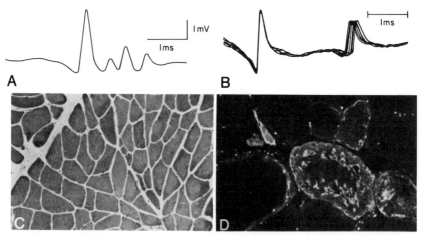

Fig 16–3.—Single-fiber electromyographic studies (**A** and **B**) and muscle biopsy histopathologic studies (**C** and **D**) of the right deltoid muscle of an asymptomatic patient aged 64 who at age 9 years had paralytic poliomyelitis involving all 4 limbs; his arms at the time of study had normal bulk and strength. **A,** 4 time-locked muscle fiber action potentials observed in determination of fiber density (mean ± SD normal value for age, 1.4 ± 0.11). **B,** 10 superimposed action-potential pairs indicating moderately increased jitter (mean consecutive difference, 74 μsec; normal for muscle, <35 μsec). **C,** hematoxylin-eosin demonstrates fiber splitting; original magnification, ×75. **D,** Neural cell adhesion molecule immunoreactivity in small diameter and large diameter muscle fibers; original magnification, ×300). (Courtesy of Cashman NR, Maselli R, Wollmann RL, et al: N Engl J Med 317:7–12, July 1987.)

had systemic fatigue. Seven patients had fasciculations at rest. Electromyography showed evidence of active denervation in 5 of 11 patients with weakness and in 4 of the 5 control patients. Immunohistochemical studies demonstrated small angulated atrophic fibers, split fibers, and nonatrophic fibers (Fig 16–3). The degree of continuing motor unit instability appeared related to the extent of past reinnervation when the patients with and those without weakness were combined.

The reinnervation of denervated muscle that occurs in paralytic poliomyelitis may be followed by late denervation of the previously reinnervated muscle fibers. Stable patients with past paralytic poliomyelitis cannot be distinguished from patients with new weakness by electromyography or muscle biopsy evidence of continuing denervation. Measures aimed at enhancing regeneration or decreasing the degeneration of terminal axons may be helpful in preventing or treating the postpoliomyelitis syndrome.

► In recent years, there have been many reports of the so-called postpoliomyelitis syndrome. Most cases have been relatively benign. This article reports that in some cases it is more severe, and may be progressive.— R.N. DeJong, M.D.

Iatrogenic Creutzfeldt-Jakob Disease
Rappaport EB (New Jersey State Dept. of Health, Trenton)
Neurology 37:1520–1522, September 1987   16–5

Creutzfeldt-Jakob disease (CJD) is a rare, transmissible, fatal neurodegenerative disorder. Iatrogenic transmission of CJD has been well documented, and CJD appears to be transmissible before overt disease manifestations. Surgical materials previously used on a patient with CJD may pose a risk to patients undergoing surgery.

Between November 1984 and April 1985, 3 young men who had received human cadaver pituitary-derived growth hormone (pit-hGH) died of CJD. Two additional patients who received pit-hGH have been documented with CJD. It would be prudent to assume that any patient exposed to pit-hGH is potentially a carrier of CJD.

The medical community must become aware of the potential infectivity of tissue and body fluids of those patients harboring CJD. Sterilization procedures of operating room materials should conform to CJD inactivation procedures. Patients exposed to pit-hGH should be followed up and, a record should be made of any surgery they undergo. Recipients of pit-hGH probably should not donate blood, tissue, or organs. The chance of using biologic products from patients contaminated with CJD should be minimized.

Encephalopathy and Myelinolysis After Rapid Correction of Hyponatraemia
Illowsky BP, Laureno R, (George Washington Univ)
Brain 110:855–867, August 1987   16–6

The recent publication of studies indicating that central pontine mye-linolysis is caused by rapid correction of hyponatremia has caused con-siderable controversy. Others have suggested instead that myelinolysis is caused by uncorrected hyponatremia, that it occurs only with overcorrec-tion of hyponatremia, or that it results from coincidental hypoxia. A se-ries of experiments was done to clarify the relationship between mye-linolysis and derangements of serum sodium and their treatment.

Fifty-five rabbits weighing 3 to 5 kg were divided into 3 groups. Severe hyponatremia was induced by injecting the rabbits with vasopressin and 5% dextrose in water. Rabbits surviving with severe uncorrected hypona-tremia for 7 to 10 days did not exhibit myelinolysis at autopsy. Myelin-otic lesions were found in 3 of 7 rabbits in the second group, in which corrective hypertonic saline solution was administered after 3 days of se-vere hyponatremia. The third group of rabbits, which received hypertonic saline within 24 hours of severe hyponatremia inducement, also showed evidence of neurologic deterioration. No lesions were noted at autopsy in the third group. None of the rabbits became hypernatremic with correc-tion.

These findings suggest that even prolonged, severe hyponatremia does not result in myelinolysis if it remains uncorrected. However, the rapid correction of hyponatremia without overcorrection can cause neurologic disease. Thus, a rapid rise in serum sodium should be avoided.

▶ These animals certainly had the neuropathologic picture of pontine and bilat-eral CNS disease from the rapid correction of low serum sodium.

Their findings are in apparent contrast to those of Worthley and Thomas (*Br Med J* 292:168–170, Jan 18, 1986), who reported fast correction of severe postoperative hyponatremia with seizures and presumed cerebral edema with a bolus of concentrated salt water followed by a diuretic.

The rapid bolus worked beautifully in 4 out of 5 patients who quickly stopped seizing and recovered without signs of CNS difficulty except for 1 who was in severe status and had been anoxic.

So giving sodium to someone with hyponatremia and possible cerebral edema without causing diuresis may be harmful unless given very slowly (Ayus et al: 1987 YEAR BOOK OF NEUROLOGY AND NEUROSURGERY, pp 196–197, but quick correction of severe hyponatremia of recent onset with seizures with an intravenous bolus of salt and nearly simultaneous diuresis does not appear to be harmful. I'm sure there will be further comments on this problem.—R.D. Currier, M.D.

Reflex Sympathetic Dystrophy: A Review
Schwartzman RJ, McLellan TL (Jefferson Med College)
Arch Neurol 44:555–561, May 1987   16–7

Reflex sympathetic dystrophy is a syndrome that includes pain, hyper-esthesia, swelling, hyperhidrosis, and trophic changes in the skin and bone of an affected extremity. Nerve injury and other conditions can precipitate the syndrome, which can then spread to uninjured areas.

The diagnosis is predominantly clinical, but roentgenography, scintigraphy, and sympathetic blockade can be used for confirmation. Treatment involves blocking sympathetic innervation, and physical therapy.

Possible explanations for reflex sympathetic dystrophy include reverberating circuits in the spinal cord that are triggered by intense pain, ephaptic transmission between sympathetic afferents, and ectopic pacemakers in the injured nerve.

▶ This article is entirely theoretical. Nowhere in it are we told what reflex sympathetic dystrophy is—if it is an entity, nor are we given an actual case report nor any neuropathology. This is an interesting review, but based entirely on hypotheses. I cannot accept it.—R.N. DeJong, M.D.

Benign Positional Vertigo: Clinical and Oculographic Features in 240 Cases
Baloh RW, Honrubia V, Jacobson K (Univ of California, Los Angeles)
Neurology 37:371–378, March 1987   16–8

Benign positional vertigo (BPV) is usually symptomatic of an inner ear disorder. It is accompanied by torsional paroxysmal positional nystagmus. Although BPV is relatively common, few large-scale studies have been done. The authors studied a homogeneous group of 240 patients with BPV and typical nystagmus.

Patients underwent electronystagmographic (ENG) examination that included positional and visual tracking tests and bithermal caloric tests, and all completed detailed questionnaires. Episodes of BPV were typically triggered by moving from prone to upright position, standing upright after bending over, or extending the neck to look up. Isolated BPV episodes seldom lasted longer than a minute; however, a series of attacks could produce lightheadedness and nausea for prolonged periods. Patients ranged in age from 11 to 84 years, and age 54 was the mean age of onset. A probable diagnosis was determined in about 50% of the patients. The most common identifiable causes were head trauma (17%) and viral neurolabyrinthitis (15%) (Fig 16–4). Fourteen patients showed evidence of central nervous system involvement. Disease in almost half of the patients was considered idiopathic. Females outnumbered males in the idiopathic group by about 2:1, suggesting a possibility of a hormonal involvement.

Clinical data strongly support a peripheral vestibular origin of BPV. Although the pathophysiology of the disorder is not clearly understood, there is a strong implication of abnormality of the posterior semicircular canal of the undermost ear. This conclusion is based on the fact that the positional nystagmus is the plane of the posterior canal, and that surgically sectioning the ampullary nerve from the posterior canal usually eliminates BPV. Idiopathic benign positional vertigo may sometimes be

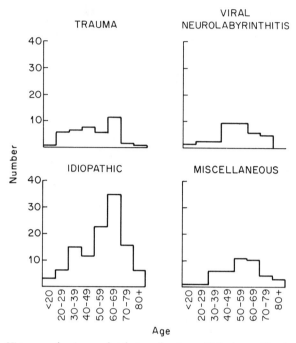

Fig 16–4.—Histograms showing age distribution of patients with benign positional vertigo in 4 major diagnostic categories. (Courtesy of Baloh RW, Honrubia V, Jacobson K: *Neurology* 37:371–378, March 1987.)

attributed to age-induced degeneration of the otolithic membrane, or may develop from damage from forgotten minor head traumas or ear infections.

▶ Benign positional vertigo is common, but it is often distressing. It usually indicates the presence of a benign inner ear disorder. These data indicate that it occurs with a peripheral posterior semicircular canal disorder.—R.N. DeJong, M.D.

HLA Antigens in Narcolepsy

Neely S, Rosenberg R, Spire J-P, Antel J, Arnason BGW (Univ. of Chicago)
Neurology 37:1858–1860, December 1987   16–9

Several studies indicate that human leukocyte antigen (HLA) DR2 and its supertypic specificity DQw1 are present in all patients with narcolepsy. Since this finding is documented in white and Japanese patients, the authors studied 18 black patients seen at a sleep clinic for excessive daytime sleepiness and daytime napping, as well as other features such as cataplexy, sleep paralysis, and hypnagogic hallucinations. Fourteen patients had multiple sleep latency tests to confirm narcolepsy.

The average sleep latency was less than 9.6 minutes. Two thirds of patients had DR2, compared with 27% of a control group, a highly significant difference. All patients had DQw1; the published frequency for American blacks is 48%. Antigen DRw52 was present in 14 subjects. There was no significant change in HLA class I antigen representation from that expected in a black American population.

It is not clear why narcolepsy should be associated with HLA-DR2/DQw1. Several HLA-associated disorders are autoimmune, but there are no firm data supporting an immune-mediated cause of narcolepsy.

▶ Not every narcoleptic has HLA-DR2, but according to these folks everyone does have DQw1. This still does not explain the relationship between an HLA type and a disease that supposedly has no immune component. There is a missing link here somewhere.—R.D. Currier, M.D.

Clinical and Neuropathological Findings in Systemic Lupus Erythematosus: The Role of Vasculitis, Heart Emboli, and Thrombotic Thrombocytopenic Purpura
Devinsky O, Petito CK, Alonso DR (New York Hosp-Cornell Univ, New York)
Ann Neurol 23:380–384, April 1988   16–10

Neuropsychiatric abnormalities are frequent in patients with systemic lupus erythematosus. Medical and autopsy findings were reviewed in 50 patients with systemic lupus erythematosus who were seen from 1968 to 1984. The 43 female and 7 male patients had a median age of 30 years at the onset of lupus. The median duration of disease was 10 years. The general clinical and laboratory findings were similar to those in other series. All patients received glucocorticoids, and 13 received azathioprine or cyclophosphamide. Three patients underwent plasmapheresis.

Three fourths of patients had psychiatric or neurologic complications or both. Five had an isolated psychiatric disorder; 17 had both types of disorder. The most frequent neurologic abnormality was tonic-clonic seizure disorder. Three patients had active systemic vasculitis, and 4 had healed arteritis. Nearly half of the patients had mitral valvulitis. Twenty-six patients had neuropathologic changes, most often embolic infarction. No patient had acute vasculitis in the brain or spinal cord. Two patients had white-matter necrosis involving the centrum semiovale, and 2 patients had myelopathy resembling that of subacute combined degeneration.

Central nervous system vasculitis is rare in patients with systemic lupus. Multiple brain infarcts may be present in patients with mitral valvulitis, particularly Libman-Sacks endocarditis. Thrombotic thrombocytopenic purpura is frequent in the terminal phase of systemic lupus, and its pathogenesis may be related to that of Libman-Sacks endocarditis.

▶ The classic teaching is apparently wrong, according to these 3 investigators. The cerebral lesions are not due to vasculitis but to embolic infarctions and infection. Terminally thrombotic thrombocytopenic purpura may develop. I hope other groups are studying this and will give us their findings. If vasculitis is not the problem, where did we get that idea in the first place?—R.D. Currier, M.D.

Treatment of Gilles de la Tourette's Syndrome: Eight-Year, Practice-Based Experience in a Predominantly Adult Population
Mesulam M-M, Petersen RC (Harvard Univ, Beth Israel Hosp, Boston)
Neurology 37:1828–1833, December 1987   16–11

Much of the literature on the treatment of Tourette's syndrome compared pharmacologic therapies, primarily in children. Such research focuses on the therapeutic agents instead of on the overall experience of individual patients. Treatment outcome in this study was described from the point of view of clinical practice rather than from pharmacologic research.

The records of all 92 patients referred for suspected Tourette's syndrome were reviewed. The syndrome was diagnosed in 80 of these patients. Of these, 58 required treatment and returned for follow-up. Forty were male and 18 were female. They ranged in age from 8 to 55 years (mean, 23 years). Mean age at onset of symptoms was 8 years, and the mean duration of symptoms was 14 years.

In more than 86%, effective pharmacologic control of symptoms was achieved for at least 3 months. Differences in response patterns were common, necessitating individualized tailoring of management. Dopamine-blocking neuroleptics were most commonly used; nevertheless, frequent mid-course changes were required as previously successful drugs stopped working or as their side effects became intolerable. Haloperidol and pimozide were used most often, but trifluoperazine and thiothixene provided superior relief in certain individuals. A combination of neuroleptics—or even a rotation from one to another—was occasionally needed. Tardive dyskinesia was not encountered in this series. Clonidine proved inferior to neuroleptics in treating motor and vocal tics but may be of use in some patients with prominent obsessive-compulsive symptomatology.

It appears that Tourette's syndrome can be treated successfully; nevertheless, it is essential that clinicians individualize therapy and be prepared for mid-course treatment changes.

▶ Not having much experience with this syndrome, I was surprised to see the high success rate. The fact that there is so far no report of tardive dyskinesia is also curious, but it may be too soon to tell.—R.D. Currier, M.D.

The Clinical Course of Spasmodic Torticollis
Lowenstein DH, Aminoff MJ (Univ of California, San Francisco)
Neurology 38:530–532, April 1988   16–12

Spasmodic torticollis is a focal dystonia characterized by tonic or intermittent neck muscle spasms that cause deviation of the head from its normal position. Most cases are idiopathic, but organic dysfunction of the extrapyramidal system is likely. Twenty-four of 36 patients referred in a 10-year period with idiopathic spasmodic torticollis were followed for longer than 1 year.

Three patients had complete or nearly complete resolution of symptoms; 8 had a partial remission. The conditions of 13 other patients were not improved at follow-up. The groups did not differ significantly in age at onset of symptoms, the duration of progression of symptoms, or the duration of peak symptoms. The overall median time from the onset to maximum disability was 3.1 years. One fourth of patients related the onset of torticollis to a specific external factor, usually trauma or stress. A minority of patients in all groups had associated movements such as head tremor or oromandibular dyskinesia. Medications failed to bring improvement and 3 unimproved patients underwent surgery without objective benefit.

These patients are readily distinguished clinically from those having more diffuse extrapyramidal syndromes. Patients whose conditions improve tend to have the onset of disease at a younger age and are less likely to have constant head deviation. There is considerable variation in the rate of progression of symptoms. Most patients find that torticollis worsens under stress or fatigue, and many find a gestural means of temporarily straightening the head.

▶ Abelardo S. Wee, Associate Professor of Neurology, University of Mississippi School of Medicine, Jackson, writes the following comment.—R.D. Currier, M.D.

▶ Although spasmodic torticollis can be relatively benign, this condition often frustrates both patient and physician. It is frequently resistant to pharmacologic or surgical treatment. In the study, the authors attempt to outline the clinical course of the disorder. This may serve to identify patients who will have a more favorable long-term outcome. Perhaps this subgroup of patients may be spared the unnecessary complications and risks of surgery and the unpleasant side effects of aggressive pharmacotherapy. Factors that tend to be unfavorable for a complete or partial remission include onset at a later age, constant neck deviation, and the presence of "geste antagonistique."

In idiopathic torsion dystonia, the onset of a focal dystonic symptom at an early age (≤20 years) usually indicates an unfavorable outcome. The majority of patients will go on to develop a generalized dystonia (Marsden et al: *Adv Neurol* 14:177–186, 1976). In the above study, the focal dystonia (torticollis) appeared during adult life, and it is interesting to note that the onset of the torticollis at a relatively later age seems to preclude a favorable prognosis.—A.S. Wee, M.D.

Benign Essential Blepharospasm Treated With Botulinum Toxin
Berlin AJ, Cassen JH, DeNelsky G, Hanson MR, Sweeney PJ (Cleveland Clinic Found, Cleveland)
Cleve Clin J Med 54:421–426, September–October 1987   16–13

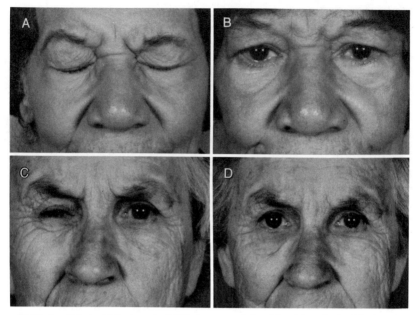

Fig 16–5.—Patient with benign essential blepharospasm before (**A**) and 1 week after injection (**B**), as well as a patient with hemifacial spasm before (**C**) and 1 week after injection (**D**). (Courtesy of Berlin AJ, Cassen JH, DeNelsky G, et al: *Cleve Clin J Med* 54:421–426, September–October 1987.)

Injection of botulinum toxin into the eyelids is designed to weaken the musculature in patients with blepharospasm. Experiences using this therapy in 9 patients with benign essential blepharospasm, 2 with hemifacial spasm, and 1 with Meige's syndrome, were reviewed. Botulinum toxin was injected subcutaneously into the lid in a dose ranging from 0.0025 μg to 0.01 gm per lid.

All patients responded to some degree, with the peak effect occurring after 3 days (Fig 16–5). One patient with hemifacial spasm also responded to injection of the orbicularis oris muscle. Three of the 5 patients with a significant personality disorder continued to have episodes of spasm, but they were less severe than before. Further injections were chosen by 9 patients after 60–90 days. One patient injected elsewhere had temporary hypertropia because of diffusion of toxin into the superior rectus muscle.

Botulinum toxin impedes conduction in the peripheral nerves by presynaptic blockade. Benign essential blepharospasm improves 2–3 months after toxin injection into the affected lids, and lasts an average of 3 months. Appropriate treatment can be selected by identifying psychological factors and excluding neurologic ones.

▶ S.H. Subramony, M.D., Associate Professor of Neurology, University of Mississippi School of Medicine, Jackson, writes the following comment.—R.D. Currier, M.D.

▶ This report agrees with results of other series that local injection of botulinum toxin in doses ranging from 6.25 to 25 units per lid gives significant symptomatic relief of this otherwise difficult to treat condition for a mean of about 12 weeks. Ocular side effects have included ptosis, changes in tear function, diplopia, and lower lid flaccidity, and they tend to be mild. Systemic side effects have not been reported, but mild neuromuscular block can be documented by single fiber EMG (Sanders et al: *Neurology* 36:545, 1986). Unanswered questions include optimal dose, the safety of repeated doses which will be required by some patients, the occurrence of an immune response to the toxin, and whether nonresponders can be weeded out by psychological testing.—S.H. Subramony, M.D.

NEUROSURGERY

ROBERT M. CROWELL, M.D.

Introduction

New technology dominated in 1988. The avalanche of papers detailing what MRI can do is testimony to the power of this new *diagnostic* modality (Abstract 17–1). Brain tumors (Abstract 19–15), cervical radiculopathy, (Abstract 22–1), lumbar arachnoiditis (Abstract 22–6)—for these MRI is now the modality of choice, and the list is constantly growing. Other diagnostic techniques, including transcranial Doppler sonography (Abstract 17–11), SPECT (Abstract 17–5), and PET scanning (Abstracts 17–9 and 17–10), are also establishing clinical roles. No less remarkable is the expansion of *interventional neuroradiology.* Balloon catheter and embolization techniques have established their pre-eminence in the treatment of carotid-cavernous fistulas (Abstract 18–2), dural arteriovenous malformations (Abstract 18–5), and vertebral arteriovenous fistulas (Abstract 18–4). There is a growing role for embolization in the therapy of intracranial arteriovenous malformations (Abstract 21–17), and even aneurysms have been obliterated with these techniques. Also advancing are techniques of stereotaxis (Abstract 18–14) and specialized radiation (Abstract 18–7), often supplanting older, more invasive pathology.

Tumor management has been advanced by correlation of stereotactic histology and MRI and CT alterations (Abstract 19–1). A host of new medical therapies has sprung up, including immunologic methodology (Abstract 19–4). Controlled studies have indicated that total resection of supratentorial gliomas leads to improved results (Abstract 19–3), and reoperation appears to hold promise in the treatment of recurrent gliomas (Abstract 19–5). In the evaluation of pituitary adenomas, magnetic resonance imaging with gadolinium will likely become the first imaging study of choice (Abstract 19–5). Inferior petrosal vein sampling in Cushing's disease is helpful in guiding the surgeon (Abstract 19–18). Magnetic resonance imaging is also extremely helpful for depiction of tumors in the internal auditory canal (Abstract 19–23). Many groups have now reported preservation of useful hearing after excision of acoustic neuroma under appropriate neurophysiologic monitoring (Abstract 19–25).

In the field of *ischemia,* computed tomographic scanning can now provide in noninvasive fashion substantial information on the carotid bifurcation (Abstract 20–1). Although some have reported declining complication rates from carotid endarterectomy (Abstract 20–4), there is great support for the North American Symptomatic Carotid Endarterectomy Trial, which is designed to evaluate in scientific fashion the benefits of carotid endarterectomy. Another important trial from the Scandinavian Stroke Study Group has failed to show a benefit for hemodilution therapy in acute stroke patients (Abstract 20–13).

Regarding *hemorrhage,* a number of important advances were reported in 1988. Intraoperative digital subtraction angiography has now reached a high point of development and can be used in the operating room to confirm the efficacy of surgery for aneurysms or arteriovenous malformations (Abstract 21–1). A deliberate policy of early operation on supratentorial aneurysms has been reported yet again to have a beneficial overall effect (Abstract 21–6). Unruptured arteriovenous malformations carry a substantial risk, and surgical correction seems warranted (Abstract 21–13). Staged treatment of arteriovenous malformations of the brain has been recommended to avoid breakthrough bleeding (Abstract 21–18). Cavernous angiomas of the brain, which carry a risk of hemorrhage, have a characteristic MRI appearance with a central zone of high signal and a periphery of low signal (Abstract 21–19).

Regarding the *spine,* surface coil MRI is just as good as myelography in the evaluation of radiculopathy (Abstract 22–1). Cervical spine stenosis resulting from ossification of the posterior longitudinal ligament is relatively common, is well demonstrated by CT, and is best treated by anterior decompression (Abstract 22–3). Intra-axial tumors of the cervical medullary junction may be removed with good results (Abstract 22–12). Magnetic resonance imaging is the study of choice for evaluation of metastatic spinal disease (Abstract 22–13); and it is also the best study for detection and follow-up of syringomyelia patients (Abstract 22–17).

In *pediatrics,* craniopagi have been classified, and modern surgical approaches defined (Abstract 24–1). The Gardner operation is advocated for treatment of hydrosyringomyelia in childhood (Abstract 24–3). Excellent results are now obtained with radical surgery for craniosynostosis (Abstract 24–4). Temporary external lumbar drainage is quite helpful in predicting the impact of shunting in patients with normal pressure hydrocephalus (Abstract 24–9).

In *functional neurosurgery,* treatment of chronic pain by deep brain stimulation is shown to have long-term effectiveness in more than half the patients so treated (Abstract 25–1). Magnetoencephalography can identify epileptogenic foci (Abstract 25–6). Psychosurgery has been continued in Scandinavia with the Gamma knife technique, obviating open surgery (Abstract 25–8). Continued studies of transplantation to the brain have indicated mixed results, and further careful controlled studies will be needed before such methods can be generally adopted.

Peripheral nerve surgery has advanced by the application of CT and MR for brachial plexopathy (Abstract 26–1). Tumors of the brachial plexus are now excised with good results, especially neurofibromas (Abstract 26–2).

A torrent of clinically relevant reports in *basic neuroscience* contains some deserving special attention. Information storage via biochemical means has been recently reviewed (Abstract 27–1). Calcium channels have been given biochemical and immunologic characterization (Abstract 27–2). Interleukin-1 receptors (Abstract 27–3) and atrial natriuretic factor (Abstract 27–4) have been identified and characterized in the brain.

Robert M. Crowell, M.D.

17 Diagnostics

Introduction

Development of *magnetic resonance* imaging continues at an impressive pace. Perhaps most exciting is the initial investigation of MR angiography of peripheral, carotid, and coronary arteries (Abstract 17–1). The current images suggest that the method is ready for testing as a noninvasive technique for imaging of the extracranial carotid bifurcation. To date, the resolution is inadequate for most intracranial problems aside from exclusion of intrasellar aneurysms, deflection of major intracranial vessels by tumors, and so forth. With the rapid improvements in MR technology, it is altogether possible that this method may provide noninvasive screening for intracranial lesions in the near future.

Magnetic resonance imaging has already established its efficacy in the evaluation of a number of CNS lesions. Studies with magnetic resonance determined the presence of intracranial sarcoidosis in 14 patients, but CT was superior in 2 (Abstract 17–4). Magnetic resonance imaging has established a place as a superior method for preoperative evaluation of pituitary adenomas (Abstract 19–15), especially when gadolinium is used (Abstract 19–16). Cervical radiculopathy is effectively evaluated with surface coil MRI (Abstract 22–1). Cervical spinal involvement in rheumatoid arthritis is beautifully imaged by MR (Abstract 22–2). Magnetic resonance imaging can diagnose lumbar arachnoiditis (Abstract 22–6). The postoperative assessment of the lumbar spine is also helped by MRI (Abstract 22–7). Physiologic support in monitoring of critically ill patients can be carried out during MRI (Abstract 17–2). Application of NMR spectroscopy is a promising approach to the metabolic, on-line evaluation of a variety of brain processes including global cerebral ischemia (Abstract 17–3).

Single-photon emission tomography (SPECT) is gaining a place in the noninvasive evaluation of cerebral hemodynamics and metabolism. For example, cerebral hemodynamics in arteriovenous malformations have been studied with this technique (Abstract 17–5), and SPECT has been used for quantitation of cobalt-57 bleomycin delivery to human brain tumors (Abstract 17–6). Changes in cerebral perfusion after acute head injury have been monitored with serial studies of ^{99m}Tc HM-PAO SPECT (Abstract 17–7). These studies are promising, but resolution requires further refinement, and correlative studies with other techniques will be needed to verify the physiologic meaning of the observed alterations.

Positron emission tomography appears to be gaining a clinical role as well as a research role. It is now possible to differentiate cerebral radiation necrosis from tumor recurrence by metabolic studies with PET (Abstracts 17–8 and 17–9). In addition, it is suggested that glucose utiliza-

167

tion by intracranial meningiomas in PET investigations may be an index of tumor aggressivity and probability of recurrence (Abstract 17–10).

Transcranial Doppler ultrasonography is carving out a place in the noninvasive extracranial evaluation of the intracranial circulation. Accuracy of the method approaches 90% compared with cerebral angiography (Abstract 17–11). The method appears to be useful for occlusive disease, arteriovenous malformations, cerebral vascular vasospasm, and assessment of collateral circulation (Abstract 17–12).

Developments in *cytology* appear to be useful diagnostic advances. Flow cytometry in cells from cerebral spinal fluid is apparently more sensitive than standard cell block cytology in the detection of tumor cells (Abstract 17–13). Monoclonal antibodies may also be used in the evaluation of cytologic specimens for greater diagnostic precision (Abstract 17–14).

Robert M. Crowell, M.D.

Magnetic Resonance

MR Angiography of Peripheral, Carotid, and Coronary Arteries
Alfidi RJ, Masaryk TJ, Haacke EM, Genz GW, Ross JS, Modic MT, Nelson AD, LiPuma JP, Cohen AM (Case Western Reserve Univ)
AJR 149:1097–1109, December 1987   17–1

Magnetic resonance (MR) angiography may provide the long-sought simple and noninvasive imaging method for atherosclerotic vascular disease. Accurate vascular imaging requires high resolution and signal-noise and contrast-noise ratios adequate for defining the vessel lumen. The use of long echo times allows correction for velocity and acceleration, and a smaller field of view. High spatial resolution with a good signal-to-noise ratio results. The problem of overlapping vessels is amenable to gated or ungated 3-dimensional subtraction processing or volume imaging.

Peripheral vessels are evaluated by an initial large-field-of-view study and then high-resolution scanning using gradient rephased/dephased sequences. Carotid imaging uses velocity-rephasing gradients to obtain improved subtraction images. Finite volume, ungated spin-echo, and ungated gradient-echo methods provide high contrast and high spatial resolution (Fig 17–1). In imaging the coronary arteries, 3-dimensional reconstruction is required to separate the coronary lumens from the cardiac chambers. Attempts at imaging the heart in vivo have been only marginally successful.

New dephasing-rephasing gradient schemes for long and short echo times are under development. Specialized surface coils might provide better signal-to-noise ratios and therefore improved spatial resolution. Very short echoes or echo-planar single-shot acquisitions might be necessary for 3-dimensional imaging of vessels.

▶ This report from Case Western Reserve University characterizes the present state of MR angiography. The published images suggest that the method is ready for testing as a noninvasive technique for imaging extracranial carotid bi-

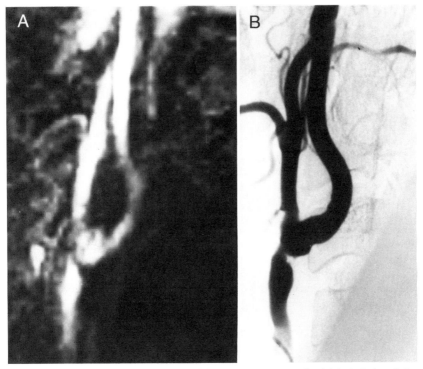

Fig 17–1.—**A,** summation image of carotid bifurcation in a patient with a left bruit. **B,** lateral view from an intra-arterial angiogram of left carotid. (Courtesy of Alfidi RT, Masaryk TJ, Haacke EM, et al: *AJR* 149:1097–1109, December 1987.)

furcation. The method must be validated against a gold standard of cerebral angiography to validate its sensitivity and specificity. It seems likely that this approach will become clinically useful, either as a unique noninvasive approach or, more likely, in conjunction with other noninvasive modalities, such as duplex Doppler. To date, the resolution is inadequate for most intracranial problems aside from exclusion of intrasellar aneurysms, deflection of major intracranial vessels by tumors, etc., a sort of depiction already quite nicely provided by static MR imaging. An improvement in resolution of very substantial degree will be required to enable MR angiography to depict intracranial aneurysm and arteriovenous malformations. With the rapid improvement of MR technology, it is altogether possible that finer resolution may permit noninvasive screening for intracranial lesions in the future.— R.M. Crowell, M.D.

Physiological Support and Monitoring of Critically Ill Patients During Magnetic Resonance Imaging
Barnett GH, Ropper AH, Johnson KA (Harvard Univ; Massachusetts Gen Hosp, Boston; Cleveland Clinic Hosp)
J Neurosurg 68:246–250, February 1988   17–2

Magnetic resonance imaging (MRI) has generally been restricted to patients who are hemodynamically and neurologically stable. The strong magnetic field and radiofrequency transmissions that are involved in MRI are possible sources of interference with monitoring equipment. A method of support and physiologic monitoring of critically ill patients undergoing MRI was developed.

Patients are imaged with a Technicare MR system, which operates at 0.6 Tesla. Mechanical ventilation is given by a Monaghan 225 ventilator, factory modified to be compatible with MRI (Fig 17−2). Because the ventilator does not use electricity or magnets, it does not produce radiofrequency waves or magnetic fields that could interfere with the imaging.

The ventilator is powered only by high-pressure oxygen supplied through high-pressure tubing. Arterial blood gas determinations are done before the patient is placed in the magnet and are repeated midway through the procedure or whenever changes in blood pressure, pulse, or intracranial pressure occur. A ventilatory pressure alarm is connected to the patient's endotracheal tube by a T-piece and high-pressure tubing. Thus, a patient's disconnection from the ventilator or loss of ventilatory pressure can be detected immediately.

Physiologic monitoring is done with a shielded electric extension cable that couples the transducer to a physiologic monitor that is placed outside the magnet room. This portable 2-channel monitor allows continuous monitoring of arterial blood pressure and intracranial pressure.

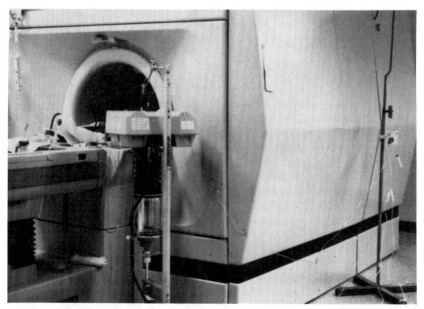

Fig 17−2.—Arrangement of ventilator and transducers in MRI suite. Transducers are clamped to nonferromagnetic pole alongside scanner at its midposition. Placing the ventilator at foot of magnet facilitates moving the patient and allows use of standard length (6-ft) ventilator tubing. (Courtesy of Barnett GH, Ropper AH, Johnson KA: *J Neurosurg* 68:246−250, February 1988.)

This method of support and physiologic monitoring of critically ill neurosurgical and neurologic patients during MRI has not caused degradation of the image attributable to electrical interference. Adequate preparation and precautions can allow many critically ill patients to safely undergo MRI.

▶ The described modifications permit safe and satisfactory MRI for critically ill patients. The addition of a factory modification for the mechanical ventilator eliminates radiofrequency and magnetic fields that could degrade image. The use of monitoring devices at a distance likewise eliminates the potential electromagnetic interference from this source.—R.M. Crowell, M.D.

Measurement of Lactate Accumulation by In Vivo Proton NMR Spectroscopy During Global Cerebral Ischemia in Rats
Richards TL, Keniry MA, Weinstein PR, Pereira BM, Andrews BT, Murphy EJ, James TL (Univ of California, San Francisco)
Magn Reson Med 5:353–357, October 1987   17–3

Intracellular lactic acidosis is a major factor in delayed cerebral tissue damage. Lactate production in vivo was evaluated noninvasively using in vivo proton nuclear magnetic resonance spectroscopy during remotely controlled global cerebral ischemia followed by reperfusion in rats. The lactate and N-acetylaspartate (NAA) peaks were monitored during both periods.

The lactate-NAA ratio correlated with survival after ischemia and subsequent reperfusion. Survival after ischemia and reperfusion was associated with a lactate/NAA ratio of 1.0 to 1.3. Based on estimates from results of in vitro studies, this corresponded to a lactate concentration of approximately 20–30 mmol.

In vivo proton nuclear magnetic resonance spectroscopy can be used to monitor cerebral lactate levels during ischemia, as well as the response during reperfusion. These results are similar to those of in vitro techniques that correlated irreversible tissue damage with levels of lactic acid accumulation.

▶ This interesting contribution indicates that noninvasive NMR spectroscopy can be used to monitor brain lactate in vivo with good correlation to outcome. Perhaps such techniques can be applied in critical neurosurgical settings for noninvasive monitoring of patients at risk for cerebral ischemia.—R.M. Crowell, M.D.

MR and CT Evaluation of Intracranial Sarcoidosis
Hayes WS, Sherman JL, Stern BJ, Citrin CM, Pulaski PD (Georgetown Univ Hosp, Washington, DC; Uniformed Services Univ of the Health Sciences, Bethesda; Magnetic Imaging of Washington, Chevy Chase; Sinai Hosp, Baltimore; Johns Hopkins Hosp, Baltimore, Md)
AJR 149:1043–1049, November 1987   17–4

Intracranial sarcoidosis occurs in approximately 5% of patients with sarcoidosis. Diagnosis is important, because complications of neurosarcoidosis account for much of the mortality and serious morbidity of the disease. Fourteen patients with neurosarcoidosis were evaluated by magnetic resonance imaging (MRI) and computed tomography (CT). Magnetic resonance images were obtained with a 0.5-T superconductive magnet with T_1- and T_2-weighted images, and CT with contrast was obtained in all patients. The granulomatous lesions were classified by location into basilar, convexity, intrahemispheric, and periventricular white-matter involvement. The presence of hydrocephalus with or without an associated lesion was also noted.

Magnetic resonance imaging studies determined the presence of disease in all patients, but was less accurate than CT in depicting disease in 2 (14%) of the patients, both of whom were undergoing high-dose steroid therapy. Contrast-enhanced CT determined the presence of disease in 12 (85%) of patients, but was less accurate than MRI in delineating hypothalamic involvement in 2 patients and periventricular white-matter involvement in 3. Hydrocephalus was equally seen with both CT and MRI, but the associated periventricular white-matter edema was better detected with MRI. Convexity involvement was well documented with both CT and MRI. There was great variability in the appearance of intracranial sarcoidosis on MRI. Three patients had lesions that were isointense or hypointense, relative to the cerebral cortex, on both T_1- and T_2- weighted images, and 9 patients had lesions that were hyperintense on T_2-weighted images.

Both MRI and CT are helpful in evaluating a patient with suspected intracranial sarcoidosis. Different but potentially complementary findings can be obtained by CT and MRI. Although MRI provides greater sensitivity than CT in evaluating hypothalamic and periventricular involvement, CT is superior to MRI in evaluating some patients undergoing high-dose steroid therapy.

Brief Notes on MRI

MRI and CSF Pulsation

The CSF flow-void sign on MRI is evidently due to the arrival of the systemic arterial pulse wave related either to a direct hydraulic effect of the venous system on the CSF or to filling an expansion of the venous system. Cardiac gating can modify this sign (Citrin CM, et al: *AJR* 148:205–208, 1987).

Cerebrospinal fluid gating may be used to improve T_2-weighted images in the spinal cord (Enzmann DR, et al: *Radiology* 162:763–767, 1987).

Moreover, for cervical spine phantom studies, CSF-gated MR imaging leads to improved quality of images (Rubin JB, et al: *Radiology* 163:784–792, 1987).

Multiphasic MR imaging may be used for direct imaging of pulsatile CSF flow (Edelman RR, et al: *Radiology* 161:779–783, 1986).

Cerebrospinal fluid pulsation leads to "ghost images." Cerebrospinal fluid without pulsation shows higher signal and may help in the diagnosis of arachnoid or intraventricular cyst, spinal stenosis, and spinal block. Abnormal patterns of CSF pulsation can cause apparent signal loss, as in patients with arachnoiditis (Enzmann DR, et al: *Radiology* 161:773–778, 1986).

Cerebrospinal fluid pulsations within nonneoplastic spinal cord cysts differentiate them from neoplastic cysts. The absence or reduction of such pulsation may be a valuable indicator of the success of the shunting procedure as evaluated by MRI (Enzmann DR, et al: *AJNR* 8:517–525, 1987).

Epidural brain compression causes changes in frequency spectrum of the CSF pulse wave (Takizawa H, et al: *J Neurol Neurosurg Psychiatry* 49:1367–1373, 1986).

Gadolinium Enhancement

In 11 cases with cerebral infarction, gadolinium-enhanced SE 500/30 images matched the contrast-material–enhanced CT scans in patterns. Small deep infarcts often did not enhance (Virapongse C, et al: *Radiology* 161:785–794, 1986).

In 23 patients with intracranial meningiomas, MRI showed on spin-echo little change relative to brain with great contrast on proton density images. In T_2 images, more than 50% showed a low signal margin between tumor and brain. After intravenous injection of gadolinium DTPA, there was marked uptake in the meningiomas (Treisch J, et al: *Fortschr Rontgenstr* 146:207–214, 1987).

Contrast enhancement with gadolinium-DTPA is greatest in acoustic neuromas (average, 310%), very high with meningiomas (180%), and least with neurofibromas, glomus tumors, and pituitary microadenomas (Breger RK, et al: *Radiology* 163:427–429, 1987).

In 15 tumor patients studied with gadolinium-DTPA, 17 of 35 lesions were detected on the T_2 but not on the post-gadolinium studies (Brant-Zawadzki M, et al: *AJR* 147:1223–1230, 1986).

Gadolinium-DTPA improves detection of metastatic foci with MR imaging (Russell EJ, et al: *Radiology* 165:609–617, 1987; Healy ME, et al: *Radiology* 165:619–624, 1987).

MRI and Metabolism

Brain water may be measured by magnetic resonance imaging and changes noted after mannitol and dexamethasone administration (Bell BA, et al: *Lancet* 1:66–69, Jan 10, 1987).

Histologic studies show that high signal on T_2 MRI in the white matter just anterior to both frontal horns is due to local increased water related to a loose network of axons, loss of ependyma, and flow of interstitial fluid (Sze G, et al: *AJR* 147:331–338, 1986).

Proton nuclear magnetic resonance spectra of 36 brain tumors showed a decreased signal intensity for *N*-acetyl aspartate (Tanaka C, et al: *Magn Reson Imaging* 4:503–508, 1986).

Fifteen cases of tuberous sclerosis were evaluated with MR. Subependymal nodules, noted in 12 of 15 patients on T_1 images, were the most specific finding. Distortion of normal cortical architecture was common with dilated ventricles in about one third, and a known astrocytoma was found in 1 case. Magnetic resonance will be at least equal to and probably superior to CT for sensitivity and specificity in this condition (McMurdo SK, Jr, et al: *AJR* 148:791–796, 1987).

Fast MR-imaging was done in 60 patients with intracerebral lesions. The gradient-echo fast MR sequence is useful in many cases, but diagnostic accuracy was low in 40%, and in 30% lesions were not detected with this method (Weiss T, et al: *Fortschr Rontgenstr* 146:214–222, 1987).

Magnetic resonance imaging of the orbit is strongly improved by surface coils (Reuther G and Requardt H. *Fortschr. Roentenstr.* 145:386–392, 1986).

Sochurek has presented a well-written account of "medicine's new vision" in *National Geographic* 171:2–41, 1987. This article explains to the intelligent layman the basis and use of CT and MRI, digital subtraction angiography, and ultrasonography. This may be useful for patients and families.— R.M. Crowell, M.D.

Single-Photon Emission Computed Tomography

Cerebral Hemodynamics in Arteriovenous Malformations: Evaluation by Single-Photon Emission CT
Takeuchi S, Kikuchi H, Karasawa J, Naruo Y, Hashimoto K, Nishimura T, Kozuka T, Hayashi M (Natl Cardiovascular Ctr, Osaka, Japan)
AJNR 8:193–197, March–April 1987   17–5

The single-photon emission computed tomographic (SPECT) technique was used to examine cerebral hemodynamics in 6 patients with supratentorial arteriovenous malformations and hemorrhage more than 1 month old. Red blood cells labeled with technetium were used, as were ^{81m}Kr and N-isopropyl-p-[^{123}I]-iodoamphetamine (Imp). Three malformations involved the basal ganglia, 2 involved the cerebral cortex, and 1 involved the cortex, subcortex, and basal ganglia.

The area of the nidus was visualized as reduced activity in iodoamphetamine studies. In Kr studies, the nidus exhibited increased activity, with a surrounding zone of lowered activity. Large and moderate-sized lesions were associated with decreased activity in the contralateral hemisphere. Increased activity in the nidus was consistently demonstrated by SPECT-technetium. Carbon dioxide reactivity during hypocapnia was preserved, except in the region of the malformation.

These SPECT studies of arteriovenous malformation demonstrate cerebral ischemia, which presumably is secondary to the cerebral steal phenomenon, especially with a large malformation. An increase in perfusion after ligation or embolization of the feeder vessels might lead to cerebral edema and even hemorrhage if systemic arterial pressure is normal. Stepwise treatment therefore is indicated, as well as barbiturate protection or controlled hypotension.

▶ Single-photon emission computed tomography can image arteriovenous malformations (AVMs), but the meaning and value of such studies is unclear. In this communication, SPECT-IMP showed decreased activity in the nidus and SPECT-Kr showed increased activity in the nidus, although both are said to reflect cerebral blood flow. The area near the nidus showed decreased activity in all studies in all cases, regardless of size. It is hard to accept a substantial steal in all cases, even in the small lesions without steal syndromes. Moreover, the resolution of the presented studies is poor. Although cerebral blood flow studies may eventually prove useful in the management of AVMs, more work will be needed to establish such a role.— R.M. Crowell, M.D.

SPECT Quantitation of Cobalt-57 Bleomycin Delivery to Human Brain Tumors

Front D, Israel O, Iosilevsky G, Even-Sapir E, Frenkel A, Kolodny GM, Feinsod M (Technion-Israel Inst of Technology, Haifa, Israel; Beth Israel Hosp, Harvard Univ)

J Nucl Med 29:187–194, February 1988   17–6

Chemotherapy that may be effective for tumors outside the central nervous system is generally useless for treating brain tumors. The blood-brain barrier is assumed to be the main limiting factor in the use of antineoplastic drugs in brain tumors. New drugs that are effective in extracerebral tumors that do not cross the blood-brain barrier are being tested. A noninvasive in vivo quantitative single-photon emission computed tomography (SPECT) was used to measure uptake of cobalt-57 bleomycin (Co-bleo) in 13 human brain tumors and uptake of [^{99m}Tc] glucoheptonate (GH) in 23 brain tumors.

The SPECT technique can characterize the blood-tissue barrier of different human brain tumors. Uptake of Co-bleo was compared with that of GH to determine whether a simple brain scanning agent could serve as an indicator of brain tumor permeability to chemotherapeutic drugs. Significant tumor uptake differences were found. Tumor concentration over time, tumor to blood ratio at 30 minutes, and tumor cumulative concentration of radioactivity showed marked differences even between tumors with the same histology. The correlation between tumor concentration of Co-bleo and GH was weak. No correlation was found between the concentration of drug in the blood and its tumor concentration.

A simple imaging agent such as GH cannot serve as an indicator of individual tumor uptake; further experience with other agents is needed. Results also suggest that the level of a drug in the blood cannot be used as a criterion of the amount of drug which will penetrate the tumor. Direct SPECT measurement of the drug concentration in the tumor itself should be performed. These results, which demonstrate marked differences in uptake between brain tumors, suggest that before chemotherapy is administered uptake of the chemotherapeutic drug in the individual tumor to be treated should be evaluated and comparisons should be made between the uptake of a series of drugs to determine which agent would be most effective on the basis of its uptake as well as its tumor cell killing potential.

▶ The use of SPECT continues to gain acceptance in a variety of diagnostic areas. In this communication, quantitation of delivery of a chemotherapeutic agent to a brain tumor has been achieved. Application of this approach may be useful in the study of a variety of chemotherapeutic and immunotherapeutic approaches.— R.M. Crowell, M.D.

Changes in Cerebral Perfusion After Acute Head Injury: Comparison of CT With Tc-99m HM-PAO SPECT

Abdel-Dayem HM, Sadek SA, Kouris K, Bahar RH, Higazi I, Eriksson S, Englesson SH, Berntman L, Sigurdsson GH, Foad M, Olivercrona H (Kuwait Univ)
Radiology 165:221–226, October 1987   17–7

Technetium-99m-hexamethyl-propyleneamine oxime (^{99m}Tc HM-PAO) with single photon emission computed tomography (SPECT) was used to evaluate 14 comatose patients after acute head injury. The SPECT findings were correlated with computed tomographic (CT) scans made within 24 hours of injury. Ten patients were studied within 72 hours of injury. Five healthy persons also were studied.

Changes in cerebral arterial perfusion were evident on SPECT study in all patients. Fifty-four lesions were demonstrated with SPECT and 22 with CT. The former study was 42% better than CT in demonstrating lesions. The true positive ratio for SPECT was 73%, but CT missed 32 lesions that were found with SPECT. Focal lesions generally appeared larger on SPECT scans. Half of the 14 patients died. Lesion size, multiplicity, and site were all significant prognostic factors.

The SPECT technique using ^{99m}Tc HM-PAO can distinguish patients with a relatively favorable outlook after serious acute head injury from those having an unfavorable prognosis. The study reflects changes in perfusion, and it demonstrates lesions more sensitively than conventional CT. In addition, lesions are demonstrated at an earlier stage by the SPECT procedure.

▶ Single-photon emission computed tomography appears to be a clinically practical method of focal cerebral blood flow determination. Disturbances of focal cerebral blood flow are known to play a major role in the evolution of acute brain injury. However, heretofore methods of blood flow determination have been too cumbersome or too unreliable to guide clinical management. Therefore, it is logical to expect that SPECT might find a clinically useful role in the management of severe head injury. The present report hints that this may be the case. Certainly the published figures indicate widespread perfusion abnormality, even in the face of restricted CT abnormalities. The method, therefore, has promise, but further experience correlating clinical developments and SPECT will be needed before the technique can be recommended for general use.— R.M. Crowell, M.D.

Brief Notes on SPECT

SPECT for Cerebral Blood Flow

SPECT with iodine-123 HIPDM can be used to evaluate regional cerebral blood flow resulting from cerebral vascular vasospasm after subarachnoid hemorrhage (Di Piero V, et al: *Clin Nucl Med* 12:395–398, 1987).

Single-photon emission computed tomography (SPECT) can demonstrate decreased intracranial blood flow in localized areas (Ueda, et al: *Neurol Med Chir, Tokyo* 26:601–607, 1986). For this quantification a tracer 123I-IMP N-isopropyl T123 iodoamphetamine) is used along with SPECT.

Long-term noninvasive single-photon emission computed tomography studies failed to show any long-lasting improvement in perfusion after EC-IC bypass surgery (DiPiero V, et al: *J Neurol Neurosurg Psychiatry* 50:988–996, 1987).

SPECT can assist in the detection of recurrent brain tumor from persistent activity at a craniotomy site (Collier BD, et al: *Clin Nucl Med* 12:226–228, 1987).

Measurement of S-phase fraction of human brain tumors in situ measured by uptake of bromodeoxyuridine may be useful in projecting the prognosis and monitoring the management of intracranial tumors.—R.M. Crowell, M.D.

Positron Emission Tomography

Differentiation of Cerebral Radiation Necrosis From Tumor Recurrence by [18F]FDG and 82RB Positron Emission Tomography
Doyle WK, Budinger IF, Valk PE, Levin VA, Gutin PH (Univ of California, Berkeley, and Univ of California, San Francisco)
J Comput Assist Tomogr 11:563–570, July–August 1987   17–8

The clinical features and natural history of cerebral radiation necrosis are similar to those of tumor recurrence. Nine radiation-treated brain tumor patients were studied by positron emission tomography (PET) in an attempt to differentiate tumor recurrence from radiation necrosis. Rubidum-82 (^{82}Rb) was used to define the region of absent or disturbed blood-brain barrier and [^{18}F]2-fluoro-2-deoxy-D-glucose ([^{18}F]FDG), a tracer of glucose metabolism, was used to evaluate the metabolic state of the lesion.

Dynamic ^{82}Rb imaging showed that the rate of ^{82}Rb accumulation was greater in tumor than in normal brain tissue. This finding alone did not differentiate tumor from necrosis, as some necrotic tissue also showed high rates of ^{82}Rb accumulation and washout kinetics were similarly nonspecific. However, a comparison of [^{18}F]FDG activity within the lesion with activity in adjacent tissue allowed the diagnosis of recurrent tumor (increased [^{18}F]FDG accumulation) in 4 patients or radiation necrosis (decreased FDG accumulation) in 3. The PET diagnosis was confirmed by histologic examination of resected tissue in 7 patients, while the other 2 who did not undergo surgery had clinical courses consistent with a PET diagnosis of radiation necrosis.

The differentiation of radiation necrosis from recurrent tumor can be made reliably by [^{18}F]FDG PET examination; the addition of ^{82}Rb PET study performed immediately before the [^{18}F]FDG injection improves the specificity and accuracy of diagnosis.

▶ In this study of 9 cases, the PET FDG image was a perfect predictor of histopathologic diagnosis: a cold image predicted a radionecrosis, a hot image predicted a recurrent tumor, and this was borne out by histology in 7 cases and in clinical course in 2. For this important clinical differentiation PET appears to have won a clinical, as opposed to a research, role.—R.M. Crowell, M.D.

Cerebral Necrosis After Radiotherapy and/or Intraarterial Chemotherapy for Brain Tumors: PET and Neuropathologic Studies

Di Chiro G, Oldfield E, Wright DC, De Michele D, Katz DA, Patronas NJ, Doppman JL, Larson SM, Ito M, Kufta CV (Natl Insts of Health, Bethesda, Md)
AJNR 8:1083–1091, November–December 1987   17–9

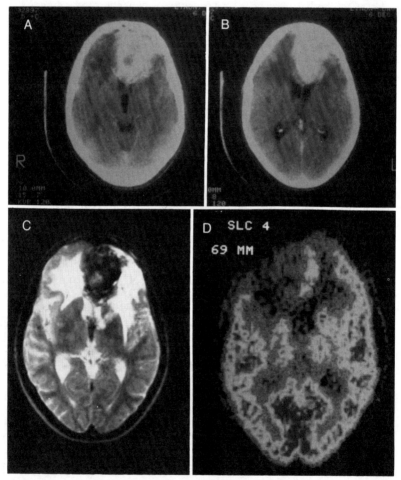

Fig 17–3.—Radiation necrosis. **A** and **B**, postcontrast axial CT scans show marked, bifrontal enhancement surrounded by hypodense halo. Lesion is larger on left. **C**, MR image (TR = 2500 msec, TE = 120 msec). Mixed-intensity signal from area corresponding to CT enhancement and high-intensity signal from surrounding edema. **D**, PET-FDG image at corresponding level. Marked hypometabolism in both prefrontal areas, larger on left, Note selective sparing of interhemispheric gray matter, which is displaced toward right. Color scale indicates range of metabolic values (in mg glucose/100 gm/minute). (On PET scan only, right side of patient is on right side of image.) (Courtesy of Di Chiro G, Oldfield E, Wright DC, et al: *AJNR* 8:1083–1091, November–December 1987.)

Cerebral necrosis after radiotherapy for brain tumors is apparently more common than previously believed. Computed tomography (CT) and magnetic resonance imaging (MRI) cannot distinguish between this iatrogenic complication and tumor recurrence. The utility of positron emission tomography (PET) with ^{18}F-deoxyglucose (FDG) in cases of cerebral necrosis after radiotherapy, intra-arterial chemotherapy, or both was explored.

The PET studies were performed with the Neuro-PET, a scanner with a full width at half maximum resolution of 6.5 mm. Using PET, 10 of 95 patients referred for the purpose of differentiating tumor recurrence from necrosis were identified. The critical PET-FDG feature was focal hypometabolism in the necrotic region, which contrasted with the hypermetabolism associated with residual or recurrent tumor (Fig 17–3). Four additional patients with cerebral necrosis after supraophthalmic, intra-arterial chemotherapy were also studied with PET-FDG. The region of chemotherapy damage was also characterized by marked hypometabolism. Histologic study revealed both similarities and differences between radionecrosis and chemonecrosis.

By using PET-FDG, a diagnosis of radiation necrosis could be reached in 10 of 95 patients referred for differentiation between tumor recurrence and necrosis. Focal hypometabolism in the area of necrosis was the critical PET-FDG feature.

▶ Positron emission tomography reliably distinguishes cerebral necrosis from residual tumor. This article demonstrates that hypometabolism ("cold") characterizes radionecrosis, whereas hypermetabolism ("hot") is typical for residual or recurrent tumor. Mixed PET metabolism studies may suggest a combination of radionecrosis and tumor. Histopathologic confirmation has been provided in a number of cases, but the study would have been more forceful if all of the histopathology had been available, at least in tabular form. The method appears to be suitable for clinical utilization after its repeated confirmation in the investigational setting.— R.M. Crowell, M.D.

Glucose Utilization by Intracranial Meningiomas as an Index of Tumor Aggressivity and Probability of Recurrence: A PET Study
Di Chiro G, Hatazawa J, Katz DA, Rizzoli HV, De Michele DJ (Natl Inst of Health, Bethesda, Md; George Washington Univ)
Radiology 164:521–526, August 1987   17–10

Positron emission tomography (PET) with fluorine-18-2-fluoro-deoxyglucose (FDG) as a tracer has made possible the in vivo measurement of glucose metabolism of brain and cerebral neoplasms. Seventeen patients with histologically proved intracranial meningiomas were studied with PET-FDG to assess the glucose utilization of these tumors. The glucose metabolic rates were correlated with tumor recurrence, tumor growth, and histopathologic findings.

Four meningiomas followed for 3–5 years after PET-FDG and surgery showed no evidence of recurrence. These tumors had significantly lower glucose utilization rates than the 11 recurrent or regrowing meningiomas. A significant negative correlation existed between glucose metabolic rates and tumor doubling time, as estimated from serial computed tomographic studies, indicating that rapidly growing meningiomas used more glucose than those that grew slowly. Histopathologically, a syncytial (atypical) meningioma had the highest glucose utilization rate, followed by papillary meningioma and an angioblastic meningioma. Individual transitional and syncytial (typical) meningiomas showed marked differences in glucose metabolism despite similar microscopic appearance. Cytologic studies showed that high cellularity and invasive features were associated with high metabolic rates.

Monitoring the glucose utilization rate with the PET-FDG technique appears to be as reliable as histologic classification and other proposed criteria in predicting the behavior and recurrence of intracranial meningiomas.

▶ This novel study indicates a clear correlation of glucose utilization on PET scanning and meningioma recurrence. In all primary meningiomas, the glucose metabolic rate was less than 3 mg/dL/min, whereas all recurrent tumors had metabolic rates above 3. (The single exception was case #11, a recurrence with metabolic rate of 2.9). Positron emission tomography criteria may be even more useful than histologic criteria in predicting recurrence. This information can be helpful in selecting patients for postoperative radiation therapy to prevent recurrence.—R.M. Crowell, M.D.

Brief Notes on PET

PET for Tumors

The metabolic rates of tissue provided by PET scanning constitute a noninvasive method of differentiating primary brain tumors (Di Chiro G: 5, *Invest Radiol* 22:360–371, 1986).

PET for Brain Metabolism

Hawkins and Phelps indicate that PET can quantify brain metabolism in various forms of dementia and steady progression in these disorders (*Curr Concepts Diagnosis Nucl Med* 3:4–13, 1986). Fluorodioxide glucose studies are usually normal in the pseudodementia of depression. In multiple infarct dementia there are multiple hypometabolic areas. In Alzheimer's disease there is a destructive pattern of hypometabolism in parietal and temporal areas. Epileptic foci have increased blood flow metabolism during seizures and decreased metabolism interictally. Use of PET can permit avoidance of depth electrode studies in search of a focus for excision.

PET in Neuropsychiatry

According to Wagner, PET is useful for the study of chemical neurotransmitters in neuropsychiatric patients. Objective assessments of the effects of such drugs as haloperidol and methadone are provided. Schizophrenic patients have increased D2-dopamine receptors in caudate and putamen. Studies show decreased glucose utilization at the locus of origin of focal epilepsy, but hypermetabolism is present during seizure. 11 C carfentanil, a potent opiate receptor binder, is less strongly bound in the thalamus of sexually aroused persons than in controls.—R.M. Crowell, M.D.

Doppler Ultrasonography

Evaluation of Cerebrovascular Disease by Combined Extracranial and Transcranial Doppler Sonography: Experience in 1,039 Patients

Grolimund P, Seiler RW, Aaslid R, Huber P, Zurbruegg H (Univ Hosp, Bern, Switzerland)

Stroke 18:1018–1024, November–December 1987   17–11

Researchers have described a method based on 2 MHz pulsed ultrasound that could be used routinely to obtain Doppler signals from the basal cerebral arteries through thin areas of the temporal and occipital bone. Because this approach gives direct access to the collateral network of the circle of Willis and cerebral end-arteries, it is a valuable supple-

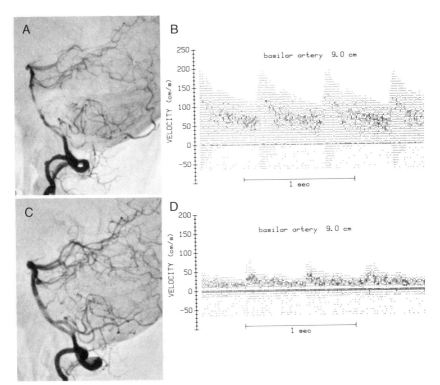

Fig 17–4.—Increased flow velocity in the basilar artery (**B**), 10 days after subarachnoid hemorrhage caused by vasospasm of this artery (**A**). Normal flow velocity in the basilar artery (**D**) after resolution of the arterial narrowing (**C**). (Courtesy of Grolimund P, Seiler RW, Aaslid R, et al: *Stroke* 18:1018–1024, November–December 1987.)

ment to Doppler examination of the extracranial arteries in patients with cerebrovascular disease. Results of 1,039 combined cervical and transcranial Doppler examinations were reported.

The patients, aged 54.7 ± 15.7 years, were examined for suspected cerebrovascular disease from 1982 to 1985. Satisfactory transcranial signals were not obtained in 2.7% of the patients. When compared with angiography, the accuracy of transcranial criteria in evaluating collateral flow over the circle of Willis was 94% for anterior circulation and 88% for posterior circulation. The method was also effective in detecting lesions of the intracranial arteries, although the number of such cases in this series was low. Arterial narrowing caused by cerebral vasospasm was diagnosed with a sensitivity of 80%. Among patients with ruptured intracranial aneurysms, an incidence of 93% arterial narrowing in basal cerebral arteries was achieved. In patients with subarachnoid hemorrhage and no aneurysm seen on angiography, arterial narrowing was observed in 56% (Fig 17–4). The time course and severity of cerebral vasospasm could be monitored. Arteriovenous malformations, characterized by Doppler findings of high velocities and low pulsatilities, were diagnosed with an accuracy of 95%.

In this study of combined cervical and transcranial Doppler examination, the transcranial Doppler approach provided technically acceptable recordings in most patients.

▶ This extensive study of transcranial Doppler sonography from Bern indicates a high sensitivity and accuracy for evaluation of the anterior and posterior circulations. Other groups, such as Hennerici and colleagues, have reported similar results. Transcranial Dopper sonography appears to be a very promising method for ongoing monitoring of the cerebral circulation in a variety of conditions in a noninvasive fashion.—R.M. Crowell, M.D.

Transcranial Doppler Ultrasound for the Assessment of Intracranial Arterial Flow Velocity: I. Evaluation of Intracranial Arterial Disease
Hennerici M, Rautenberg W, Schwartz A (Univ Med School, Düsseldorf, West Germany)
Surg Neurol 27:523–532, June 1987   17–12

Transcranial pulsed Doppler ultrasound studies were carried out in 71 patients with extracranial and intracranial cerebrovascular disorders to assess flow velocity within the basal intracranial arteries. Twenty-seven patients had had stroke, and 12 reported transient ischemic attacks. Continuous-wave Doppler studies were performed to evaluate the carotid and vertebral arteries, and duplex system studies were performed to visualize the extracranial carotid system. The basal arteries were examined with a transcranial directional pulsed-wave device operating at 2 MHz.

Twenty-two patients had significant obstructive lesions of the intracranial basal cerebral arteries (Fig 17–5). Abnormalities of the fast-Fourier

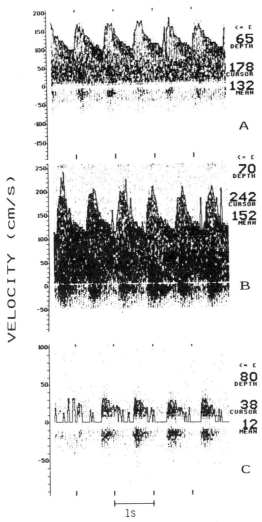

Fig 17–5.—Transcranial Doppler spectra recorded stepwise at different depths from a stenosis of the basilar artery. Note the increase of flow velocity at 65 mm (**A**) and particularly at 70-mm depths, associated with incidence of bidirectional high-amplitude but low-flow velocity signals at the major site of the lumen narrowing (**B**). Distal to the latter (**C**) (80 mm) pronounced reduction of faint Doppler signals is seen. (Courtesy of Hennerici M, Rautenberg W, Schwartz A: *Surg Neurol* 27:523–532, June 1987.)

transformed Doppler spectra served to detect and classify obstructive lesions as well as ectatic arteriopathies. Functional stenosis secondary to a large shunting volume was diagnosed in patients with arteriovenous malformation and significant collateralization of extracranial obstructive lesions. The development and resolution of vasospasm secondary to subarachnoid bleeding were observed in several cases.

Transcranial Doppler ultrasound is a means of obtaining real-time assessment of flow velocity patterns in the basal cerebral arteries. It may be used noninvasively to follow the course of cerebrovascular disease with or without treatment.

▶ The use of transcranial Doppler ultrasound to detect occlusive disease has been validated by several groups (Aaslid R, et al: *Neurosurgery* 60:37–41, 1984). The present report indicates good correlation with cerebral angiography for stenotic or occlusive lesions of the middle cerebral, basilar, and vertebral arteries (only a branch occlusion of the middle cerebral artery was missed). Detection of small changes over time may be less reliable, however. Transcranial Doppler seems likely to achieve an important position in the diagnosis and follow-up of occlusive intracranial cerebrovascular disease, including vasospasm.—R.M. Crowell, M.D.

Brief Notes on Doppler Ultrasonography

There was variability in transcranial Doppler findings and regional cerebral blood flow during carotid endarterectomy in 8 patients (Halsey JH, et al: *Stroke* 17:1206–1208, 1986).

Ultrasonic diagnosis is possible for isolated fourth ventricle, which is always secondary to a shunt procedure. (Couture A, et al: *Ann Radiol* 29:345–352, 1986).

Cytology

Detection of DNA Abnormalities by Flow Cytometry in Cells From Cerebrospinal Fluid

Cibas ES, Malkin MG, Posner JB, Melamed MR (Mem Sloan-Kettering Cancer Ctr; Cornell Univ, New York)
Am J Clin Pathol 88:570–577, November 1987   17–13

Cytologic examination of cerebrospinal fluid (CSF) is a common means used to detect malignant cells, and although several studies have attested to its high specificity, the technique is only moderately sensitive. A prospective study of the diagnostic value of DNA/RNA flow cytometry (FCM) was undertaken to compare it with cytology in an attempt to extend the sensitivity of these examinations. The DNA and RNA content of cells were measured in 223 CSF samples of 17 controls with nonmalignant disorders and 147 patients with solid tumors or lymphomas.

Results in the 17 control samples were all reported negative by cytologic examination. Of the 216 specimens from patients with malignant tumors, 27 were suspicious, 163 negative, and 26 specimens from 16 patients were positive by cytology. Twenty-eight samples from 19 patients with malignancies were abnormal by FCM. Twenty specimens showed an abnormal peak distinct from a coexisting diploid peak, and 8 had no distinctly abnormal peak, but an increased number of cells in the S and G_2M phases of the cell cycle. Of these 28 positive FCM samples, cytologic results were positive in 18, suspicious in 3, and negative in 7. Compared with cytology, the sensitivity of FCM was 69% and the specificity was 95%, calculated by considering negative and suspicious cases together as nondiagnostic.

Eight of the 9 patients with 10 cytologically negative or suspicious specimens positive by FCM had other laboratory and/or radiographic supporting evidence of leptomeningeal metastasis within 1 week of the FCM, so the specificity of FCM may actually be higher.

Eight specimens from 7 patients that were FCM negative were cytologically positive; abnormalities of the RNA content were not of diagnostic help in identifying these samples. There was a significant difference in the proportion of tumor cells to reactive inflammatory cells in cytologically positive samples that were positive vs. negative by FCM.

Because the cells present are already in fluid suspension and minimal sample preparation is required, CSF is almost ideally suited for evaluation by FCM. A total cell count less than 500 on FCM examination correlated strongly with the absence of tumor. More important than absolute cellularity is the proportion of tumor cells to reactive cells in the specimen; a high percentage of malignant cells favors the detection of abnormalities in cellular DNA content. Flow cytometry was especially sensitive in detecting lymphomatous involvement of CSF. The intrinsic strength of conventional cytology is its ability to recognize and identify frankly malignant cells, even if they are not present in large numbers.

▶ Flow cytometry is clearly more sensitive than standard cytologic examination in the search for malignant cells in CSF. The method shows great promise in the identification of patients with a high risk of delayed seeding from medulloblastoma. Flow cytometry seems likely to establish a standard place in the diagnostic armamentarium.—R.M. Crowell, M.D.

The Use of a Panel of Monoclonal Antibodies in the Evaluation of Cytologic Specimens From the Central Nervous System
Vick WW, Wikstrand CJ, Bullard DE, Kemshead J, Coakham HB, Schlom J, Johnston WW, Bigner DD, Bigner SH (Duke Univ; Inst of Child Health, London; Frenchay Hosp, Bristol, England; Natl Cancer Inst, Bethesda, Md)
Acta Cytol 31:815–824, November–December 1987   17–14

The role of cytopathology is becoming more important in the diagnosis of intracranial masses. Monoclonal antibody technology is a means of generating reagents with single epitope specificity, reproducible reliability, and capacity for large supply. A panel of 4 monoclonal antibodies was tested immunohistochemically to determine the efficacy of such reagents in distinguishing among metastatic carcinoma, lymphoma, leukemia, and primary brain tumors.

The antibodies used were a cocktail comprised of 3 antiglial fibrillary acidic protein antibodies (α-GFAP); UJ13A, a pan-neuroectodermal antibody; B72.3, which recognizes a carcinoma-distinctive tumor-associated glycoprotein complex; and 2D1, a pan-leukocyte antibody. Fifty-three specimens were obtained from 21 gliomas, 2 meningiomas, 1 pineoblas-

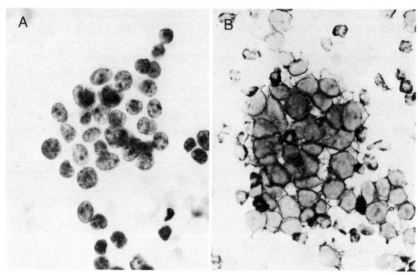

Fig 17–6.—Needle washing specimen obtained from a 4-year-old girl with a pineoblastoma. **A,** Papanicolaou-stained cytocentrifuge preparation reveals tumor cells with a high nuclear-cytoplasmic ratio (original magnification, × 1,000). **B,** air-dried cytospin preparation stained with UJ13A reveals tumor cells showing intense staining of thin cytoplasmic rims (original magnification, × 680). (Courtesy of Vick WW, Wikstrand CJ, Bullard DE, et al: *Acta Cytol* 31:815–824, November–December 1987.)

toma, 11 metastatic tumors, 3 lymphomas, 1 leukemia, and 14 patients without tumor. The specimens were 21 cerebrospinal fluids, 1 ventricular fluid, 2 brain cyst fluids, 12 needle washings, 15 imprints, 1 subdural fluid, and 1 postshunt fluid. The α-GFAP stained all gliomas and all specimens containing reactive brain fragments. The UJ13A had a reactivity pattern comparable to that of α-GFAP but also stained the meningiomas, pineoblastoma (Fig 17–6), oat-cell carcinoma, and embryonal rhabdomyosarcoma. The B72.3 stained all the adenocarcinomas and the large cell carcinoma. The 2D1 stained the lymphoma and leukemia, all inflammatory cells, and 4 of the 12 glioblastomas.

Four monoclonal antibodies were tested to ascertain the utility of such reagents in distinguishing among metastatic carcinoma, lymphoma, leukemia, and primary brain tumors. Although no single antibody was diagnostic of a specific tumor type, the panel of 4 accurately differentiated among most primary brain tumors, metastases, leukemias, and lymphomas.

▶ A panel of antibodies can be used for diagnosis of intracranial tumors by testing CSF or other small specimens. Although the panel as yet cannot distinguish between certain types of tumors (for example, adenocarcinoma from a breast primary as opposed to a lung primary), ongoing research in this area is likely to increase the diagnostic specificity of such examinations. This is especially important in this area of increasing utilization of CT-guided stereotactic biopsy.—R.M. Crowell, M.D.

Brief Notes on Cytology

Cerebrospinal fluid may be screened for carcinoembryonic antigen (CEA). Sixteen of 18 meningeal carcinomatosis cases were positive, although only 47% of intraparenchymal carcinomas were detected. Seven of 54 primary brain tumors were positive for CEA. (Jacobi C, Felgenhauer K: *J Neurol* 233:358–361, 1986).

The monoclonal antibody Ki-67 appears to be a useful technique for identification of proliferating tumor cells (Burger PC, et al: 10:611–617, 1986).

Immunoperoxidase labeled antibody is useful in the differential diagnosis of CNS hemangioblastoma and renal cell carcinoma (Andrew SM, Gradwell E: *J Clin Pathol* 39:917–919, 1986).

A brain protein has been cloned identified with autoantibodies for a patient with paraneoplastic cerebellar degeneration (Dropcho EJ, et al: *Proc Natl Acad Sci USA* 84:4552–4556, 1987).

Both S-100 and GFAP were demonstrated in retinoblastomas (Schroder HD: *Virchows Arch* A 411:67–72, 1987).—R.M. Crowell, M.D.

18 Techniques

Introduction

Balloon catheters have evolved with remarkable rapidity and increasing clinical efficacy. At a recent course at New York University, Hieshima and colleagues from the University of California, San Francisco, described experience with more than 200 cases of intra-aneurysmal silicone balloon obliteration of intracranial aneurysms. An experience of more than 600 cases has been accumulated with intra-aneurysmal detachable balloon obliteration of aneurysms by Shcheglov in Kiev, with preservation of 80% of the parent intracranial arteries. Schmidek and colleagues intend to evaluate this Kiev system in North America. Although the results are promising, careful validation of these techniques, with meticulous reporting of both successes and complications, will be necessary to establish this methodology for widespread use in this country.

Percutaneous transluminal angioplasty of subclavian arteries has been achieved successfully with balloon catheters (Abstract 18–1). Balloon catheter technology has also been used successfully for the treatment of carotid-cavernous fistula (Abstract 18–2), dural fistulas involving the cavernous sinus (Abstract 18–3), and vertebral arteriovenous fistulas (Abstract 18–4). Preoperative balloon occlusion of feeders to arteriovenous malformations has facilitated surgical excision of these lesions (Abstract 18–5). Experimental studies have shown that injection of fibrin sealant can occlude experimental aneurysms in the rabbit, and present catheter systems could conceivably deliver such obliterating substances in human aneurysms (Abstract 18–6).

Radiation therapy has been applied in new ways. Follow-up data indicate the efficacy of radiation therapy in the treatment of partially resected meningiomas (Abstract 18–7) and acoustic neurilemomas (Abstract 18–8). Primary radiotherapy of prolactinomas produced encouraging results (Abstract 18–9). Stereotactic intercavitary irradiation for acystic craniopharyngiomas has posted encouraging results (Abstract 18–10). Brachytherapy of recurrent tumors of the skull base and spine with iodine-125 sources seems a promising method of treating otherwise incurable recurrent neoplasms (Abstract 18–11). However, radiation can occasionally produce neoplasms of the brain (Abstract 18–12). In addition, focused-beam stereotactic radiation of the brain may induce radiation changes in the brain, some reversible and some permanent. An in vitro model for the response to irradiation of different types of human intracranial tumors has been developed and may be useful in the specific tailoring of radiation treatment plans for individual patients (Abstract 18–13).

Stereotactic surgery has advanced in several areas. Transcerebellar biopsy in the posterior fossa has been performed in 29 cases over 12 years using the Leksell system (Abstract 18–14). CT-stereotactic drainage of colloid cyst in the foramen of Monro and third ventricle has been reported in 12 successful cases (Abstract 18–15).

In other technical studies, transoral dural closure is facilitated by a fibrin glue patch (Abstract 18–16). New techniques are described for the closure of extensive and complicated laminectomy wounds (Abstract 18–17).

Robert M. Crowell, M.D.

Balloon Catheters

Percutaneous Transluminal Angioplasty of Subclavian Arteries

Burke DR, Gordon RL, Mishkin JD, McLean GK, Meranze SG (Univ of Pennsylvania, Philadelphia; Hadassah Med Ctr, Hebrew Univ of Jerusalem, Israel)
Radiology 164:699–704, September 1987   18–1

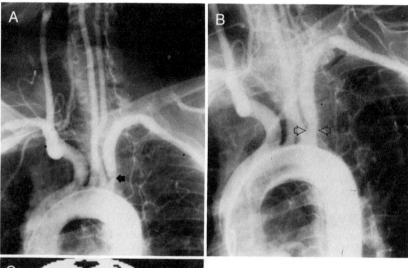

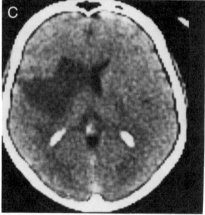

Fig 18–1.—Images of a 49-year-old man with ischemic symptoms in the left arm. *Arrows* indicate stenotic lesion. **A,** aortogram demonstrates left subclavian artery stenosis with separate origin of the left vertebral artery. **B,** post-percutaneous transluminal angioplasty (PTA) angiogram reveals excellent results, but the patient sustained a right hemispheric stroke immediately after angiography. **C,** head computed tomography scan 3 days after PTA demonstrates stroke in right middle cerebral distribution. (Courtesy of Burke DR, Gordon RL, Mishkin JD, et al: *Radiology* 164:699–704, September 1987.)

Thirty subclavian angioplasties were attempted in 27 patients. Eight patients had neurologic symptoms only, 6 had arm symptoms, and 9 had both. Two other patients had leg claudication, 1 had angina, and 1 had no symptoms. Dizziness and vertigo were the most prevalent neurologic symptoms. All subclavian artery stenoses were proximal to the vertebral artery origin. Angioplasty was done from either a femoral or axillary approach. Heparin was used in 9 instances before balloon inflation.

Three procedures failed, all involving high-grade stenoses at the left subclavian origin. Two patients had embolic complications (Fig 18–1). Two procedures were considered clinical failures. Presenting symptoms were completely relieved after angioplasty in 17 patients and 2 others improved significantly. Patients remained well on follow-up for 3 years, except for 1 with a stroke and another with labyrinthitis. The outcome was not related to the degree of stenosis, lesion length, or the postangioplasty angiographic appearance.

Percutaneous angioplasty and the subclavian artery is a technically feasible and relatively safe treatment where flow is compromised. Long-term symptomatic improvement is expected.

► This report sustains enthusiasm for angioplasty of subclavian stenosis (Motarjeme: *Radiology* 155:612–613, 1985; Ringelstein B: *Neuroradiology* 26:189, 1984). There were 3 technical failures and 2 embolic complications, 1 leading to a permanent left hemiplegia. Twenty-five of 28 noted immediate relief of symptoms, with late recurrence in only 2.

Thus, the method appears to have a low morbidity and no mortality with a high rate of clinical effectiveness. The precise impact of the procedure remains unknown because of the protean nature of clinical symptomatology in patients with varied collateral circulatory patterns. However, the major alternative therapy, carotid subclavian bypass, although highly effective, carries a significant morbidity and mortality (Herring M: *Am Surg* 43:220–228, 1977). Thus, angioplasty is probably the initial procedure of choice for symptomatic subclavian stenosis.—R.M. Crowell, M.D.

Indications for Treatment and Classification of 132 Carotid-Cavernous Fistulas
Debrun GM, Viñuela F, Fox AJ, Davis KR, Ahn HS (The Johns Hopkins Med Insts, Baltimore, Md; Univ of California, Los Angeles; Univ Hospital, London Ont; Harvard Univ)
Neurosurgery 22:285–289, 1988   18–2

Angiographic classification of carotid-cavernous fistulas (CCFs) depends on the velocity of blood flow through the shunt and the anatomical origin of the arteries supplying the cavernous sinus fistula. Barrow and coworkers identified 4 categories of CCFs on the basis of these criteria and on etiology, traumatic or spontaneous. Their classification was used for indications for treatment in 132 patients with CCFs.

According to the Barrow classification, type A patients have fast flow fistulas that are manifest by a direct connection between the internal carotid arterial siphon and the cavernous sinus through a single tear in the arterial wall. The best therapy is obliteration of the connection by a detachable balloon; 92 of 95 patients with traumatic CCFs were treated in this fashion. Direct surgical exposure of the cervical or cavernous internal carotid artery was performed in the remaining 3 patients, who had undergone unsuccessful surgical trapping. Three ruptured cavernous aneurysms and 2 spontaneous CCFs also had type A connections. Slow flow, spontaneous dural arteriovenous malformations are classified as types B, C, and D on the basis of arterial supply. Four type C cases were identified in the 37 patients with spontaneous CCFs. All were in patients aged younger than 30 years and were shunts between the middle meningeal artery and the cavernous sinus. There were 28 cases of type D CCFs, which possess meningeal feeders from both the internal and external carotid arteries, often from both sides. Several embolizations of the external carotid branches were performed, but the fistula was only eradicated in 12 of 25 patients; 3 cured spontaneously.

▶ For high flow spontaneous carotid-cavernous fistulas (Barrow type A), detachable balloon occlusion of the fistula, with preservation of the carotid, is highly effective and safe. For slow flow lesions, (Barrow types B–D), this approach is significantly less effective. For the majority of these lesions, balloon treatment by an experienced interventionist is the treatment of choice. Only occasionally will surgical intervention be needed for exposure of the carotid artery above a previous occlusion, or for exposure of the cavernous sinus intracranially.— R.M. Crowell, M.D.

Dural Fistulas Involving the Cavernous Sinus: Results of Treatment in 30 Patients
Halbach VV, Higashida RT, Hieshima GB, Reicher M, Norman D, Newton TH (Univ of California, San Francisco; Radiology Med Group, San Diego)
Radiology 163:437–442, May 1987   18–3

Indirect carotid cavernous fistulas (CCFs) are communications between the dural branches of the internal and external carotid artery and cavernous sinus. They occur most often in elderly women and generally cause fewer symptoms than direct CCFs. However, some indirect CCFs may have more severe symptoms. The results of treatment of 30 indirect CCFs were reported.

The CCFs occurred in 22 women and 8 men, aged 22–75 years (mean, 47 years). All patients were followed up at 1 month, 6 months, and yearly intervals after treatment. A variety of treatment modalities were used. Combined carotid artery and jugular vein compression completely cured 7 of 23 patients, or 30%, and improved 1 patient's condition. No complications were associated with this treatment. Patients in whom carotid jugular compression therapy failed or who had corticol venous drainage or visual decline were treated with intravascular embolization.

Embolization completely cured 17 of 22, or 77%, and improved 4 additional patients' conditions. One patient needed surgical excision of the involved dura after embolization to achieve complete cure. The 1 permanent complication that occurred was stroke, resulting in mild weakness caused by clot formation on a catheter.

In this series, carotid compression therapy resulted in complete cure in 30% of patients treated. This modality can also be used as an adjunct to subtotal embolization to obtain further thrombosis.

▶ This communication throws further light on the problem of low flow carotid cavernous fistulas. These lesions show only a small amount of arteriovenous shunting, which may come from the external carotid or internal carotid arteries draining into the cavernous sinus. Carotid compression therapy is an interesting concept and deserves further study. However, there are certainly hazards to this practice, including embolization from carotid occlusive disease. In addition, it is possible that these lesions would have thrombosed without such therapy, and the efficacy of this method is not established by this communication. The authors are certainly correct to emphasize the relatively benign nature of the lesion and therefore the appropriateness of low-risk therapy, which may not achieve complete angiographic obliteration.—R.M. Crowell, M.D.

Treatment of Vertebral Arteriovenous Fistulas

Halbach VV, Higashida RT, Hieshima GB (Univ of California, San Francisco)
AJR 150:405–412, February 1988   18–4

Vertebral arteriovenous fistulas, abnormal connections between the extracranial vertebral artery or its branches and neighboring veins, are uncommon lesions. These fistulas are usually caused by penetrating neck injuries. The results of treatment of 20 patients with vertebral arteriovenous fistulas by transvascular embolization techniques were reported.

Of the fistulas treated, 8 were spontaneous; 6, traumatic without vertebral artery transection; and 6, traumatic with vertebral artery transection. Transvascular embolization techniques resulted in complete fistula closure in all patients. The fistulas were at C-1–C-2 in 45% of the cases, C-2–C-3 in 25%, C-4–C-5 in 15%, C-5–C-6 in 10%, and C-6–C-7 in 5%. Thirty percent were caused by knife wounds, 20% by gunshot wounds, and 10% by blunt trauma. Two of the 8 spontaneous fistulas were associated with fibromuscular dysplasia. Three patients with large, long-standing fistulas developed neurologic deficits coincident with the abrupt closure of the fistula, which resolved with reestablishment of fistula flow. Two of these patients were treated by staged closure, and the third was treated by gradual closure. Complete fistula closure without neurologic complications resulted in all 3 cases. The remaining spontaneous fistulas were closed by balloon embolization with preservation of vertebral artery and no deficits. The 6 patients with traumatic fistulas without transection were treated with balloon embolization without deficits.

Vertebral flow was preserved in 4. The remaining 6 patients with traumatic fistulas with transection were cured by balloon embolization, with flow preservation in 2. Four patients needed bilateral approaches to the fistula to achieve complete fistula closure. Only one complication occurred—a mild residual Wallenberg syndrome after occlusion of the posterior inferior cerebellar artery in the treatment of a transection at CT.

Transvascular balloon embolization is recommended as the treatment of choice for vertebral fistulas. It is often possible to preserve vertebral arterial flow in patients with spontaneous or traumatic fistulas without transections. Patients with long-standing fistulas may be at risk for neurologic deficit if occlusion is abrupt. In patients with transection, a trapping procedure is often needed to achieve complete fistula closure.

▶ Results of treatment in 20 patients indicate that transvascular balloon embolization is the treatment of choice for vertebral fistulas. In patients without transections, preservation of the parent vertebral artery is often possible. In patients with long-standing fistulas, staged vascular occlusion may be necessary to avoid neurologic deficit.—R.M. Crowell, M.D.

Preoperative Balloon Occlusion of Arteriovenous Malformations
Halbach VV, Higashida RT, Yang P, Barnwell S, Wilson CB, Hieshima GB (Univ of California, San Francisco, Univ of Arizona, Tucson)
Neurosurgery 22:301–308, 1988   18–5

Many materials have been used to embolize cerebral arteriovenous malformations (AVMs) before surgery. Specific vascular anatomy with large feeding vessels deep to the nidus or aneurysms in feeding arteries are better treated with detachable balloons than with other embolic agents. Such balloons permit test occlusion of a vascular pedicle before permanent occlusion and can obliterate aneurysms in feeding arteries. A study was done to define the unique situations in which preoperative balloon embolization is advantageous and to summarize the results of 36 feeder arterial balloon occlusions performed.

From 1980 to 1986, 31 patients with AVMs underwent 36 feeder arterial occlusions by transvascular balloon techniques. The patients were 15 females and 16 males, aged 11–60 years. Twenty-nine patients subsequently underwent surgical resection. None of the patients developed normal perfusion pressure breakthrough or needed blood transfusions. The neurosurgeon judged the preoperative balloon occlusion to decrease significantly the difficulty in surgical resection of the malformation. The remaining 2 patients had embolization before radiosurgery. One had aneurysms in the feeding artery, which was balloon-occluded to reduce the risk of hemorrhage. Two neurologic deficits and 3 asymptomatic arterial dissections were related to the balloon procedure. Illustrative case examples were given (Fig 18–2).

Balloon occlusion of arteries supplying AVMs was found to be a useful technique preoperatively. Using this technique is especially appropriate

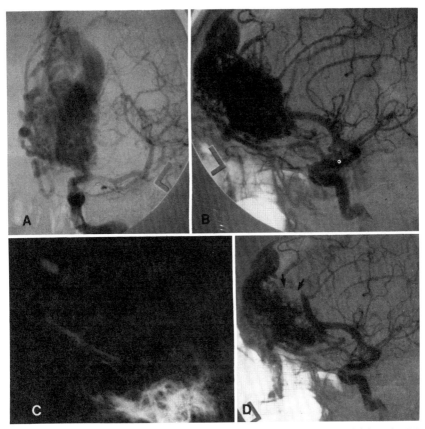

Fig 18–2.—A 19-year-old woman with a parenchymal hemorrhage secondary to a left frontal AVM. Left internal carotid artery injection, anteroposterior (**A**) and lateral (**B**) view, shows a large frontal lobe AVM with anterior venous drainage to the superior sagittal sinus and mass effect secondary to the recent hemorrhage. A plain film in a lateral (**C**) view during test occlusion of the frontopolar branch of the anterior cerebral artery shows the inflated balloon attached to the microcatheter. Left internal carotid injection, lateral view (**D**) post embolization, shows that the frontopolar artery has been occluded by a balloon *(arrows)*, with decreased supply to the AVM. (Courtesy of Halbach VV, Higashida RT, Yang P, et al: *Neurosurgery* 22:301–308, 1988.)

when surgical ligation of the arterial supply is difficult or normal perfusion breakthrough is possible.

▶ This report from the University of California, San Francisco, demonstrates the utility of preoperative arterial feeder occlusion with balloon catheters. Thirty-six arterial feeders were occluded in 31 patients with significant decrease in the difficulty of surgical resection in 29 cases. Two neurologic deficits and 3 asymptomatic arterial dissections were related to the balloon procedure. Normal pressure perfusion breakthrough and blood transfusion were avoided in these cases.

This technique is particularly appropriate in cases inappropriate for particle embolization because of large feeders. Inoperable lesions destined for radiosurgical treatment may also be prepared in this fashion. Obviously, an expert team of interventional radiologists and neurosurgeons is necessary for this type of management.— R.M. Crowell, M.D.

Experimental Aneurysms in the Rabbit: Occlusion by Intrasaccular Injection of Fibrin Sealant

Moringlane JR, Grote R, Vonnahme FJ, Mestres P, Harbauer G, Ostertag CB (Univ of the Saarland, Saar, West Germany)
Surg Neurol 28:361–366, 1987   18–6

Studies have shown that acrylate injection produces good results in the treatment of aneurysms. However, this treatment is associated with the danger of embolization into the parent vessel and many other disadvantages. The fibrin sealant Tissucol may be a more suitable substance for the study of aneurysm thrombosis. A study was done to investigate the sequential changes of a fibrin clot in experimentally induced aneurysms.

Twenty-nine aneurysms were produced in 29 rabbits using the microsurgical technique of grafting a venous sack onto the artery in the neck of the rabbits after the removal of an elliptical piece of arterial wall. Twenty-five aneurysms were occluded with Tissucol. On microscopic examination, complete resorption of the fibrin clot and the formation of dense granulation tissue within the aneurysm, which was covered with a layer of endothelial cells after 2 weeks, were observed (Fig 18–3).

In this study, resorption of the fibrin tissue adhesive injected into the experimental aneurysms occurred. It was replaced by a dense granulation tissue delineated by an endothelial cell layer, irrespective of whether the occlusion of the aneurysm was complete or partial. The results of this study are only tentative and further research is needed.

▶ In animal studies, experimental aneurysms were occluded in 25 of 29 cases by direct injection of a fibrin sealant that was replaced with granulation and endothelial cells after 2 weeks. With the rapid effective development of catheter systems for percutaneous entry into aneurysms, the potential for utilization of such a tissue sealant comes closer to reality. Further experimental studies will be needed to demonstrate whether such an approach can be effective and safe in patients.— R.M. Crowell, M.D.

Detachable Balloons for Aneurysms

The group from London, Ontario, has reviewed their experience with proximal balloon occlusion of carotid or vertebral artery in 68 cases with inaccessible aneurysm. Thrombosis of the aneurysm was achieved in 76.9%. There was delayed ischemia in 12.3%, but medical hyperperfusion almost always eliminated the deficits (1.5% residual). The use of cerebral blood flow studies to guide therapy, mannitol to increase CBF, and heparin to minimize embolization may further improve results of blood occlusion for aneurysm.

Hieshima and colleagues recently reported successful obliteration of a

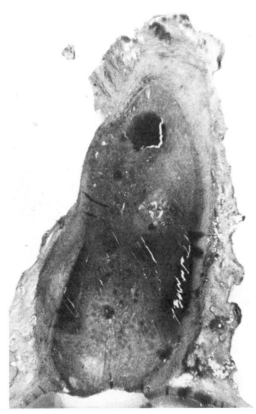

Fig 18–3.—Longitudinal section of the aneurysm after occlusion with a fibrin clot. Height, 7 mm; width, 4 mm. (Courtesy of Moringlane JR, Grote R, Vonnahme FJ, et al: *Surg Neurol* 28:361–366, 1987.)

large mid-basilar aneurysm. This approach requires transvascular introduction of detachable balloons into the aneurysm, test balloon occlusion of brain arteries in awake patients, and utilization of solidifying polymers to preclude deflation. At a recent symposium on interventional radiology at New York University, discussants presented complications such as aneurysmal rupture, balloon embolization, and vascular occlusion with symptomatic infarction.

Although these complications are impressive, several groups have achieved striking success with intra-aneurysmal balloon obliteration. Leading the way is Shcheglov of Kiev, who has utilized this method in more than 600 cases. American visitors have been impressed by what they have seen at the clinic in Kiev. It seems likely that intra-aneurysmal balloon treatment will be advanced in the near future.

Balloon catheter treatment is clearly a group activity. This method is a radiologic technique closely related to catheter angiography. But the patient also needs a neurosurgeon to assess treatment options (including surgery), to participate in decision making on all aspects including balloon occlusion, to treat complications, and to interact with family regarding the complex illness.

Brief Notes on Balloon Catheters

Forty-three cases of pure dural arteriovenous fistulas of the lateral sinus were treated by a percutaneous embolization technique. The benign nature of these lesions should be emphasized (Fermand M, et al: *Neuroradiology* 29:348–355, 1987).

For traumatic carotid-cavernous fistula with failure of transvascular detachable balloons, intraoperative angiography and open ICA catheterization aided successful occlusion of the fistulas with subtemporal transdural insertion of detachable balloons into the fistula with preservation of carotid patency (Batjer HH, et al: *Neurosurgery* 22:290–296, 1988).

In the treatment of dural arteriovenous malformation, transvascular occlusion of the malformation is recommended, with venous graft between the lateral sinus and the internal jugular vein in case of lateral sinus thrombosis (Convers P, et al: *Neurochirurgie* 32:495–500, 1986).—R.M. Crowell, M.D.

Radiation

Radiation Therapy in the Treatment of Partially Resected Meningiomas
Barbaro NM, Gutin PH, Wilson CB, Sheline GE, Boldrey EB, Wara WM (Univ of California, San Francisco)
Neurosurgery 20:525–528, April 1987   18–7

Meningiomas constitute 15% to 20% of all intracranial neoplasms. The recurrence rate of these lesions is significant, especially when the location of the lesion precludes total resection. Although early reports stated that radiation therapy was not effective in treating meningiomas, a growing body of evidence suggests that irradiation delays recurrence of partially resected lesions. To determine whether radiation therapy is beneficial in managing partially resected meningiomas, experience with meningiomas in a 10-year period was reviewed.

The records of all patients admitted to 1 institution between 1968 and 1978 who had a diagnosis of intracranial meningioma were reviewed. Fifty-one patients had gross total resection and did not receive radiation therapy, 30 had subtotal resection and no radiation therapy, and 54 had subtotal resection and radiation therapy. The patients in the 2 groups undergoing subtotal resection were similar in average age, gender ratio, and tumor location. Follow-up ranged from 5 to 15 years, with an average of 78 months. The overall recurrence rate was 27%. Of the patients whose tumors were totally excised, 2 (4%) had a recurrence. Sixty percent of the patients who had subtotal resections and no radiation therapy suffered recurrences, whereas 32% of those undergoing subtotal resection and radiation therapy had recurrences. The median time to recurrence was found to be significantly longer in the irradiated group than in the nonirradiated group. No complications related to radiation therapy were noted.

These findings provide convincing evidence that radiation therapy is beneficial in treating patients with partially resected meningiomas. Total excision afforded the greatest likelihood of curing a patient with an intracranial meningioma. When total excision was not possible, radiation therapy prevented or delayed recurrence of the lesion in most patients.

▶ This contribution adds further support for radiation therapy of partially resected meningiomas. There are methodologic problems with a study that includes potential confounding variables in matching the 2 groups as well as the use of clinical progression as the definition of recurrence (in some cases radiation itself could cause symptomatic deterioration). Nevertheless, this report, combined with others, suggests that localized radiation therapy for residual meningioma is probably of value to the younger patient (Wara et al: *AJR* 123:453–458, 1975; Carella RJ, et al: *Neurosurgery* 10:332–339, 1982). Radiation therapy is probably best deferred until after postoperative edema has subsided, perhaps 3 months. Parenthetically, this report does not support the notion that patients with totally excised meningioma should receive radiation.— R.M. Crowell, M.D.

Efficacy of Irradiation for Incompletely Excised Acoustic Neurilemomas
Wallner KE, Sheline GE, Pitts LH, Wara WM, Davis RL, Boldrey EB (Univ of California, San Francisco)
J Neurosurg 67:858–863, December 1987   18–8

It is not always possible to remove an acoustic neurilemoma totally, making it necessary to decide whether to recommend postoperative irradiation or to withhold further treatment in the absence of progression. Thirty-one of 124 patients received radiotherapy as part of their primary treatment for acoustic neurilemoma between 1945 and 1983. Sixty-two patients definitively treated surgically had total resection, and 15 others had near-total resection. Twenty-five patients received planned postoperative irradiation, 20 after subtotal resection and 3 after biopsy only.

Two patients (3%) had recurrences after presumed total resection. Six of 13 patients had recurrence after subtotal resection without irradiation, but only 1 of 17 patients given more than 45 Gy postoperatively had recurrent disease. Survival was higher after radiotherapy when data were adjusted for deaths caused by intercurrent disease (Fig 18–4). Smaller doses appeared ineffective. Three of 7 patients irradiated for postsurgical recurrence were well at long-term follow-up.

Postoperative irradiation lowers the risk of local progression after subtotal removal of an acoustic neurilemoma. It also may be effective after biopsy, but is not worthwhile when a tumor is totally or nearly totally removed.

▶ This important report documents the utility of postoperative radiation after subtotal excision of acoustic neuromas. Postoperative radiation decreases the

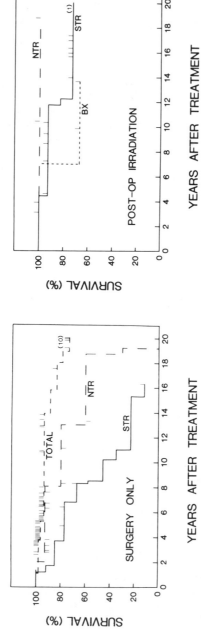

Fig 18–4.— Survival curves for each entire group, not corrected for death caused by intercurrent disease. Three patients treated with irradiation of less than 45 Gy were excluded. NTR, nearly total resection; STR, subtotal resection; BX, biopsy. (Courtesy of Wallner KE, Sheline GE, Pitts LH, et al: *J Neurosurg* 67:858–863, December 1987.)

recurrence rate after subtotal resection from 46% to 6%. The effective dosage appears to be 50–55 Gy, and less than 50 Gy is apparently ineffective. Remarkably, no evidence of complications from radiation therapy were recorded. It may be concluded that for patients with subtotally resected acoustic neuroma, postoperative radiation of 50–55 Gy is strongly recommended.

Ancillary points regard less thoroughly treated subjects: among 6 patients undergoing preoperative radiation for highly vascular tumor, the vascularity was found to be remarkably reduced in all cases, suggesting the utility of this approach. In 3 cases receiving biopsy followed by radiation, none showed progression of disease at 7, 10, and 14 years after irradiation.

The message is clear: neurosurgeons must be aware of the utility of orthovoltage irradiation techniques in the preoperative and postoperative care of patients with acoustic neuroma. Whether stereotactic radiosurgical techniques will have anything to offer beyond this level of efficacy and safety remains to be seen.—R.M. Crowell, M.D.

Primary Radiotherapy of Prolactinomas: Eight- to 15-Year Follow-up
Mehta AE, Reyes FI, Faiman C (Univ of Manitoba; Health Sciences Ctr, Winnipeg, Man)
Am J Med 83:49–58, July 1987   18–9

Little is known about the long-term effects of primary radiotherapy of prolactin-producing pituitary tumors. Eight women with amenorrhea, galactorrhea, and hyperprolactinemia were followed for 8–15 years after primary irradiation. Six had macroadenomas and 2 had microadenomas. The patients received conventional cobalt treatment to the pituitary through 6 portals, to total doses of 4,400–5,000 rad over 4–5 weeks.

Five patients gained normal prolactin values after radiotherapy, but in widely varying periods. Galactorrhea ceased in all patients a median of 2 years after treatment. Four of the 5 patients who became normoprolactinemic had ovulatory menses a median of 4 years after treatment. Hypopituitarism developed in 1 patient; the prolactin returned to the high-normal range in this case. Four patients were considered cured on long-term follow-up. One other patient had remission. Two patients had control of growth; 1 had a recurrence requiring surgical treatment. All patients have retained normal visual fields.

Radiotherapy should be considered as primary treatment of prolactinoma, especially a macroadenoma in an older patient or in a patient who does not immediately wish to conceive. Addition of dopamine agonist treatment after irradiation may be useful in patients with microadenomas.

▶ Mehta and colleagues present detailed data regarding long-term effects of orthovoltage radiotherapy for prolactinomas, with encouraging results. Although the number of cases is relatively small (8 women), the overall results are excellent, with no major complications. Obviously, this approach cannot be offered for patients with pre-existing visual field loss, in which case prompt surgical decompression is required. The method is particularly attractive for the older patient, and the addition of bromocriptine therapy during the period of waiting for radiation effect offers a significant adjunct.—R.M. Crowell, M.D.

Stereotaxic Intracavitary Irradiation for Cystic Craniopharyngiomas

Pollack IF, Lunsford LD, Slamovits TL, Gumerman LV, Levine G, Robinson AG
(Univ of Pittsburgh)
J Neurosurg 68:227–233, February 1988   18–10

Craniopharyngiomas are histologically benign but clinically treacherous lesions. Their attachment to critical cerebral, endocrine, and vascular structures makes radical excision very difficult.

Nine patients with cystic craniopharyngiomas were treated with stereotaxic intracavitary irradiation and instillation of phosphorus-32 (32P) colloidal chromic phosphate.

The 6 female and 3 male patients were aged 3.5–72 years. Serial neurologic, ophthalmologic, neuroendocrinologic, and radiologic assessments were performed before and after treatment. Dosimetry was based on a computed tomographic (CT) estimation of tumor volume, and was calculated to provide a tumoricidal dose of 200–300 Gy to the cyst wall. The follow-up period ranged from 14 to 45 months. After therapy, all patients showed improvement in symptoms and radiologic evidence of cyst regression. Because of an expanding solid component producing recurring symptoms, 1 patient required a craniotomy 14 months after isotope instillation. Three of 5 patients with impaired visual acuity before operation had significant improvement in acuity after ^{32}P therapy. In 4 of 8 patients, preoperative visual field defects improved after ^{32}P treatment. One of 7 patients with preoperative endocrine abnormalities had almost complete normalization, and another had improved endocrine function. Patients who had residual neuroendocrine function before isotope instillation developed no significant deterioration in endocrine status during follow-up.

These results suggest that stereotactic intracavitary irradiation is safe and effective and should be considered as the initial surgery for patients with cystic craniopharyngiomas.

▶ Intracystic P-32 led to improvement in symptoms and radiographic studies in all 9 patients so treated. No significant complications were noted. The reported efficacy and safety in this group of patients corroborates previous encouraging reports of this approach. The method should be considered as the initial treatment for patients with cystic craniopharyngioma.—R.M. Crowell, M.D.

Brachytherapy of Recurrent Tumors of the Skull Base and Spine With Iodine-125 Sources

Gutin PH, Leibel SA, Hosobuchi Y, Crumley RL, Edwards MSB, Wilson CB, Lamb S, Weaver KA (Univ of California, San Francisco)
Neurosurgery 20:938–945, June 1987   18–11

Postoperative radiotherapy can prevent or delay the recurrence of meningiomas, pituitary adenomas, and chordomas. When tumor does recur, however, it can be difficult to treat. Brachytherapy with iodine-125 (^{125}I) sources was used for the reirradiation of aggressively recurrent skull base and spine tumors, or for augmentation of primary conventional teletherapy in 13 patients with rapidly growing, life-threatening extra-axial tumors. All patients had received conventional teletherapy, and most had had multiple resections. Computed tomography was used to confirm accurate placement of the ^{125}I source, and a computer program was used to plan dosing (Fig 18–5). Brachytherapy was used to augment conventional treatment in 2 patients with meningioma.

Implantation of radioiodine sources into basal tumors was technically difficult. Three of 5 chordomas stabilized or regressed, and 2 patients with recurrent malignant meningioma had long-term remission following brachytherapy.

Interstitial brachytherapy for recurrent tumors at the skull base or spine required aggressive surgical exposure of the affected area. It might

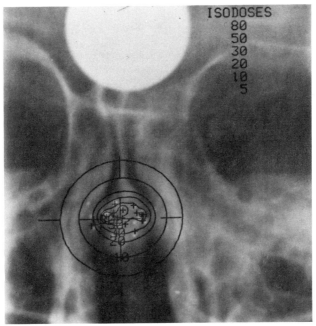

Fig 18–5.—Isodose curves superimposed on an anteroposterior roentgenogram show distribution of radiation doses around sources implanted in the cavity created by resection of the recurrent clivus chordoma. *Curves* represent the total dose delivered from implanted sources. Values for the isodoses are given in gray (1 Gy equals 100 rad). (Courtesy of Gutin PH, Leibel SA, Hosobuchi Y, et al: *Neurosurgery* 20:938–945, 1987.)

be useful to implant a source for a "boost" dose, either microsurgically at initial resection or stereotactically after conventional teletherapy. This approach may be most useful for controlling potentially devastating tumors, such as chordomas and malignant melanomas.

▶ Implanted ^{125}I sources may help to control recurrent skull base tumors. The experience at UCSF with 15 life-threatening tumors was somewhat encouraging, but with the varied histology and tumor burden, the results are hard to interpret. Further work is needed and should be confined to centers experienced in this specialized and potentially dangerous methodology.— R.M. Crowell, M.D.

Radiation-Induced Neoplasms of the Brain
Kumar PP, Good RR, Skultety FM, Leibrock LG, Severson GS (Univ of Nebraska)
Cancer 59:1274–1282, April 1, 1987   18–12

Radiation-induced tumor is a rare but serious complication of therapeutic radiation. Two patients were seen with radiation-induced neoplasms that resulted from therapeutic craniospinal axis irradiation for medulloblastoma.

Case 1.—Girl, 11 months, was seen initially because of irritability, lethargy, and increased difficulty in walking. After discovery of a large midline tumor of the vermis of the cerebellum, craniotomy and partial tumor resection were performed; a medulloblastoma was observed. Postoperatively, the patient received a total of 4,000 rad of cobalt therapy. Twelve years later a secondary neoplasm— an atypical meningioma—was discovered within the original field of irradiation. The radiation-induced malignancy was histologically distinct from the primary medulloblastoma. The patient could not be treated with further external beam radiotherapy, so she received 10 iodine-125 (^{125}I) seeds of 0.34 mCi/seed activity within tissue-absorbable Vicryl Suture placed in the tumor bed. However, the tumor was not controlled with the ^{125}I implant, and she subsequently died.

Case 2.—Boy, 6 years, had a medulloblastoma of the right cerebellar hemisphere. A soft tumor was removed, and the patient received a course of 4,000 rad of cobalt. He remained well until age 29 years, when computed tomographic (CT) examination and subsequent surgery revealed a polymorphous cell sarcoma within the original field of irradiation. The radiation-induced malignancy was histologically distinct from the primary medulloblastoma. Because of initial radiation therapy, this patient could not be treated with further external beam radiotherapy. He received a single high-activity ^{125}I seed in the region of the progressing residual tumor. In this patient, follow-up CT scan at 10 months indicated that the tumor had disappeared and showed no evidence of edema or necrosis in the area of the permanent seed. At 27-month follow-up, the tumor had not recurred. Thus, long-term tumor control was achieved with permanent implant of high-activity [125]I.

It appears that the endocurietherapeutic technique of permanently implanting high-activity ^{125}I can be useful to patients with radiation-induced neoplasms who cannot receive external beam radiotherapy or undergo surgical resection.

▶ This interesting presentation demonstrates radiation-induced neoplasms in 2 cases. The frequency of this occurrence, however, must be very low. Only population studies could provide relevant risk information. Whether implanted I-125 seeds of radioactivity actually help in such cases will also require further validation.— R.M. Crowell, M.D.

In Vitro Model for the Response to Irradiation of Different Types of Human Intracranial Tumors
Fischer H, Hartmann GH, Sturm V, Schwechheimer K, Krauss O, Schakert G, Kunze S (Univ of Heidelberg)
Acta Neurochir (Wien) 85:46–49, 1987   18–13

The wide range of radiosensitivity of tumors of the same type creates problems in designing radiotherapy for brain tumors. An in vitro study of tumor radiosensitivity was carried out in 27 cases of low-grade and high-grade gliomas and 5 cases of meningioma. Tumor specimens were cultured in vitro as tissue cells, tumor cells, or both, and cell survival or growth was used as a measure of radiation response after exposure to 15-MeV x-rays. Radiation effects were evaluated by light microscopy 18–30 days after exposure.

The meningiomas were resistant to doses of 10–30 Gy, but 3 of 5 glioblastomas were reactive to the 20-Gy and 30-Gy doses. Grades II and III astrocytomas and glioblastomas exhibited individual patterns of radiosensitivity ranging up to 90 Gy (Fig 18–6).

Gross differences in radiosensitivity between various types of brain tumors can be demonstrated by this in vitro culture technique. Radiation responses among high-grade astrocytomas and glioblastomas differ widely in individual patients.

▶ The radiobiology of gliomas remains poorly understood (Hochberg FH, Pruitt A: *Neurology* 30:907–911, 1980). These laboratory investigations of tumor radiosensitivity in tissue culture are welcome. The remarkable variability of response can in part be related to sampling problems, in that individual tumors may contain heterogeneous zones of tumor tissue. Whether these methods can be used to guide clinical radiation therapy remains to be proved.— R.M. Crowell, M.D.

Brief Notes on Radiation

Specialized Radiation

A helium-ion beam for stereotactic radiosurgery of CNS disorders is described by the group at the University of California, Berkeley. This unit uses a 230-MeV helium ion beam with uniform field up to 40 mm in diameter and variable depth of penetration from 40 to 140 mm (Lyman JT, et al: *Med Phys* 13:695–698, 1986).

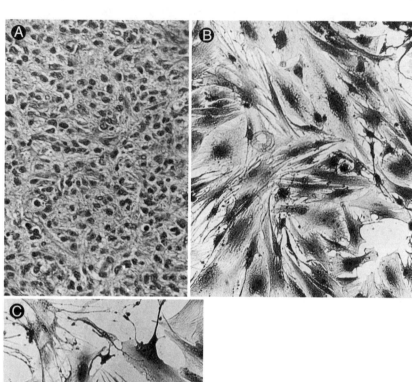

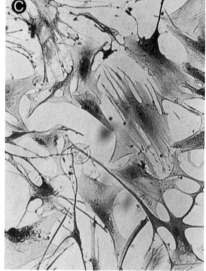

Fig 18–6.—Histology and morphology of cells of a glioblastoma. **A,** section of the original tumor tissue; **B,** tissue culture obtained from a specimen of the same glioblastoma; and **C,** response seen on microscopic evaluation after a dose of 90 Gy, fixed and stained 27 days after irradiation. (Courtesy of Fischer H, Hartmann GH, Sturm V, et al: *Acta Neurochir (Wien)* 85:46–49, 1987.)

Good results in the treatment of Cushing's disease are reported after stereo-tactic radiosurgery to the pituitary gland (Degerblad M, et al: *Acta Endocrinol.* 112:310–314, 1986).

Computed tomography scans show a change in tumor size in 49% of patients after 30 Gy of radiation (Tellkamp VH, et al: *Fortschr Rontgenstr* 147:379–385, 1987).

Complications of Radiation

Four cases are presented with histologically documented glioma in the irradiation field of a previously treated malignancy of a different cell line (Marus G, et al: *Cancer* 58:886–894, 1986).

Magnetic resonance demonstrates radiation effects in cerebral white matter as periventricular symmetric high signal foci mimicking infarction (Tsuruda JS, et al: *AJR* 149:165–171, 1987).

Progressive impairment in hypothalamic-pituitary function occurs after cranial irradiation and can be demonstrated as early as 1 year after RT (Lam KSL, et al: *J Clin Endocrinol Metab* 64:418–424, 1987).

Depression of cerebral blood flow correlates with CNS symptoms brought on by x-ray therapy of tumors (Hylton PD, et al: *Neurosurgery* 21:843–848, 1987).

In 35 cases, radiation therapy of pituitary adenoma was studied. After 4–5 years, this treatment frequently produces deficiencies of pituitary hormones (Snyder PJ, et al: *Am J Med* 81:457–462, 1986).

Forty-nine children with cranial radiation therapy were evaluated by CT. Generalized volume loss was seen in 51%, with calcification in 28%, and white matter abnormalities in 26% (Davis PC, et al: *AJR* 147:587–592, 1986).

In 2 cases of pediatric radiotherapy, pontine calcification could be demonstrated by CT scanning (Price DB, et al: *J Comput Assist Tomogr* 12:45–46, 1988).—R.M. Crowell, M.D.

Stereotaxis

Transcerebellar Biopsy in the Posterior Fossa; 12 Years Experience
Mathisen JR, Giunta F, Marini G, Backlund EO (Univ of Bergen, Norway; Civil Hosp, Brescia, Italy)
Surg Neurol 28:100–104, August 1987   18–14

Many stereotactic systems make it difficult to approach the intracranial compartment from behind. The Leksell system has been used for a transcerebellar approach to biopsy of posterior fossa lesions. Twenty-nine patients underwent this procedure in a 12-year period; 12 were children. General anesthesia was used only for pediatric patients. Transcerebellar biopsy was performed with the awake patient sitting upright; in anesthetized patients, the head was supported by hand or with a clamp or skull traction tongs (Fig 18–7).

More than 1 specimen was obtained from each biopsy target. In only 1 case was there difficulty in interpreting the preparations. Most procedures went smoothly, without serious side effects. One child had more marked hemiparesis after the procedure. An adult patient in whom the burr hole was too close to the transverse sinus suffered a small sinus tear when the dura mater was cut; an episode of air embolism may have occurred without permanent sequelae.

The transcerebellar approach to biopsy of posterior fossa lesions, using the Leksell stereotactic system, is a direct and safe approach to obtaining representative tissue samples. Any intracranial region can safely be approached for stereotactic biopsy if an appropriate technique is used.

▶ Transcerebellar biopsy of posterior fossa lesions appears safe and effective in this relatively large series (29 patients). Even brain stem lesions have been

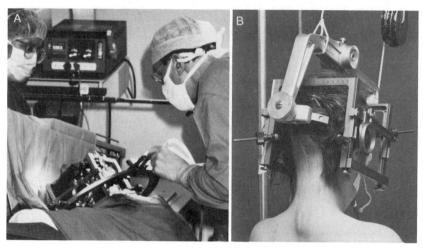

Fig 18–7.—The Leksell system offers alternative positioning of the patient during the biopsy procedure. **A,** awake patient can sit upright, with the surgeon sitting or standing behind. **B,** for children and other patients in need of general anesthesia, the head is supported by a Mayfield clamp. (Courtesy of Mathisen JR, Giunta F, Marini G, et al: *Surg Neurol* 28:100–104, August 1987.)

sampled with good results. This experience is similar to that of Coffey and Lunsford (*Neurosurgery* 17:12–19, 1985).

A transcerebral-transtentorial trajectory may be more risky, but a transcerebral approach avoiding the tentorium has been used with good results (Hood TW, et al: *J Neurosurg* 65:172–176, 1987). The authors stress the need for preoperative angiography to avoid injury to major vessels, and the use of transcerebral trajectories for supratentorial brainstem targets. Although some surgeons prefer to omit stereotactic biopsy when the lesion is highly vascular, the described procedure appears to remove the last barrier to deep brain biopsy for a suspected intracranial tumor.—R.M. Crowell, M.D.

CT-Stereotaxic Drainage of Colloid Cysts in the Foramen of Monro and the Third Ventricle

Mohadjer M, Tashmar E, Mundinger F (Univ Hosp, Freiburg, West Germany)
J Neurosurg 67:220–223, August 1987   18–15

Colloid cysts of the foramen of Monro and third ventricle are rare space-occupying lesions. Twelve cases were diagnosed and treated by a computed tomographic (CT) stereotactic approach. Five patients had an enlarged ventricular system with occlusion of the foramen of Monro resulting from hydrocephalus. Surgery was done under local anesthesia, locating the target point by a CT-stereotactic approach. After the cyst wall had been punctured and biopsies had been obtained for histologic confirmation, the cystic contents were aspirated, and the capsule was irrigated and evacuated. The cyst was periodically demonstrated radiographically with air and contrast medium.

Nine patients had complete evacuation of the cyst, and 3 had partial removal. No complications occurred, and no patient had a worse deficit after surgery. No recurrences were seen during an average follow-up of 42 months after complete evacuation. One of the other patients had a repeat procedure. Increased intracranial pressure resolved rapidly in all cases. One abscess was stereotactially punctured and evacuated.

This is a relatively safe and accurate method of puncturing deep-seated tumors and cysts. Evacuation of colloid cysts now is possible with substantially less risk than before. The procedure is done under local anesthesia. In most instances a shunt procedure is not necessary.

▶ The team from Freiburg reports excellent results with CT stereotactic drainage of colloid cysts of the third ventricle. Evacuation (partial in 3) was achieved in all 12 cases without complications, and no patients required shunting. Surely these results will be hard to beat by direct intracranial attack. If other series are confirmatory, this approach may become the treatment of choice.

Mohadjer et al. report that 12 colloid cysts were drained stereotactically without complications (*J. Neurosurg* 67:220–223, 1987).—R.M. Crowell, M.D.

Brief Notes on Stereotaxis

Stereotactic localization using MRI and CT is better than 2 mm with exception of the Z coordinate (2.3 mm) Wyper DJ, et al: *J Neurol Neurosurg Psychiatry* 49:1445–1448, 1986).

Among 750 stereotactic biopsies, 6 deaths occurred, 3 of which were with pinealoblastoma. (Peragut JC, et al: *Neurochirurgie* 33:23–27, 1987).

Among 35 patients with epilepsy alone and nonenhancing low density lesion on CT, CT-guided stereotactic biopsy yielded the diagnosis in 97% of the patients (Wilden JN, Kelly PJ: *J Neurol Neurosurg Psychiatry* 50:1302–1305, 1987).

Among 45 patients with metastatic intracranial tumors, resection by computer-assisted stereotactic technique led to gross total removal without postoperative mortality. Nine of 10 patients who were normal preoperatively remained so (Kelly PJ, et al: *Neurosurgery* 22:7–17, 1988).

A stereotactic frame is described that is compatible with CT, MR, and DSA for clinical utilization (Peters TM, et al: *Radiology* 161:821–826, 1986).

A 3-dimensional digitizer (neuronavigator) has been described for assisting the operator during CT-guided stereotactic surgery (Watanabe E, et al: *Surg Neurol* 27:543–547, 1987).

Experience with 77 cases suggests that CT-guided stereotactic biopsy was just as effective as stereotactic biopsy (Goldstein S, et al: *J Neurosurg* 67:341–348, 1987).

Cytologic results of 34 fine needle aspiration biopsies of CNS lesions were obtained at the time of craniotomy. Tissue was analyzed using direct smear preparations. Sensitivity of the procedure was 90.7%, specificity 100%, positive predictive value 100%, and efficacy 91%. There were no false positive diagnoses and 3 false negative diagnoses. These results suggest the effectiveness of the approach and its possible utilization by burr hole stereotactic technique (Silverman JF, et al.: *Cancer* 58:1117–1121, 1986).—R.M. Crowell, M.D.

Other Techniques

Comparative Transoral Dural Closure Techniques: A Canine Model

Hadley MN, Martin NA, Spetzler RF, Sonntag VKH, Johnson PC (Barrow Neurological Inst, Phoenix)

Neurosurgery 22:392–397, February 1988   18–16

A water-tight dural closure is difficult to accomplish after transoral-transclival operation for ventral intradural lesions at the craniocervical junction. Such procedures have high morbidity and mortality from cerebrospinal fluid (CSF) fistula, meningitis, and abscess. Three different dural closure techniques were compared to determine whether any technique provides a superior water-tight dural closure after transoral-transclival surgery.

Twenty-two adult greyhound dogs were used. The three dural closure techniques investigated were primary suture closure, laser patch welding, and fibrin glue patch. The primary suture closure technique was found to be inadequate. All 8 leaked CSF during surgery, and 5 had radiographic leaks and were incompetent at autopsy. All 7 of the laser closures were noted to leak CSF at operation, although only 1 was incompetent at autopsy. The fibrin glue technique was superior to both. It provided a solid seal at operation, even with repeated Valsalva maneuvers to 40 mm Hg (Fig 18–8). The immediate, persistent seal at operation was clinically significant because it may prevent CSF leak, meningitis, and abscess in human patients after transoral surgery.

Fibrin glue is an excellent material for patch repairing complex dural defects, especially those created during the transoral-transclival approach to intradural lesions. Fibrin glue was recommended for evaluation in controlled clinical trials.

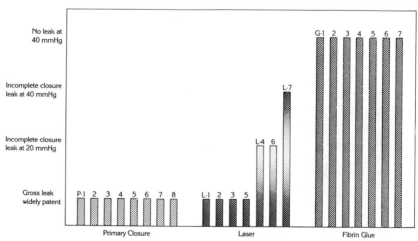

Fig 18–8.—Graphic representation of competence of the dural closure at operation. (Courtesy of Hadley MN, Martin NA, Spetzler RF, et al: *Neurosurgery* 22:392–397, February 1988.)

▶ Fibrin glue was effective in a laboratory setting for dural closure. Extensive experience in Britain reported by Crockard (Am Assn. of Neurologic Surgeons Annual Meeting, Toronto, May 1988) indicates the suitability of this approach in the operating room.— R.M. Crowell, M.D.

Closure of Extensive and Complicated Laminectomy Wounds: Operative Technique
Zide BM, Wisoff JH, Epstein FJ (New York Univ Med Ctr, New York)
J Neurosurg 67:59–64, July 1987   18–17

Radical resection of tumor in previously irradiated patients with intramedullary spinal cord neoplasms can produce a high incidence of wound complications. At 1 center, 9 of 21 such patients developed cutaneous cerebrospinal fluid (CSF) and large pseudomeningoceles after re-exploration. Thus, an alternative method of wound closure was developed.

The success of closure depends on the surgeon's ability to mobilize local muscle and maintain the quality of the muscle fascia. The back was subdivided into zones, and the method of obtaining the layers required for closure at each level was described. Because an irradiated scarred dural closure cannot prevent CSF leakage, closure above the dura must be water-tight. Musculofascial flap layers are mobilized for tension-free clo-

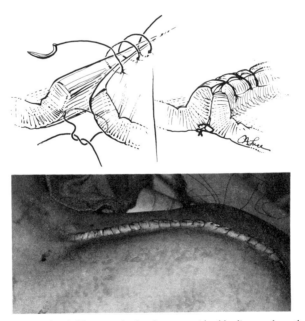

Fig 18–9.—A large absorbable suture is placed at a considerable distance from the undermined wound edges to evert the edges. This provides maximal dermis-to-dermis contact in the event of a cerebrospinal fluid leak to the subcutaneous space. (Courtesy of Zide BM, Wisoff JH, Epstein FJ: *J Neurosurg* 67:59–64, July 1987.)

sure, and permanent 2-0 Prolene sutures are placed interrupted in a modified figure-of-eight fashion. Protruding vertebral spines have to be removed at the upper and lower wound limits to permit proper soft tissue approximation. Prominent transverse processes that may subsequently produce a pressure sore should be removed. The most competent musculofascial layer must be tested by injecting saline through a catheter placed subjacent to this layer. A suction drain should be inserted subcutaneously through a stab incision outside the irradiated field. Large permanent sutures are then placed along the drain track and at the egress site to block the drainage channel after the drain is removed. Skin closure should be greatly hypereverted to maximize dermis-to-dermis contact in the event of CSF leakage into the subcutaneous area (Fig 18–9). This decreases the chances of a CSF cutaneous fistula. These techniques were used successfully in 52 patients to provide closure of difficult wounds. The complications experienced were minor.

A high incidence of postoperative cutaneous CSF fistulas and large pseudomeningoceles after routine closure prompted the development of an alternative technique of wound closure using mobilized musculofascial flaps. The surgical techniques and pitfalls to be avoided during the closure of complicated laminectomy wounds were described.

▶ The NYU Group, with very substantial experience in intramedullary spinal cord tumors, has evolved an approach to successful closure of complex laminectomy wounds. A crucial step is the development of a solid musculofascial layer that can be closed in a water-tight fashion. The authors describe technical pointers that have been successful toward this end.—R.M. Crowell, M.D.

Brief Notes on Other Techniques

Neodymium-YAG laser was used in 42 cases and found to be of value in the treatment of vascular intracranial tumors and metastatic lesions of the spine (Wirth FP, et al: *Neurosurgery* 21:867–871, 1987).—R.M. Crowell, M.D.

19 Tumors

Introduction

Glioma investigations have advanced understanding and management of these common tumors. Stereotactic histologic correlations with computed tomography (CT) and magnetic resonance (MR) abnormalities help the clinician to understand the meaning of alterations in preoperative studies (Abstract 19–1). Further studies of monoclonal antibodies against human astrocytomas indicate the complexity of tumor immunology and the difficulties it faces in clinical application (Abstract 19–2). An antitransferrin receptor antibody-ricin immunotoxin offers encouraging results in the treatment of human gliomas (Abstract 19–4). A controlled study suggests that total surgical resection of supratentorial gliomas leads to improved survival and quality of life (Abstract 19–3). Reoperation appears to hold promise in the treatment of recurrent intracranial malignant gliomas (Abstract 19–5). Implantation of autologous killer lymphocytes seems hopeful in the salvage immunotherapy of malignant glioma (Abstract 19–6). An amplified, highly expressed gene has been identified in human glioma (Abstract 19–8). Synaptophysin appears to be a reliable marker for medulloblastomas (Abstract 19–9). Controversy exists about the effectiveness of radiation therapy for oligodendroglioma (Abstracts 19–10 and 19–11). There is significant controversy regarding the utilization of radiation and surgery in the management of optic nerve glioma (Abstracts 19–12 and 19–13).

In the management of *adenocarcinoma* of the ethmoid sinus, preliminary results indicate relatively successful outcomes for a radical combined ENT and neurosurgical approach (Abstract 19–14).

In the evaluation of *pituitary adenomas*, MRI has proved superior to CT (Abstract 19–15), although CT is sometimes more useful (Abstract 19–16). Gadolinium is likely to make MR the study of choice for pituitary adenoma (Abstract 19–17). Inferior petrosal vein sampling in Cushing's disease is very helpful in guiding the surgeon to the side of the lesion (Abstract 19–18). Growth hormone dynamics and somatomedin-C levels are helpful in predicting the long-term benefit after transsphenoidal surgery for acromegaly (Abstract 19–19). Preoperative bromocriptine treatment does not hamper surgical outcome for prolactin-secreting adenomas (Abstract 19–20). Giant invasive prolactinomas are best managed by debulking and postoperative radiotherapy (Abstract 19–21). Radical resection of craniopharyngioma carries a substantially higher perioperative morbidity compared with conservative surgery (Abstract 19–22).

Regarding *acoustic neuromas,* MRI is very effective for detection of tumor in the internal auditory canal (Abstracts 19–23 and 19–24). With suboccipital craniectomy and meticulous technique under electrophysiologic monitoring, hearing may be preserved after surgical removal of acoustic neuromas (Abstracts 19–25 and 19–26). This approach is not associated with an increased frequency of tumor recurrence (Abstract 19–27). The underlining genetic defect of bilateral acoustic neurofibromatosis has been identified (Abstract 19–28).

Cavernous sinus *meningiomas* are best treated by local resection and postoperative radiation (Abstract 20–1). The histologic and clinical features of malignant and atypical meningiomas have been reviewed (Abstract 20–2).

Robert M. Crowell, M.D.

Gliomas

Stereotactic Histologic Correlations of Computed Tomography- and Magnetic Resonance Imaging-Defined Abnormalities in Patients With Glial Neoplasms

Kelly PJ, Daumas-Duport C, Scheithauer BW, Kall BA, Kispert DB (Mayo Clinic, Rochester, Minn.)
Mayo Clin Proc 62:450–459, June 1987   19–1

The findings on computed tomographic (CT) and magnetic resonance (MR) imaging were correlated with those of serial stereotactic biopsy in 39 patients with previously untreated brain tumors. Twenty-one patients had astrocytomas, whereas 9 each had oligoastrocytomas and oligodendrogliomas. The tumors were classified as type I, consisting only of circumscribed neoplastic tissue; type II, with isolated tumor cells as well; or type III, with intact parenchyma infiltrated by isolated tumor cells. The mean age of the patients was 43 years.

One patient had a type I tumor, 26 had type II lesions, and 11 had type III tumors. Biopsy sampling was inadequate in one instance. Contrast-enhancing areas seen on CT reflected both tumor tissue proper and infiltration of residual brain tissue by isolated tumor cells (Table 1). Hypodensity on CT most often corresponded to edematous parenchyma, usually permeated by tumor cells. The MR abnormalities were more marked than the zone of hypodensity on CT. Tumor tissue, isolated tumor-cell infiltration, and sometimes edema alone served to prolong both T_1- and T_2-weighted MR images (Table 2).

TABLE 1.—Correlation of Histopathologic and Computed Tomographic Findings in 177 Biopsy Specimens From 39 Patients With Glial Neoplasms*

Histopathologic finding	No. of biopsy specimens	Contrast-enhanced computed tomographic finding		
		Isodense	Hypodense	Hyperdense
Tumor tissue	33	2	12	19
Isolated tumor cells	122	34	74	14
Necrosis	7	...	6	1
Normal or edema	15	9	6	...

*(Courtesy of Kelly PJ, Daumas-Duport C, Scheithauer BW, et al: *Mayo Clin Proc* 62:450–459, June 1987.)

TABLE 2.—Correlation of Histopathologic and Magnetic Resonance Imaging Findings in 177 Biopsy Specimens From 39 Patients With Glial Neoplasms*

Histopathologic finding	No. of biopsy specimens	Magnetic resonance imaging finding		
		Short	Normal	Prolonged
T1 studies				
Tumor tissue	29	1	...	28
Isolated tumor cells	108	3	16	89
Necrosis	5	...	...	5
Normal or edema	10	...	7	3
T2 studies				
Tumor tissue	33	...	...	33
Isolated tumor cells	122	1	4	117
Necrosis	7	...	...	7
Normal or edema	15	...	6	9

*T1 values were not available for 5 patients (25 biopsy specimens).
(Courtesy of Kelly PJ, Daumas-Duport C, Scheithauer BW, et al: *Mayo Clin Proc* 62:450–459, June 1987.)

Detection of tumor boundaries on CT and MR imaging and examination of serial stereotactic biopsy specimens are necessary to demarcate glial neoplasms and assess isolated tumor-cell volumes, as well as to determine the spatial extent of each component of a neoplasm. All these data are important in planning appropriate treatment. Solid tumor-tissue components of type I and type II tumors can be resected stereotactically. At present, only external irradiation and chemotherapy are available for treating the infiltrative portions of type II and type III neoplasms.

▶ Contrast enhancement usually indicates tumor; infiltrated parenchyma is hypodense on CT with prolonged T_1 and T_2 on MR. This information is quite helpful in interpreting CT and MR in patients with tumors. However, only tissue sampling can definitively diagnose neoplasm, and serial, multitrajectory biopsies are needed to define lesions for appropriate therapy. Excision is appropriate for an isolated tumor mass, and irradiation or chemotherapy are most appropriate for infiltration. This landmark communication serves to put tumor radiology and therapy on a more sound scientific basis. In a related study, impedance measurements during stereotactic biopsy were correlated with CT scans and showed decreased impedance with low-density regions and increased impedance for enhancing lesions (Bullard DE, Makachinas TT: *J Neurol Neurosurg Psychiatry* 50:43–51, 1987).—R.M. Crowell, M.D.

Monoclonal Antibodies Against Human Astrocytomas and Their Reactivity Pattern

Stavrou D, Keiditsch E, Schmidberger F, Bise K, Funke I, Eisenmenger W, Kurrie R, Martin B, Stocker U (Technical Univ of Munich; Univ of Munich; Marburg, West Germany)
J Neurol Sci 80:205–220, September 1987
19–2

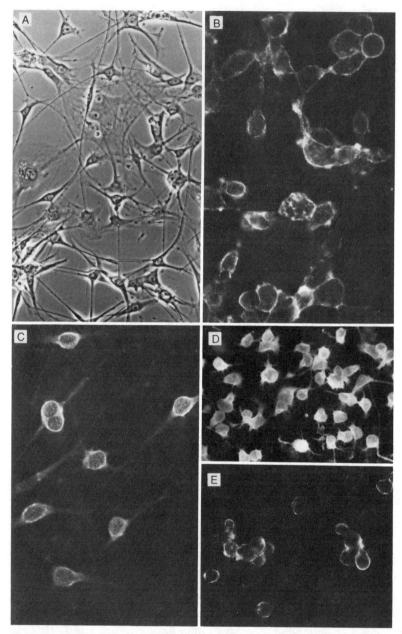

Fig 19–1.—Glioma cell line derived from a human astrocytoma grade III consists entirely of bipolar or stellate cells (**A**). Binding capacity of MUC 2-63 and MUC 8-22 monoclonal antibodies to glioma cells by indirect immunofluorescence staining under different conditions (**B–E**). The unfixed cells (**B**: monolayer; **E**: cytospin preparation) show binding for MUC 2-63 on the cell membrane. Acetone-fixed glioma cells (**C**: monolayer; **D**: cryosection) tested for reactivity with MUC 8-22 antibody demonstrate fluorescent structures mainly in the cytoplasm. (**A–C**: original magnification, ×200; **D, E**: original magnification, ×125). (Courtesy of Stavrou D, Keiditsch E, Schmidberger F, et al: *J Neurol Sci* 80:205–220, September 1987.)

Immunoglobulin-secreting hybridomas were established using cultured and uncultured human astrocytoma cells as antigen to produce molecules for typing intracranial malignancies. Hybridomas were established after fusion of X63-Ag8.653 mouse myeloma cells and splenocytes from BALB/c mice hyperimmunized against human astrocytomas. The animals were primed with either chemically modified or cultured glioma cells, and they received an intrasplenic booster injection 6 weeks after the last immunization and 3 days before spleen cells were prepared for fusion.

Seven hybridoma products reacted with gliomas (Fig 19–1), neuroblastomas, and melanomas, as well as with embryonic and fetal cells. They did not recognize nonneurogenic tumors. Variable antigenic profiles were identified among glioma-cell preparations, using monoclonal antibodies of IgG_1 and IgG_{2a} isotypes.

Distinct antigenic heterogeneity is evident among and within brain tumors, and patterns of antigen expression can change continuously. Monoclonal antibodies that recognize these antigens facilitate the objective typing of intracranial tumors. It is possible that these antibodies could serve as carriers for radionuclides and cytostatic or cytotoxic agents.

▶ The specificity of antibody for antigen has for some time made immunologic approaches attractive for the diagnosis and treatment of brain tumors. However, these efforts have been thwarted by the complexity and diversity of tumor immunology: gliomas carry a wide spectrum of antigens, and the antigenic profile changes continuously. These features of tumor immunology are well demonstrated in the present report. The principle strategy for immunologic management of tumors is the development of correspondingly complex immunologic probes for diagnosis and treatment. Instead of using a single probe or carrier immune complex, panels of monoclonal antibodies may serve as carriers for agents to detect and destroy tumors.—R.M. Crowell, M.D.

Effect of the Extent of Surgical Resection on Survival and Quality of Life in Patients With Supratentorial Glioblastomas and Anaplastic Astrocytomas

Ammirati M, Vick N, Liao Y, Ciric I, Mikhael M (Evanston Hosp, Northwestern Univ, Chicago)
Neurosurgery 21:201–206, August 1987   19–3

The overall median survival of patients with supratentorial glioblastomas or anaplastic astrocytomas is not satisfactory. Such patients are usually treated with surgery followed by radiation therapy and chemotherapy. Thirty-one patients undergoing surgery for these lesions were studied to determine the effect of the extent of surgical resection on the length and quality of survival.

The patients were 20 men and 11 women, aged 23 to 82 years. Twenty-one patients had glioblastoma multiforme; 10 had anaplastic astrocytoma. The tumor was in the frontal lobe in 11 patients, the temporal lobe in 15, and the parietal lobe in 5. The median Karnofsky rating before surgery was 80. Early postoperative enhanced CT determined the extent of tumor resection. Nineteen patients had gross total tumor resection; 12 had subtotal resection. These 2 treatment groups were comparable in age, sex, pathologic condition, preoperative Karnofsky rating, tumor location, postoperative radiation therapy, and postoperative chemotherapy. Median survival for all 31 patients was 53 weeks. Patients undergoing gross total resection had a median survival of 90 weeks, whereas those who had subtotal resection had a median survival of 43 weeks. The 2-year survival rate among those with gross total resection was 19% and 0% for the subtotal resection group: 6 of the 31 patients survived. Three of the long-term survivors had glioblastoma multiforme, and 3 had anaplastic astrocytoma. The mean functional ability measured by the Karnofsky rating was significantly increased postoperatively in the gross total resection group, but not in the subtotal resection group. Patients who had gross total resection spent significantly more time after surgery in an independent status compared with those who had subtotal resection, with a median of 185 and 12.5 weeks, respectively.

This study demonstrated that gross total resection of supratentorial glioblastomas and anaplastic astrocytomas is feasible and directly associated with longer and better survival when compared with subtotal resection.

▶ This paper presents solid data supporting radical excision of malignant gliomas. The authors document a significantly longer survival in patients undergoing gross total resection of tumor; in addition, the functional capacity of these patients was significantly greater. Therefore, a strong argument is made for radical resection of these tumors wherever possible. This recommendation presumably would also extend to many cases that would otherwise undergo only stereotactic biopsy. It should be noted that the present report refers only to supratentorial lesions, and not those involving the posterior fossa or brain stem. Other recent reports bolster this proposal (Shapiro WR: *Ann Neurol* 12:231–237, 1982; Salcman M: *Neurol Clin* 3:831–842, 1985).—R.M. Crowell, M.D.

Potent and Specific Killing of Human Malignant Brain Tumor Cells by an Anti-Transferrin Receptor Antibody-Ricin Immunotoxin

Zovickian J, Johnson VG, Youle RJ (Natl Inst of Neurological and Communicative Disorders and Stroke, Bethesda, Md)
J Neurosurg 66:850–861, June 1987   19–4

Primary malignant brain tumors still have a dismal prognosis, partly because physicians are unable to direct treatment specifically to the tumor. Immunotoxins are hybrid molecules combining the selectivity of monoclonal antibodies with the potent toxicity of tumor-active agents. An immunotoxin made from a murine monoclonal antibody against the human transferrin receptor (TR) and the plant toxin ricin was evaluated in vitro. The SNB75 cell line, from primary explants of a glioblastoma mutliforme, was used in testing.

Highly potent, cell type-specific killing of glioblastoma cells was observed. Cells of the K562 human erythroleukemia cell line also were killed. The immunotoxin destroyed more than half the "target" cells at a concentration of 5.6×10^{-13}M after 18 hours of incubation with the ionophore monensin. The ratio of target-cell to nontarget-cell killing was at least 150. Radioimmunoassay demonstrated significantly higher levels of TR in the glioblastoma cells (as well as surgical samples of glioblastoma and medulloblastoma) than in normal brain tissue.

Immunotoxins targeted to the transferrin receptor may be specific enough to be of therapeutic value in the management of CNS neoplasms involving compartments where transvascular transport would not be necessary. Intrathecal, intraventricular, or cystic lesions therefore may be treatable in this way. Certain tumors, including glioblastoma medulloblastoma, and leukemia, contain abundant transferrin receptors.

► This innovative report presents encouraging data for the use of monoclonal antibody-carrying toxins to brain tumors. An antitransferrin receptor was selected, and since glioblastoma is rich in transferrin, the monoclonal preparation could be delivered to tumors via the cerebrospinal fluid.—R.M. Crowell, M.D.

Reoperation in the Treatment of Recurrent Intracranial Malignant Gliomas
Ammirati M, Galicich JH, Arbit E, Liao Y (Northwestern Univ; Mem Sloan-Kettering Cancer Ctr, New York)
Neurosurgery 21:607–614, November 1987   19–5

Intracranial malignant gliomas generally recur 8–11 months after initial treatment with surgery, radiation therapy, and chemotherapy. Recurrent tumor treatment consists almost exclusively of steroids, additional chemotherapy, and more radiation therapy. Reoperation has been proposed only in selected patients, although its value has never been thoroughly studied. The authors present the results of 55 consecutive patients who were reoperated on for recurrent intracranial malignant gliomas.

The patients underwent reoperation at 1 center between 1972 and 1983. Patients were aged 10 to 70 years, with a median of 48 years. Sixty-four percent of the patients had glioblastoma multiforme, and 36% had anaplastic astrocytoma. The median interval between the first and second operations was 43 weeks. Karnofsky ratings before reoperation ranged from 40 to 90 (median, 70). Twenty percent of the patients had more than one reoperation. The mortality rate was 1.4% per procedure, and the morbidity rate was 16% per procedure. After reoperation, 75% of the patients had chemotherapy and/or radiation therapy. The overall median survival was 92 weeks. The median survival after reoperation was 36 weeks. Patients with Karnofsky scores of 70 or greater, anaplastic astrocytomas, or in whom gross total removal of the tumor was done lived longer than their respective counterparts. The most important inde-

Comparisons Between Pairs of Survival Curves After
Reoperation

Groups	No.	Median Survival (wk)	P^a
Male	34	37.1	0.149
Female	21	34.0	
Age[b] ≥ 40 yr	36	30.2	0.285
Age[b] < 40 yr	19	49.0	
Interval[c] ≥ 6 mo	44	32.9	0.045
Interval[c] < 6 mo	11	64.8	
Interval[c] ≥ 6 mo	44	32.9	0.140
Interval[c] < 6 mo	7[d]	62.0	
Right hemisphere	34	36.0	0.876
Left hemisphere	20[e]	42.4	
Karnofsky rating[f] ≥ 70	40	48.5	<0.001
Karnofsky rating[f] < 70	15	19.0	
Gross total resection	32[g]	51.2	0.006
Subtotal resection	19[g]	23.3	
Anaplastic astrocytoma	20	61.1	0.024
Glioblastoma multiforme	35	29.0	

[a]Comparison between 2 survival curves using the Lee-Desu statistic.
[b]Age at reoperation.
[c]Interval between the first and second operations.
[d]Four patients with an interoperative interval of no more than 8 weeks were excluded.
[e]One patient had a posterior fossa tumor.
[f]Karnofsky rating before reoperation.
[g]Information on the extent of the surgical resection was not available for 4 patients.

(Courtesy of Ammirati M, Galicich JH, Arbit E, et al: *Neurosurgery* 21:601–614, November 1987.)

pendent factors related to survival after reoperation were the prereoperative Karnofsky rating and the extent of surgical resection (table). Forty-six percent of the patients had improved Karnofsky ratings after reoperation, and the 32 patients who were independent after reoperation were able to remain so for longer than 6 months of their survival time.

Reoperation for recurrent intracranial malignant gliomas is feasible, with acceptable mortality and morbidity. When such tumors recur, the combined use of reoperation and adjuvant therapy can prolong good quality life. Patients with prereoperation Karnofsky ratings of 70 or greater in whom extensive resection of tumor is done will have better outcomes after reoperation.

▶ Similar reports from the University of Maryland and the University of California, San Francisco, indicate encouraging results with reoperation for recurrent malignant glioma. In this study, 46% of patients had improvement in Karnofsky performance status, and only 25% of the patients became worse. These results are related to preoperative status of the patient as well as to meticulous radical tumor removal at the time of surgery. Indications for such surgery would appear to be clinical or radiographic worsening in patients with Karnofsky ratings of 70 or above.—R.M. Crowell, M.D.

Salvage Immunotherapy of Malignant Glioma
Ingram M, Jacques S, Freshwater DB, Techy GB, Shelden CH, Helsper JT (Huntington Med Research Insts and Huntington Mem Hosp, Pasadena, Calif)
Arch Surg 122:1483–1486, December 1987   19–6

Malignant gliomas are invariably fatal. Various therapeutic regimens have been developed as adjuvant therapy; at best, however, these regimens have only been modestly successful at extending survival. The preliminary results of a phase I clinical trial of adoptive immunotherapy for recurrent or residual malignant gliomas were studied. The treatment protocol involved surgical debulking followed by implantation into the tumor bed of autologous lymphocytes that were stimulated with phytohemagglutinin-P and then cultured in vitro in the presence of interleukin 2. Fifty-five patients with a mean Karnofsky rating of 64 were treated between February 1985 and March 1987. On the basis of the Kernohan classification, 3 patients had grade II and the others had grade III or IV tumors.

No significant toxic effects were associated with immunotherapy. Fifty patients showed positive initial response, 9 had early recurrences, 5 did not respond to therapy, and 22 patients died. A cohort of 19 patients treated during the first year (February 1985 through February 1986) was available for follow-up. As of April 1987, the mean survival for all patients was 51.0 weeks, and response rates and survival times were substantially greater for patients with a Karnofsky rating of 60 or greater.

These preliminary results of adoptive immunotherapy for patients with recurrent or residual malignant gliomas are encouraging. In contrast to patients treated with lymphokine-activated cells in conjunction with systemically administered interleukin 2, the direct delivery of cells into the target tissue does not allow immediate systemic circulation of cells, thereby accounting for absence of toxicity. In addition, the stimulated autologous lymphocytes represent a much broader range of lymphocytes than does the lymphokine-activated-cell population. During culture, the cytotoxic/suppressor subset (T4−T8+) outgrows the helper/inducer (T4+T8−) and other subsets so that the helper/suppressor ratio is markedly altered after culture.

▶ This represents another preliminary report suggesting a beneficial effect for lymphokine-activated killer cell treatment of malignant glioma (see also Jacobs SK, et al: *Cancer Res* 46:2101–2104, 1986). Certainly, much more detailed and controlled investigations will be needed to establish a place for such novel therapy in the treatment of malignant gliomas.— R.M. Crowell, M.D.

Familial Glioma: Occurrence Within the "Familial Cancer Syndrome" and Systemic Malformations

Vieregge P, Gerhard L, Nahser HC (Klinikum der Gesamthochschule, Essen, West Germany)
J Neurol 234:220–232, May 1987   19–7

Nervous system tumors occur in a familial pattern in the phakomatoses, and a group of hereditary gliomas has been proposed apart from these neuroectodermal syndromes. Data on family of 8 generations were reviewed because of the association of osteochondrodysplasia and other skeletal abnormalities, familial glial tumors in a father and son, and colonic and other adenomatous disease. Pigment changes also were present. The tumor in the father and in the son contained fibrillary astrocytes. Spindle-shaped "sarcoma-like" cells in the arachnoid part of the tumors were shown to be of astrocytic origin. Tumor vessels were abnormal in both cases and caused hemorrhage in 1 of these patients.

This cluster of abnormalities is considered a dysontogenetic process with blastomatous features. It may be classed with the phakomatoses. Dysraphic conditions are about threefold more common in relatives of glioma patients than in controls. The histologic features of the present gliomas did not differ substantially from those of gliomas not associated with neurocutaneous abnormalities.

Some reported "familial gliomas" are associated with other malformations and may be considered examples of phakomatosis. Others occur in the form of a "familial cancer syndrome." The rarity of familial gliomas may reflect the difficulty of determining "formes frustes" in the phakomatoses.

▶ Such a hereditary pattern of brain tumor adds to evidence that genetic defect may underline intracranial tumor, as in the phakomatoses. The detailed biochemical and genetic understanding of the mechanisms of tumor production are particularly well understood for bilateral acoustic neurofibromatosis, where the specific chromosome abnormality has been identified, and it is likely that such approaches will provide further understanding of the genetic mechanisms involved in the production of gliomas as well. One looks forward to chromosomal and genetic studies in these familial glioma cases.— R.M. Crowell, M.D.

Identification of an Amplified, Highly Expressed Gene in a Human Glioma

Kinzler KW, Bigner SH, Bigner DD, Trent JM, Law ML, O'Brien SJ, Wong AJ, Vogelstein B (Johns Hopkins Univ; Duke Univ; Univ of Arizona, Tucson; Univ of Colorado, Denver; Natl Cancer Inst, Frederick, Md)
Science 236:70–73, April 3, 1987   19–8

One of the challenges of current cancer research is to identify additional genes that are genetically altered in human cancers. This study reports on the isolation of a novel gene, termed *gli*, that was amplified more than 50-fold in a malignant glioma.

The tumor was a malignant glioma removed from a karyotypically normal male. Chromosome analysis of the primary tumor and of the cell line established from it, D-259 MG, revealed numerous double minute chromosomes, suggesting the presence of gene amplification. The plasmids pKK380 and pKK354 were used as probes in the Southern blot analysis to estimate the level of amplification in the D-259 MG cell line and in the original tumor. The amplification unit was repeated approximately 75 times per haploid genome in the derived cell line as well as in the original tumor. The gene was located at chromosome 12 position (q13 to q14.3). A large part of the amplification unit was cloned.

A genomic library was constructed from D-259 MG DNA by means of a cosmid vector and screened for cosmids containing amplified sequences that used DNA isolated from double minute chromosomes as a hybridization probe. Of the 48 cosmids isolated, only 4 cosmids contained expressed sequences, and each of these cosmids detected transcripts of the same size in Northern blot experiments. The subclone pKK36P1, which contained the transcribed sequences, detected the transcripts in the D-259 MG cell line grown in vitro or as xenograft in a nude mouse. These transcripts were not found in cell lines from 2 malignant gliomas, a neuroblastoma, a pancreatic carcinoma, and small cell lung carcinoma.

The gene detected by the pKK36P1 clone will be termed *gli* (for glioma). The *gli* gene is a member of a select group of cellular genes that are genetically altered in primary human tumors.

▶ This contribution illustrates the use of modern basic science techniques in human brain tumor research. First, the investigators used chromosome analysis to identify specific sites of chromosomal abnormality. Then, on the basis of these changes, they selected gene probes to further investigate the nature of the genetic abnormality. Further studies come down on a novel gene, which they have termed *gli*. Further studies of this type are likely to expand our understanding of mechanisms of tumor production by alteration of genome.—R.M. Crowell, M.D.

Synaptophysin: A Reliable Marker for Medulloblastomas
Schwechheimer K, Wiedenmann B, Franke WW (Inst. für Neuropathologie der Universität, Heidelberg, West Germany)
Virchows Arch [A] 411:53–59, April 1987   19–9

Synaptophysin is an acidic membrane glycoprotein of presynaptic vesicles that is found in various neurons and neuroendocrine cells and in tumors derived from them. The material is detectable in pheochromocytomas, paragangliomas, ganglioneuroblastomas, islet cell tumors of the pancreas, carcinoid tumors, and medullary thyroid carcinomas. Indirect

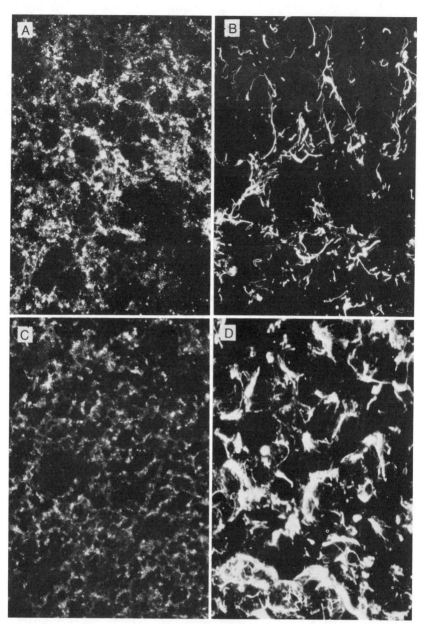

Fig 19–2.—Immunofluorescence microscopy of different types of medulloblastomas. **A, B,** neurofilament-positive medulloblastoma: **A,** synaptophysin immunoreactivity showing punctate patterns; **B,** neurofilament-L immunoreactivity **C, D,** vimentin-positive medulloblastoma: **C,** synaptophysin immunoreactivity with small fluorescent spots; **D,** immunoreactivity for vimentin; original magnification, ×500. (Courtesy of Schwechheimer K, Wiedenmann B, Franke W: *Virchows Arch [A]* 411:53–59, April 1987.)

immunofluorescence microscopy of cryostat sections was carried out using the monoclonal antibody SY 38. Material was obtained from 6 medulloblastomas, 3 neuroblastomas, 1 ganglioneuroma, and 1 glioneuronal hamartoma.

Synaptophysin immunoreactivity was found in all the medulloblastomas (Fig 19–2), typically in a granular cytoplasmic pattern. Immunoreactive neurofilaments were absent in 5 medulloblastomas. Synaptophysin immunoreactivity in neuroblastomas was consistent, and usually strong. In the ganglioneuroma, synaptophysin-positive spots were seen around large ganglion cells, and strong activity was present in the so-called glioneuronal hamartoma. The presence of synaptophysin in the medulloblastomas was confirmed by the immunoblot technique.

Synaptophysin is a marker for both differentiated and undifferentiated neuronal tumors, such as medulloblastomas and neuroblastomas. It is especially useful in diagnosing medulloblastoma, in view of the inconsistent patterns of intermediate-sized filament protein in these lesions.

▶ Immunocytochemical fluorescence for synaptophysin reliably identifies medulloblastomas. The present report, with 6 of 6 histologically verified tumors positive, confirms previous work (Wiedenmann B, et al: *Proc Natl Acad Sci USA* 83:3500–3504, 1986). The presence of synaptophysin in medulloblastomas bolsters the inclusion of these tumors amongst the primitive neuroectodermal tumors (Rubinstein LJ: *J Neurosurg* 62:795–805, 1985).—R.M. Crowell, M.D.

Oligodendroglioma: An Analysis of the Value of Radiation Therapy
Bullard DE, Rawlings CE III, Phillips B, Cox EB, Schold SC, Jr, Burger P, Halperin EC (Duke Univ)
Cancer 60:2179–2188, November 1, 1987   19–10

Significant controversy exists over the role of radiation therapy in the postoperative treatment of patients with oligodendrogliomas. Seventy-one patients with histologically proved oligodendrogliomas were evaluated prospectively. Statistical analysis of population and prognostic factors failed to reveal any significant differences between 34 patients who were treated with surgery alone and 37 patients treated with both surgery and radiotherapy.

There were no significant differences between the groups for symptom-free intervals, time until tumor recurrence, and survival times, nor did radiation appear beneficial for any subgroup. Radiation parameters, including field size, total dosage, and orthovoltage vs. megavoltage treatment, were evaluated for impact on survival, and none proved significant.

For diagnosis and initial treatment, all patients were operated on; 4 patients had total resection of tumor and 67 had partial resection. Eighteen patients had a second operation and 3 had a third. No patient underwent biopsy alone. One or more courses of postoperative radiotherapy was given to 37 patients. The median time until clinical deterioration was 39 months vs. 27 months; the median time until documented tumor recurrence was 27 vs. 28 months; and the median survival time was 4.5 vs. 5.2 years for nonirradiated vs. irradiated patients. Demographic, clinical, and radiographic variables by multivariate statistical analysis showed a poorer prognosis associated with persons of increased age, black persons, and those with papilledema, hemiparesis, intellectual deficits, and necrosis.

Difficulties in evaluating all treatment modalities for oligodendrogliomas include the relative rarity of the tumor, its long natural history, the heterogeneity of the patient population, and the retrospective nature of the comparison. Many previous studies are difficult to interpret because of failure to show that the clinical, radiologic, histologic, and treatment characteristics of the groups were similar. Because of the size, close clinical follow-up, and extensive statistical analysis of the groups, the authors were partially able to obviate these deficiencies. A statistical benefit to radiotherapy for either prolonged disease-free interval or survival was not shown, although the percentage of patients in the irradiated group surviving was consistently higher for the first 5 years after initial treatment.

▶ This study did not indicate a beneficial effect for radiation in oligodendroglioma. In order to adequately assess this question by modern means, a prospective randomized clinical trial will be required.— R.M. Crowell, M.D.

Statistical Analysis of Clinicopathological Features, Radiotherapy, and Survival in 170 Cases of Oligodendroglioma

Lindegaard K-F, Mørk SJ, Eide GE, Halvorsen TB, Hatlevoll R, Solgaard T, Dahl O, Ganz J (Univ of Oslo; The Norwegian Radium Hosp, Oslo; Univ of Bergen; Ullevål Hosp, Oslo; Regional Hosp, Trondheim, Norway)
J Neurosurg 67:224–230, August 1987   19–11

The sensitivity of cerebral oligodendrogliomas to radiation therapy is difficult to assess because of the limited number of cases reported. Thus, the question of whether postoperative radiation therapy should be given to such patients has not been unequivocally answered. All histologically verified oligodendrogliomas in Norway in a 25-year period were analyzed.

Of 208 patients with cerebral oligodendrioglioma treated from 1953 to 1977, 175 had postoperative survivals of more than 1 month. The extent of surgery was known to be subtotal in 126 patients and total in 43 patients. Of this group, 52 patients had subtotal surgery only. Seventy-four had subtotal surgery plus postoperative radiation therapy, and 34 had total surgery plus postoperative radiation thearpy. Radiation doses were known in 66 cases. Survival times were significantly prolonged if postoperative radiation therapy was done. The median survival times of patients with and without radiation therapy were 38 and 26.5 months, respec-

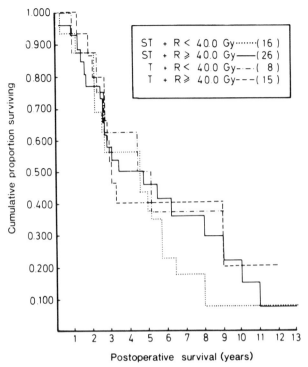

Postoperative survival (years)

Fig 19-3.—Cumulative survival rates for patients with total *(T)* or subtotal *(ST)* surgery correlated with "adequate" (≥ 40 Gy) or "inadequate" (< 40 Gy) irradiation. Median survival times: total resection group with high-dose irradiation (T + R), 36.5 months; total resection group with low-dose irradiation, 60 months; subtotal resection group with high-dose irradiation (ST + R), 57 months; and subtotal resection group with low-dose irradiation, 54 months. (Courtesy of Lindegaard KF, Mørk SJ, Eide GE, et al: *J Neurosurg* 67:224-230, August 1987.)

tively. Five-year survival rates were 27% and 36%, respectively. After 8 years, the respective survival rates were 14% and 17%. Irradiation did not appear to be of benefit after total removal (Fig 19-3). Irradiation doses between 40 and 50 Gy were as effective as doses between 50 and 60 Gy in increasing the probability of surviving 5 years after subtotal tumor resection.

Postoperative radiation therapy significantly prolongs the median survival time but does not influence the cure rate in patients with oligodendroglioma after subtotal surgery. Radiation therapy is not indicated after total surgical removal of the lesion and, after subtotal resection, the radiation dose given should be more than 40 Gy.

▶ This important study adds to the information that supports radiotherapy for patients with subtotally resected oligodendroglioma. The number of cases is substantial (175), the follow-up extensive, and the statistical reporting careful. However, uncontrolled variables such as extent of resection detract from the validity of the study. Only a properly constructed, controlled randomized study with appropriate follow-up can firmly establish the role of radiotherapy in these cases.—R.M. Crowell, M.D.

Controversy in the Management of Optic Nerve Glioma
Weiss L, Sagerman RH, King GA, Chung CT, Dubowy RL (SUNY Health Science Ctr at Syracuse)
Cancer 59:1000–1004, March 1, 1987   19–12

The natural history and best form of treatment of optic nerve gliomas are controversial issues. The records of 16 patients with optic nerve glioma treated between 1961 and 1984 were reviewed. All but 2 patients had extension of tumor beyond the chiasm to the hypothalamus, adjacent brain, and/or along the posterior optic tract. Eleven cases were biopsy proved. In 2 craniotomy and visual inspection were performed but no biopsy was obtained. Biopsy was not diagnostic in 2. Fourteen patients received megavoltage radiation therapy, usually consisting of 50 Gy in 5 weeks (range, 40–56 Gy), 1 patient received chemotherapy only, and 1 had surgical excision only. Follow-up ranged from 1 to 20 years (mean, 7.7 years).

Of the irradiated patients, 7 were alive, 3 died of the disease at 3, 6, and 9 years posttreatment, respectively, 1 died of intercurrent disease at 5.5 years, and 3 were unavailable for follow-up. Overall vision was improved in 5 patients and was stable in 7. Five patients had recurrences, including 1 who was retreated with 30 Gy in 3 weeks and remained free of disease at 20 years. Another patient received no treatment for recurrent disease and had no change in vision or appearance of the mass during the next 10 years. The 3 other patients with recurrence died of progressive disease. The patient treated with chemotherapy showed regression of tumor at 15 and 42 months following therapy. The patient treated surgically had incomplete removal of the tumor and an enlarging mass was observed; enucleation was performed.

Although optic gliomas have been considered benign, congenital, self-limited tumors, they also have a potential for aggressive growth, particularly with the more extensive, posterior tumors. Radiation therapy should be undertaken in tumors with extension beyond the chiasm at the time of presentation, rather than waiting for increasing symptoms, because any vision lost may not be recovered. Treatment with 50 Gy in 5 weeks is effective in halting disease progression in most patients. Chemotherapy needs to be investigated further, but holds promise especially for the younger children.

▶ This series of 16 patients with optic nerve glioma demonstrates that in some cases, particularly those with more posteriorly placed lesions, a progressive downhill course may be experienced. This type of development justifies aggressive radiotherapy. This experience is in line with a more recent review of the experience at the University of California, San Francisco.—R.M. Crowell, M.D.

Optic Gliomas: A Reanalysis of the University of California, San Francisco Experience

Wong JYC, Uhl V, Wara WM, Sheline GE (Univ of California, San Francisco)
Cancer 60:1847–1855, Oct 15, 1987   19–13

The best management of optic gliomas is uncertain. Most reports indicate that these tumors are not self-limiting. Twenty-four of 38 patients seen between 1953 and 1984 underwent megavoltage radiotherapy. Eight patients—all younger than age 10 years—had stigmata of neurofibromatosis. Twenty-seven patients had tumor biopsy, and 3 others underwent exploratory craniotomy. Twenty chiasmal tumors and 4 optic nerve tumors received a mean dose of 4,800 cGy. The mean follow-up was 9.4 years.

One of 4 irradiated patients with optic nerve tumors failed to respond and was salvaged by surgery. Only 9 of 20 irradiated patients with chiasmal tumors failed to respond, compared with 6 of 7 unirradiated patients. Overall actuarial survival at 10 years was 87%, and the relapse-free survival rate was 55%. Radiotherapy improved relapse-free survival with the difference approaching statistical significance, but did not affect actuarial survival (Fig 19–4) (p. 230). Chiasmal gliomas had a poorer prognosis than optic nerve tumors, independent of invasion into adjacent brain tissue. Among patients with chiasmal tumors, those older than 20 years of age had a worse outlook. Only 1 of 5 nonirradiated patients with optic nerve tumors failed to respond.

Optic nerve gliomas carry a relatively good prognosis of survival, whereas many patients with recurrent chiasmal tumors eventually die. Radiotherapy appears to be helpful to patients with chiasmal glioma, and it can lead to improved vision and fewer relapses. A dose of 50–60 Gy to mature brain in 5–6½ weeks is recommended. Tumors confined to 1 optic nerve may be resected.

▶ This report emphasizes that optic gliomas are progressively enlarging lesions with declining clinical status. Although this is not a randomized, controlled study, the presented data suggest improved relapse-free survival with radiotherapy for optic chiasmal tumors. The report lacks modern data with MR scanning. Nonetheless, any alternative treatment program must demonstrate a superior track record as compared with these results.—R.M. Crowell, M.D.

Brief Notes on Gliomas

Glioma Biology

Expression of 3 viral oncogenes has been demonstrated in primary human brain tumors of neuroectodermal origin (Fujimoto M, et al: *Neurology* 38:289–293, 1988).

Intrinsic deficiencies in lymphocytes from patients with malignant gliomas are apparently the basis for failure of mitogen to induce blastogenesis in these cells (Elliot L, et al: *JNCI* 78:919–922, 1987).

Iodine-131 metaiodobenzylguanidine concentrates in neuroblastoma and ma-

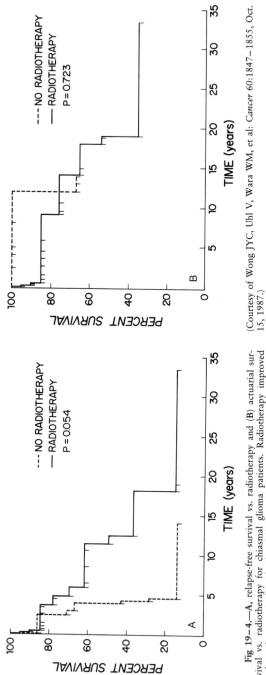

Fig 19–4.—A, relapse-free survival vs. radiotherapy and (B) actuarial survival vs. radiotherapy for chiasmal glioma patients. Radiotherapy improved relapse-free survival with the difference approaching statistical significance. (Courtesy of Wong JYC, Uhl V, Wara WM, et al: *Cancer* 60:1847–1855, Oct. 15, 1987.)

lignant pheochromocytoma, for both diagnosis and treatment of these lesions (Hoefnagel CA, et al: *J Nucl Med* 28:308–314, 1987).

Jacobsen et al. describe 4 permanent cell lines established from human gliomas, with 3 exhibiting striated muscle differentiation (*J Neuropathol Exp Neurol* 46:431–450, 1987).

DNA analysis of glioblastoma multiforme indicates that (1) small anaplastic cells that appear to represent the most aggressive population in glioblastomas have a DNA content diploid–near diploid, and (2) in malignant gliomas the degree of aneuploidy of the main stem line is not related to the biologic behavior of the neoplasm (Giangaspero F, et al: *Cancer* 60:59–65, 1987).

Cerebral endothelial cell growth in vitro is markedly reduced by steroids but not by heparin (Beck DW, et al: *J Neuropathol Exp Neurol* 45:503–512, 1986).

In studies of human brain tumors, both primary and metastatic, excellent correlation was found between the degree of macrophage infiltration on immunoperoxidase staining and peritumoral edema on CT scan (Shinonaga M, et al: *J Neurosurg* 68:259–265, 1988).

Chemotherapy

BCNU and cisplatin cause ischemic damage and are toxic to both retinal and neural tissues in patients with gliomas (Kupersmith MJ, et al: *Neurology* 38:284–289, 1988).

In 81 patients with anaplastic supratentorial gliomas, multiple-agent chemotherapy was not superior to single chemotherapeutic regimens (Mahaley MS, Jr, et al: *Surg Neurol* 27:430–432, 1987).

Chemotherapy is recommended for intracranial endodermal sinus tumor, a highly malignant radioresistant pineal-area neoplasm (Anderson B: *Can J Neurol Sci* 14:166–171, 1987).

A nonrandomized phase II study with a 7-drug chemotherapy protocol indicated median time to tumor progression was 42 weeks, a modest improvement in patients with glioblastoma multiforme (Levin VA, et al: *Cancer Treat Rep* 70:739–743, 1986).

Hematoporphyrin derivative in tissue culture shows almost complete cytotoxicity against human brain tumors at minimum effective concentration (Cohen AM, et al: *J Surg Res* 41:81–83, 1986).

Three patients are reported with sudden onset of blindness after treatment with oral CCNU and low-dose cranial irradiation (Wilson WB, et al: *Cancer* 59:901–907, 1987).

Results of a pilot study suggest that eflornithine and mitoguazone may have a role in the treatment of recurrent primary brain tumors (Levin VA, et al: *Cancer Treat Rep* 71:459–464, 1987).

Supraophthalmic intracarotid infusion of BCNU is said to prevent ocular toxicity (Chrousos et al: *Ophthalmology* 93:1471–1475, 1986).

Wolpert et al. have described a new catheter system for chemotherapeutic infusions distal to the ophthalmic artery (*Radiology* 166:547–549, 1988).

Other Glioma Treatments

Both bromodeoxyuridine labeling indices and flow cytometry of brain tumors can be predictive of biological malignancy of individual brain tumors (Nagashima T, et al: *J Neurosurg* 68:388–392, 1988).

Immunoelectronmicroscopy was used to study S-100 protein positive cells in olfactory neuroblastoma (Choi H-SH, Anderson PJ: *J Neuropathol Exp Neurol* 45:576–587, 1986).

Chemotherapy with procarbazine followed by radiation therapy and hydroxy-urea during radiation was well tolerated and may permit reduction of radiation doses outside the posterior fossa (Levin VA, et al: *J Neurosurg* 68:383–387, 1988).

In a study of 70 pediatric patients with primary thalamic and brain stem tumors, statistical analysis showed survival to be influenced by primary site of disease, extent of surgery, race, cranial nerve paresis at diagnosis, and dose of radiation. Only total radiation dose and race were of prognostic significance (Grigsby PW, et al: *Cancer* 60:2901–2906, 1987).

Previously untreated germinoma is highly chemosensitive. Patients with complete responses to chemotherapy tolerate a significant reduction in radio-therapy dosage without compromising long-term survival (Allen JC, et al: *J Neurosurg* 67:65–70, 1987).

In 4 patients with intracranial tumors, the initial presentation was diabetes in-sipidus, which only later was diagnosed by imaging technique and found to be related to an intracranial tumor (Sherwood MC, et al: *Arch Dis Child* 61:1222–1235, 1986).

Retreatment of pediatric brain tumors with radiation and misonidazole re-sulted in substantial nausea and vomiting and peripheral neuropathy in 21%. Median time to progression was 5 months, and median survival was 13 months. More effective treatment is clearly needed (Wara et al: *Cancer* 58:1636–1640, 1986).

Oligodendroglioma

In 42 cases of oligodendroglioma, only 10 patients survived 5 years; younger patients tended to survive longer than older patients. Focal neurologic deficit at diagnosis and presence of nuclear pleomorphism both were bad prognostic signs (Wilkinson IMS, et al: *J Neurol Neurosurg Psychiatry* 50:304–312, 1987).

Four cases of oligodendroglioma of the lateral ventricle presented with a CT picture of midline nodular intraventricular mass with punctate calcifications and cysts and slight to marked enhancement after infusion of contrast material (Hasuo K, et al: *J Comput Tomogr* 11:376–382, 1987).

The histologic features of necrosis and mitotic count can be used to identify the anaplastic oligodendroglioma (Burger PC, et al: *Cancer* 59:1345–1352, 1987).—R.M. Crowell, M.D.

Other Malignancies

A Combined ENT and Neurosurgical Approach in the Treatment of Adeno-carcinoma of the Ethmoid Sinus: Preliminary Results in 15 Cases
Brasnu D, Roux FX, Fabre A, Menard M, Manolopoulos L, Chodkiewicz JP, Lac-courreye H (Hôpital Laënnec, Ctr Hospitalier Sainte-Anne, Paris)
Ann Oto-Laryngol Chir Cervico Fac (Paris) 104:347–351, 1987   19–14

Because the 5-year survival rate for adenocarcinoma of the ethmoid si-nus using current therapeutic modalities is at most 50%, using more drastic surgical procedures to treat these cases appears to be well justified.

Of 13 male and 2 female patients, aged 50–72 years, with adenocarcinoma of the ethmoid sinus, 11 underwent primary operation and 4 underwent reoperation because of tumor recurrence. Thirteen of the patients were woodworkers. An identical treatment protocol was followed in all 15 patients. Before operation, 3 courses of induction chemotherapy were administered at 21-day intervals. The operation combined a paralateronasal approach to the ethmoid sinus with a bifrontocoronal incision to perform a bilateral ethmoidectomy and reconstruct the anterior base of the skull. All patients received prophylactic antibiotics, which were continued during the postoperative recovery period. Two patients received postoperative radiation therapy.

One patient died of pulmonary embolism 3 weeks after operation. Four patients had postoperative meningitis, but all of them recovered without neurologic sequelae. None of the patients had clinical rhinorrhea. Eleven patients showed excellent recovery after 10 months of follow-up, and 7 patients had excellent recovery after 1 year of follow-up. Three patients underwent reoperation because of tumor recurrence. The survival rate at 1 year was 84% for the newly diagnosed cases.

The preliminary results of this study demonstrate that a combined surgical approach to adenocarcinoma of the ethmoid sinus is justifiable.

▶ This report illustrates a logical neurosurgical and ENT approach to adenocarcinoma of the ethmoid sinus. Although the survival rate of 84% at 1 year is encouraging, significant complications occurred, including meningitis and recurrence in 3. Further data will be needed to substantiate the use of this radical approach.—R.M. Crowell, M.D.

Brief Notes on Other Malignancies

Craniofacial Tumors

Rhabdomyosarcoma of the head and neck has been imaged by CT scanning with resulted improvement in surgical results. The MRI seems promising, but the exact role is as yet unknown (Latack JT, et al: *AJNR* 8:353–359, 1987).

Radical surgery can achieve cure of rhabdomyosarcoma of the pterygoid fossa. A wide bicoroneal exposure down to the mandible preserves the facial nerve within the continuous flap and gives wide exposure at the lateral skull base. Temporary removal of the zygomatic arch provides access to the pterygoid fossa. Skull, mandibular, and maxillary bone adjacent to tumor is readily and safely resected. Craniotomy bone is harvested and split into inner and outer tables to reconstruct bony defects. Morbidity and mortality are low with an experienced craniofacial team (Albin RE, et al: *Cancer* 58:163–168, 1986).

In 24 patients with resection of cranial base tumors, resultant defects have been reconstructed with local fascial flaps, transposition of local muscle, and microsurgical transfer of free muscle flaps (Jones NF, et al: *Br J Plast Surg* 40:155–162, 1987).

The frontalis galea may be used for a myofascial flap in craniofacial reconstructive surgery (Jackson IT, et al: *Plast Reconstr Surg* 77:905–910, 1986).

Studies of the Johns Hopkins Oncology Center indicate that neurologic problems will soon be the most common reasons for hospital admission in patients with disseminated cancer (Gilbert MR, Grossman SA: *Am J Med* 81:951–954, 1986).

Primary Lymphoma

In 23 years, 19 patients with primary malignant lymphoma of the CNS were seen at McGill University Hospitals. All 4 patients who underwent surgery alone died within 2 months of diagnosis. Of 12 patients with surgery and radiotherapy, 11 died at a median of 12 months. The usual cause of death was tumor at brain sites other than those originally involved (Freeman CR, et al: *Cancer* 58:1106–1111, 1986).

Spontaneous clinical and radiologic remission may occur temporarily in primary CNS lymphoma (Rubin M, et al: *Can J Neurol Sci* 14:175–177, 1987).

Thirty-six of 355 patients with non-Hodgkin's lymphoma developed CNS involvement. In 9 patients, extradural tumor compressed brain or spinal cord. Half of these responded well to treatment. In 27 patients, infiltration of the CNS was associated with a poor prognosis (Mead GM, et al: *Q J Med* 231:699–714, 1986).

In 15 patients with histologically proved primary CNS lymphoma, 7 had AIDS. Computed tomogram observations in non-AIDS patients showed hyperdense or isodense masses with contrast enhancement and surrounding edema. In AIDS patients, ring enhancement was often seen. A few cases showed multiple infiltrative nonnodular solid enhancement with extensive edema (Lee Y-Y, et al: *AJR* 147:747–752, 1986).

Central nervous system lymphoma was identified in 96 patients with non-Hodgkin's lymphoma at Sloan-Kettering Cancer Center, and 68 other patients without CNS disease received CNS prophylactic chemotherapy. Cytologic study of CSF was the most sensitive and specific laboratory test. Lymphoma was treated in 85 patients, 46 with intracranial cannulae, and 81% improved. Median survival after diagnosis of CNS disease was 4 months, but there were 7 long-term disease-free survivors, and CNS disease contributed to death in only 14%. Prophylaxis was with methotrexate or cytosine arabinoside, usually by lumbar puncture (Recht L, et al: *Am J Med* 84:425–435, 1988).

Despite surgery, radiotherapy, and chemotherapy, all 6 patients with primary CNS lymphoma died in less than 2 years. (Grant JW, et al: *Arch Pathol Lab Med* 110:897–901, 1986).

Metastases

Fifty of 100 patients treated with chemotherapy showed regression of brain metastases in breast carcinoma (Rosner D, et al: *Cancer* 58:832–839, 1986).

Blood-stain barrier modification can increase delivery of tumor-specific monoclonal antibodies to metastatic melanoma in the brain (Neuwelt, EA et al: *Neurosurgery* 20:885–895, 1987).

Two cases are presented in which CT was superior to MR in imaging metastatic lesions of the brain (Goldstein S, Neuwelt EA: *Neurosurgery* 20:959–962, 1987).

Jacobs et al. present controlled data regarding a possible role for prophylactic cranial radiation in adenocarcinoma of the lung (*Cancer* 59:2016–2019, 1987).

Leptomeningeal metastasis may not be apparent on MR imaging (Davis PC, et al: *Radiology* 163:449–454, 1987).

In small cell lung cancer, brain metastases found at diagnosis did not affect survival statistics (Giannone L, et al: *Ann Intern Med* 106:386–389, 1987).

The high probability of brain metastasis from superior sulcus tumors, regardless of histology, suggests that prophylactic cranial irradiation could probably contribute favorably (Komaki R, et al: *Cancer* 59:1649–1653, 1987).—R.M. Crowell, M.D.

Parasellar Tumors

Comparison of Magnetic Resonance Imaging and Computed Tomography in the Preoperative Evaluation of Pituitary Adenomas

Nichols DA, Laws ER, Jr, Houser OW, Abboud CF (Mayo Clinic and Found, Rochester, Minn)
Neurosurgery 22:380–385, February 1988   19–15

Radiologic assessment of pituitary adenomas can be difficult because these lesions may become manifest clinically when the tumor is still small. Computed tomography (CT) has proved useful in evaluating pituitary tumors before operation, but it has limitations. Magnetic resonance imaging (MRI) has several theoretical advantages over CT.

An experience with high-field-strength MRI and CT in the preoperative evaluation of 20 patients with pituitary adenomas was described. In the study there were 11 microadenomas, 4 macroadenomas, 2 recurrent microadenomas, and 3 recurrent macroadenomas.

Nine of the microadenomas were adequately detected and localized with MRI and 10 were adequately detected and localized with CT. Computed tomography was superior to MRI in detecting a 3-mm-ACTH-secreting microadenoma in 1 patient. Magnetic resonance imaging and CT were equivalent in detecting pituitary stalk displacement and demonstrating cystic degeneration in an 8-mm invasive prolactin-secreting microadenoma.

Both MRI and CT failed to demonstrate the cystic nature of a 9-mm cystic ACTH-secreting microadenoma. Both techniques showed bony erosion that was associated with an invasive prolactin-secreting microadenoma. Magnetic resonance imaging demonstrated invasion of the cavernous sinus better than CT.

Microadenomas were best shown on the T_1-weighted coronal images as focal areas of signal hypointensity. In patients with macroadenomas, MRI and CT were equivalent in detecting the lesions and pituitary stalk displacement, but MRI was superior in characterizing the extrasellar extent.

Coronal T_1- and T_2-weighted images were especially helpful in showing cavernous sinus displacement or invasion (Fig 19–5). Sagittal T_1-weighted images were most useful in showing suprasellar extent and

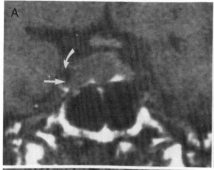
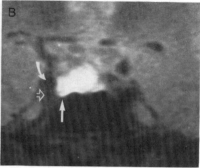
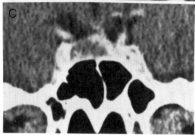

Fig 19–5.—Appearance of an ACTH-secreting macroadenoma. **A,** T_1-weighted coronal image (TR 500, TE 20) demonstrating lateral extension of hypointense adenoma into right cavernous sinus (confirmed at operation). Hypointense adenoma is located inferior *(straight arrow)* to intracavernous carotid artery *(curved arrow)*. **B,** T_2-weighted coronal image (TR 2,000, TE 60) located just anterior to **A.** There are intensity differences among hyperintense adenoma *(arrow)*, slightly hypointense cavernous sinus *(open arrow)*, and very hypointense intracavernous carotid artery *(curved arrow)*. **C,** contrast-enhanced coronal CT scan. Compared with MRI scans (**A** and **B**), cavernous sinus invasion is more difficult to demonstrate. (Courtesy of Nichols DA, Laws ER, Jr, Houser OW, et al: *Neurosurgery* 22:380–385, February 1988.)

displacement of optic pathways. Both MRI and CT adequately demonstrated cystic components of a large glycoprotein macroadenoma.

Both techniques failed to demonstrate a 6-mm recurrent microadenoma that was situated posteriorly, but they adequately showed another 5-mm recurrent microadenoma. Recurrent macroadenomas were adequately detected by MRI and CT, but MRI characterized extrasellar extent better than CT in all 3 cases.

Magnetic resonance imaging was comparable to CT in detecting pituitary adenomas greater than 3 mm in diameter, and MRI may become as good as or better than CT in detecting small microadenomas with the future use of Gd-DTPA. Magnetic resonance imaging was shown to be superior to CT in detecting and characterizing the extrasellar extent of adenomas.

▶ According to these data, MRI is almost always as good as CT in detection of pituitary adenomas. Tiny lesions (3 mm or less) may occasionally show up better in CT, but the addition of Gd-DTPA is likely to make MRI as good as or better than CT even for these lesions. Magnetic resonance is as good as CT for recurrence and better for detection and characterization of extrasellar extent. Kulkarni et al. found that of 37 patients suspected of pituitary tumor, MR detected a focal pituitary abnormality in 83% and CT detected a focal abnormality in 42%. Magnetic resonance is superior to CT in detecting microadenoma (Kulkarni MV, et al: *AJNR* 9:5–11, 1988). Lanzieri et al. report that to differentiate meningioma from pituitary adenoma in the suprasellar zone, evaluation of the superior contour is a reliable sign. A single upward convexity correlated with meningioma (15 of 19 cases), and a multiple upward convex curve correlated with pituitary adenoma (19 of 23 cases) (Lanzieri CF, et al: *J Comput Tomogr* 10:215–220, 1986). Kaufman et al. found that MRI has a high sensitivity for detection of abnormality in the size and configuration of the pituitary gland, but specificity of differentiation of lesion has not been accomplished (*J Lab Clin Med* 109:308–319, 1987).—R.M. Crowell, M.D.

MR Imaging of Pituitary Adenoma: CT, Clinical, and Surgical Correlation
Davis PC, Hoffman JC Jr, Spencer T, Tindall GT, Braun IF (Emory Univ)
AJR 148:797–802, April 1987   19–16

Both computed tomography (CT) and magnetic resonance (MR) imaging were carried out in 25 patients suspected of having pituitary adenoma. Sixteen patients were hyperprolactinemic, and 4 had increased adrenocorticotropin levels. Four patients had symptoms of hypopituitarism or optic chiasm compression or both. One patient had an elevated growth hormone level. High-resolution CT was performed with intravenous contrast enhancement. Coronal MR images were obtained by spin-echo sequencing.

Nine patients underwent transsphenoidal surgery, and 3 of them had a documented reduction in lesion size when given bromocriptine. It was found that CT was more sensitive than MR imaging in detecting focal lesions and erosion of the sellar floor (table), but that MR imaging was better for identifying infundibular abnormalities, focal changes in the sellar diaphragm, cavernous sinus invasion, and optic chiasm compression.

In this study, CT and MR imaging were of comparable value in identifying and localizing pituitary macroadenomas. Currently, CT is better for identifying focal lesions, but the sensitivity of MR imaging may improve if slice thickness is reduced or paramagnetic contrast agents are employed. The advantage of MR imaging is that it requires no irradiation

MR Imaging and CT Findings in Proved Cases of Pituitary Adenoma*

	Focal Lesion		Sellar-Floor Erosion		Infundibulum Abnormality		Diaphragma Sellae Abnormality		Cavernous[†] Sinus Invasion		Optic[†] Chiasm Compression	
	MR	CT[‡]	MR	CT	MR	CT	MR	CT	MR	CT	MR	CT
Microadenoma (n = 4)	1	2	0	1	1	1	1	0	—	—	—	—
Macroadenoma (n = 6)	0	0	4	6	4	4	5	5	3	2	3	0

Proof of diagnosis was based on surgical findings or decrease in size of mass with bromocriptine therapy. Not included are data on 2 patients who underwent exploratory surgery for suspected microadenoma and who had normal MR, CT, and surgical findings.

†Cavernous sinus invasion and optic chiasm compression were not confirmed surgically because of difficulty in visualizing these structures via a transsphenoidal approach.

‡One focal lesion on CT was opposite the adenoma at surgery.

(Courtesy of Davis PC, Hoffman JC Jr, Spencer T, et al: *AJR* 148:797–802, April 1987.)

or iodinated contrast medium; CT, however, remains the choice when microadenoma is suspected.

▶ Both MRI and CT continue to have drawbacks in the diagnosis of pituitary adenoma: MRI may miss a small or calcified lesion, and CT does not often detect cavernous sinus invasion or chiasmal compression. According to the surgical correlations presented, MRI and CT were of comparable value for localizing macroadenomas, but CT was superior for showing microadenomas. The latter point may be questioned, because there were only 4 confirmed microadenomas and CT indicated 1 on the wrong side. Magnetic resonance was better for identifying infundibular displacement (a highly reliable sign), as well as cavernous sinus invasion and chiasmal compression, both signs of great clinical significance.

With the addition of thinner sections and gadolinium contrast enhancement, MRI seems highly likely to be the study of choice in the future, but confirmatory data are needed.— R.M. Crowell, M.D.

Gadolinium-DTPA and MR Imaging of Pituitary Adenoma: A Preliminary Report

Davis PC, Hoffman JC, Jr, Malko JA, Tindall GT, Takei Y, Avruch L, Braun IF (Emory Univ)

AJNR 8:817–823, September–October 1987   19–17

Gadolinium (Gd) diethylenetriamine pentaacetic acid (DTPA)/ dimeglumine is a valuable paramagnetic contrast agent in the enhancement of tissue abnormalities, such as tumor, inflammation, and infarcts, by shortening the T_1 (spin-lattice) relaxation time of hydrogen nuclei. To assess the role of Gd-DTPA magnetic resonance imaging (Gd-MRI) in the diagnosis of pituitary adenoma, Gd-MRI, unenhanced MRI, and contrast-enhanced computed tomographic (CT) studies were compared prospectively in 6 patients with surgically-confirmed pituitary adenomas and 3 patients without sellar pathology.

In the 3 patients without sellar pathology, the pituitary gland, cavernous sinus, and infundibulum increased in intensity with T_1 shortening after Gd injection. Three microadenomas were recognizable with contrast-enhanced CT, but 1 was not detected with Gd-MRI. The 2 focal lesions detected by Gd-MRI became isointense with normal gland on delayed images, indicating that the earliest short repetition-time sequence performed after Gd injection was best for focal lesion detection. Three macroadenomas were studied. Contrast-enhanced CT, Gd-MRI, and plain MRI were equally able to identify gland enlargement, sellar floor erosion, and abnormalities of the diaphragm sellae. Infundibulum displacement was better seen with contrast-enhanced CT, but unenhanced and Gd-MRI were better than enhanced CT for demonstrating chiasmal compression. Gadolinium enhancement of both the normal cavernous sinus and adenoma made the identification of cavernous sinus extension of adenoma difficult.

Gadolinium-DTPA MRI is a promising technique for the evaluation of pituitary adenomas. However, further modifications are necessary to improve focal lesion detection. These include thinner slices and immediate scanning after Gd injection.

▶ This study indicates that gadolinium-DTPA is a quite promising adjunct for depiction of pituitary adenoma. The authors' suggestion that thinner slices and early scanning times be utilized seems logical and probably will lead to this being the method of choice for depiction of most pituitary tumors. In questionable cases, CT remains a useful method.—R.M. Crowell, M.D.

Usefulness of Preoperative Inferior Petrosal Vein Sampling in Cushing's Disease
Snow RB, Patterson RH, Jr, Horwith M, Saint Louis L, Fraser RAR (Cornell Univ)
Surg Neurol 29:17–21, January 1988   19–18

It often is difficult to localize the pituitary as the source of elevated adrenocorticotropic hormone (ACTH). Preoperative bilateral inferior petrosal venous sampling was evaluated in 10 patients having typical clinical and biochemical features of Cushing's disease, with normal or indefinite thin-slice computed tomography studies. Three patients had normal magnetic resonance scans.

In all patients but 1, petrosal vein sampling showed a gradient between pituitary and peripheral ACTH levels, confirming the pituitary etiology of hypercortisolism. The petrosal sinus/peripheral blood ratio exceeded 2.5 in these cases. The patient without a gradient had received cyproheptadine before sampling; this apparently can suppress ACTH release by pituitary adenomas. Seven studies localized the tumor to 1 side of the pituitary, and this was confirmed in all 6 cases in which a tumor was identified. Eight patients were cured postoperatively. In 1 other case, the pituitary adenoma probably was an incidental tumor.

Inferior petrosal venous sampling for ACTH is useful in diagnosing pituitary-dependent Cushing's disease and in lateralizing a small microadenoma. More efficient removal should be possible as a result.

▶ This report supports the contention of Oldfield and others at the NIH (*N Engl J Med* 312:100–103, 1985) that inferior petrosal sinus sampling can help lateralize pituitary microadenomas. It is useful to know that cyproheptadine may confound this examination. Recent unpublished work from Milwaukee indicates that the sensitivity of the test may be enhanced yet further by the use of stimulation with intravenously administered corticotropin releasing factor.—R.M. Crowell, M.D.

Value of Growth Hormone Dynamics and Somatomedin C (Insulin-like Growth Factor I) Levels in Predicting the Long-term Benefit After Transsphenoidal Surgery for Acromegaly

Arafah BM, Rosenzweig JL, Fenstermaker R, Salazar R, McBride CE, Selman W (Case Western Reserve Univ)

J Lab Clin Med 109:346–354, March 1987   19–19

The role of dynamic human growth hormone (hGH) studies in assessing the outcome after removal of hGH-secreting pituitary adenomas was examined in a series of 43 patients with acromegaly, 22 men and 21 women with a mean age of 42 years at diagnosis. The mean duration of symptoms was about 8 years. Eleven patients had been treated elsewhere. The mean basal hGH level was 66.5 ng/ml. Levels were not suppressed during an oral glucose tolerance test in about half the patients, but one third had a paradoxical increase. The serum concentration of insulinlike growth factor I (IGF-I) was increased in 27 of 29 patients, as was the serum PRL level in 13 of 41 patients.

Basal serum hGH levels were higher than 5 ng/ml in 30% of the patients 3 months after surgery, but these patients had lower levels than before surgery. The serum IGF-I concentration was normal in most patients with normal basal hGH levels and low in 2 patients with hypopituitarism. Of 9 patients with normal basal hGH levels but abnormal dynamics, 7 tested had normal serum IGF-I levels postoperatively (table). Five of these patients had recurrent acromegaly. The remaining patients had persistently elevated basal hGH levels and increased IGF-I levels.

Dynamic hGH testing is helpful in predicting the long-term outcome of acromegalic patients who are treated surgically. Levels of IGF-I alone are not sufficiently predictive. The findings are consistent with a pituitary origin of hGH-producing adenomas, although hypothalamic dysfunction cannot be ruled out in some cases.

▶ Dynamic testing of GH and somatomedin C predicts the clinical course of acromegaly (see the Table, in which group I indicates normal basal hGH and dynamics; group II, hypopituitarism, with no recurrence; group III, normal basal hGH and abnormal dynamics, with 5 of 9 recurrence; and group IV, persistently elevated levels of basal hGH). It is not enough to monitor basal hGH or so-

Postoperative Levels of IGF-I* in Patients With Acromegaly

	Groups			
	I (n = 19)	II (n = 2)	III (n = 9)	IV (n = 13)
Mean postoperative IGF-I levels (ng/ml)	227 ± 21	124 ± 26.2	296 ± 62.5	536 ± 38.9
No. tested	12	2	8	8
No. of patients with normal IGF-I levels	12/12	0/2*	7/8	0/8

*IGF-I, insulin-like growth factor I.
†Both values were below lower limits of normal.
(Courtesy of Arafah BM, Rosenzweig JL, Fenstermaker R, et al: *J Lab Clin Med* 109:346–354, March 1987.)

matomedin C levels. Careful follow-up in coordination with the neuroendocrine service is imperative.— R.M. Crowell, M.D.

Prolactin-Secreting Adenomas: The Preoperative Response to Bromocriptine Treatment and Surgical Outcome

Hubbard JL, Scheithauer BW, Abboud CF, Laws ER, Jr (Mayo Clinic, Rochester, Minn)
J Neurosurg 67:816–821, December 1987   19–20

Prolactin-secreting adenomas are common pituitary tumors that usually are successfully treated by transsphenoidal microsurgery. Although bromocriptine has gained widespread use since its introduction for the treatment of prolactin-secreting adenomas, controversy still exists over the effect on surgical outcome after preoperative bromocriptine treatment. The authors' 4-year experience with 55 patients with confirmed prolactin-secreting pituitary adenomas who underwent transsphenoidal microsurgery after bromocriptine pretreatment was reviewed.

The study population included 39 female and 16 male patients (aged 8–72 years) who had been treated with bromocriptine at various doses and for variable durations before operation. Basal prolactin levels before bromocriptine treatment ranged from 38–100 ng/ml in 11 patients and 101–200 ng/ml in 12 patients, and more than 200 ng/ml in 29 patients. Postoperative prolactin levels returned to normal in 54% of those in the first group, 58% of those in the second group, and 38% of those in the third group.

Twenty-one (68%) of 31 patients with microadenomas, 2 (17%) of 12 patients with diffuse microadenomas, and 2 (17%) of 12 patients with grossly invasive adenomas were cured after operation. Postoperative prolactin levels were normal in 9 (50%) of 18 patients who had responded to preoperative bromocriptine treatment and in 9 (31%) of 29 patients

Outcome by Prolactin Response to Preoperative Bromocriptine*

Outcome	Responder		Hyporesponder		Unknown: Total†
	Total	M:F	Total	M:F	
normalized	9	2:7	9	0:9	7
recurrent	5	1:4	5	1:4	0
persistent	4	3:1	15	9:6	1
total cases	18	6:12	29	10:19	8
cure rate	50%		31%		87%

*Normalized: normalized responders—those whose prolactin levels returned to normal after bromocriptine administration; recurrent: prolactin level rose after initially normalizing; persistent: prolactin level always abnormal; cure rate: prolactin normalization.
†All patients in whom the postbromocriptine prolactin levels were unknown were female.
(Courtesy of Hubbard JL, Scheithauer BW, Abboud CF, et al: *J Neurosurg* 67:816–821, December 1987.)

who had shown only a partial response to preoperative bromocriptine administration (table).

When the data of this study were compared with those in 26 control patients with prolactinomas who had not been treated preoperatively with bromocriptine, no significant differences were observed in the frequency or extent of fibrosis, calcification, or prolactin immunoreactivity.

Short-term preoperative bromocriptine administration does not adversely affect surgical outcome and surgical outcome cannot be predicted on the basis of response or lack of response to preoperative bromocriptine treatment.

▶ This report documents no difference in outcome in patients undergoing transsphenoidal hypophysectomy for prolactin-secreting adenomas with or without preoperative bromocriptine treatment. Although other investigators have reported worse surgical results after bromocriptine treatment (Landolt et al: *Lancet* 2:657–658, 1982), the results are in agreement with the experience in another large series (Marcovitz S, Hardy J: *Semin Reprod Endocrinol* 2:73–81, 1984). In the present study, histologically demonstrated fibrosis and difficulty of surgery were also unaffected by previous bromocriptine therapy.—R.M. Crowell, M.D.

Giant Invasive Prolactinomas
Murphy FY, Vesely DL, Jordan RM, Flanigan S, Kohler PO and John L McClellan (Univ of Arkansas Mem VA Hosp, Little Rock)
Am J Med 83:995–1002, November 1987   19–21

Although no rigid criteria exist for classifying large pituitary tumors, the term giant has been suggested for any pituitary tumor larger than 4 cm in diameter. Two patients were seen with the largest prolactinomas ever documented. Follow-up of 9 and 10 years, respectively, demonstrated how aggressive these tumors may become and how difficult invasive prolactinomas are to treat.

CASE 1.—Man, 44, had a very large prolactinoma that invaded the internal auditory canals, causing sensorineural deafness and simultaneously grew inferiorly, forcing the patient to use both hands to hold his head up. When the patient was admitted to the hospital in 1978, laboratory evaluation revealed a serum prolactin level greater than 5,000 ng/dl (normal, up to 15 ng/dl). One week after pituitary surgery, he had a generalized seizure, and phenytoin therapy was initiated. His prolactin level remained elevated. Bromocriptine therapy was begun because of progressive deafness and seizures and there was a gradual lowering of his prolactin levels with increasing doses. No measurable reduction of the tumor mass was seen on computed tomography (CT) until that time. Slow shrinkage continued until 1985, when the amount of decrease appeared to have leveled off.

CASE 2.—Man, 64, had a prolactinoma that had invaded the sphenoidal, ethmoidal, and cavernous sinuses as well as the clivus and petrous bone. Laboratory results obtained on admission in March 1976 revealed a serum prolactin level of

5,600 ng/ml. He had pituitary surgery followed by radiation. He was relatively asymptomatic until July 1982. Computed tomography revealed a massive pituitary tumor invading the bony structure around it and a subdural hematoma on the right side that caused a 1.3 cm shift of the midline to the left, which was not present on previous CT scans. The subdural hematoma was surgically removed; at that time, his prolactin level was 6,047 ng/dl. Bromocriptine therapy was initiated, resulting in a decrease in his prolactin level to 1,900 ng/dl after 1 month.

There has been no evidence of regrowth or enlargement of the prolactinoma in either patient. In patient 1, the absolute value of prolactin did not correlate directly with tumor size. Even though the serum prolactin level decreased from more than 5,000 ng/dl to less than 200 ng/dl (> 95%), the tumor mass decreased by only 20%. Patient 2 had marked tumor reduction and complete normalization of serum prolactin levels with only 7.5 mg of bromocriptine per day. Computed tomography is also necessary to follow up patients with invasive prolactinomas and their response to therapy. Initial treatment of patients with this condition should be with dopamine agonists, although surgery and radiotherapy may be necessary in many patients.

► Two case reports demonstrate the utility of bromocriptine therapy for giant invasive prolactinomas. Transsphenoidal decompressive surgery is sometimes useful in this situation for patients with chiasmal compression (Black PMcL, Zervas NT, Condia G: *Surg Neurol* 29:443–447, 1988). In addition, radiation, either as standard orthovoltage radiation or as radiosurgery, has an established place in the management of these difficult tumors.—R.M. Crowell, M.D.

Perioperative Morbidity Associated With Operative Resection of Craniopharyngioma: A Review of Ten Years Experience

Bucci MN, Chin LS, Hoff JT (Univ of Michigan Hosp, Ann Arbor)
Neurochirurgia 30:135–138, 1987   19–22

The management of craniopharyngioma is a difficult and controversial issue. Eradication of this tumor is fraught with postoperative disability and frequent tumor recurrence. Little is known about metabolic dysfunction and perioperative morbidity related to the extent of surgical resection. In a 10-year review of data on patients with craniopharyngioma, metabolic dysfunction and major complications were compared with the extent of resection.

From 1974 to 1983, 23 patients underwent 34 operations. The patients were divided into 2 groups: those who had at least 95% resection, and those who had partial resection. A significant difference was found in both high and low sodium values between the 2 groups that correlated with a significant difference in the change in sodium between the groups. Glucose values tended to be significantly higher in the 95% or greater resection group. A significant increase in high temperature readings in the postoperative period was noted in the 95% or greater resection group

---

Perioperative Morbidity and Mortality

	95% or > Resection (N = 16)	Partial Resection (N = 18)	χ^2 (Chi-Square)
Diabetes Insipidus	13	3	P < .05
Major Complications	10	2	P < .005
Death	3	0	P > .05

*N = number of operations. Death: 30-day postoperative period.
(Courtesy of Bucci MN, Chin LS, Hoff JT: *Neurochirurgia* 30:135–138, 1987.)

---

compared with the partial resection group. The overall change in temperature in the first group was significant as well. Low glucose and low temperature for both groups were not significant. Perioperative morbidity, including diabetes insipidus and major complications, was significantly increased in the 95% or greater group (table). The only postoperative deaths occurred in the 95% or greater group; however, the difference between groups was not statistically significant. Careful assessment of surgical morbidity is warranted in patients with craniopharyngioma.

▶ This substantial experience from the University of Michigan suggests that radical resection of craniopharyngioma is associated with substantial morbidity and mortality. Although the study suffers from drawbacks of mixed ages of patients, various surgeons, various surgical techniques, with some cases being done microsurgically, nonetheless the series may be taken to represent the efforts of a major neurosurgical American center over some period of time on a difficult problem. With a perioperative mortality of 18% in the radical resection group and nil in the limited resection group, a very significant concern arises about radical resection in this setting. This is particularly true since the less aggressive approach may have good results. Baskin and Wilson (*J Neurosurg* 65:22–27, 1986) noted an approximately 90% remission following subtotal resection and postoperative radiotherapy. Several groups have now reported excellent results with instillation of P-32 into cystic lesions. Radiosurgery has posted good results in this group of patients. Therefore it is mandatory to consider less aggressive methods of treatment for certain patients with craniopharyngioma.—R.M. Crowell, M.D.

Brief Notes on Parasellar Tumors

ACTH and Tumors

In 35 patients with ACTH-secreting adenomas, coronal CT scans had a sensitivity of 63%, a specificity of 62.5%, and an overall accuracy rate of 62.8% (Marcovitz S, et al: *AJNR* 8:641–644, 1987).

Cushing's disease may present with avascular necrosis of the femoral heads complicated by pituitary apoplexy (Wicks IP, et al: *Ann Rheum Dis* 46:783–786, 1987)

Cushing's disease recurred in childhood in a case of radiation-induced remission (Cappa M, et al: *Am J Dis Child* 141:736–740, 1987).

After pituitary surgery, a morning serum cortisol level 2 days postoperatively and 24 hours after discontinuation of hydrocortisone accurately predicts postoperative corticotropin reserve (Watts NB, Tindall GT: *JAMA* 259:708–711, 1988).

Gadolinium is helpful in identifying pituitary adenomas with Cushing's disease: positive images were obtained in 10 of 12 surgically treated and histologically verified patients (Dwyer AJ, et al: *Radiology* 163:421–426, 1987).

Growth Hormone and Tumors

Somatostatin receptors may be visualized with autoradiography and immunohistochemistry for correlation with growth hormone and prolactin in pituitary adenomas, indicating different tumor subclasses (Reubi JC, et al: J Clin Endocrinol Metab 65:65–73, 1987).

Immunohistochemistry has been used to demonstrate colocalization of growth hormone and alpha subunit in human GH-secreting pituitary adenomas (Osamura R, Watanabe K: *Virchows Arch [A]* 411:323–330, 1987).

Serial CT and endocrinologic studies in 23 untreated patients with acromegaly were carried out for 2–13 years. Results show that GH-secreting pituitary tumors may remain stationary for extended periods of time and that complete or partial disappearance occurs frequently, probably as a result of infarction with development of empty sella or sellar cyst (Bjerre P, et al: *J Clin Endocrinol Metab* 63:287–295, 1986).

After transsphenoidal removal of pituitary adenoma, restoration of growth hormone levels to normal does not necessarily restore normal responses to insulin tolerance test and oral glucose tolerance test (Karashima T, et al: *Clin Endocrinol* 25:157–163, 1986).

Alpha subunit is a tumor marker for gonadotropin-producing pituitary adenomas (Demura R, et al: *J Clin Endocrinol Metab* 63:564–569, 1986).

Growth hormone secreting pituitary adenomas are heterogeneous in cell culture and commonly secrete glycoprotein hormone alpha subunit (White MC, et al: *Clin Endocrinol* 25:173–179, 1986).

Enolase subunits may be useful markers for diagnosing and monitoring patients with neuroendocrine tumors (Iwase K, et al: *J Clin Endocrinol Metab* 63:94–101, 1986).

In 58 patients operated on by Hardy for pituitary somatotroph adenomas, the preoperative coronal CT scan correctly localized 81% of microadenomas and 94% of macroadenomas (Marcovitz et al: *AJNR* 9:19–22, 1988).

SMS 201-995, a long-acting somatostatin analogue, is promising in the medical treatment of acromegaly (George SR, et al: *Clin Endocrinol* 26:395–405, 1987).

Studies of the somatostatin analogue SM 201-995 have been carried out on the prolactin/ACTH-secreting pituitary tumor 7315A in rats. Studies show that the SMS 201-995 inhibits the growth of the pituitary tumor. This effect shows tachyphylaxis. In addition, high glucocorticosteroid levels reduce the number of somatostatin receptors diminishing any tumor effect of the drug (Lamberts SWJ et al: *Endocrinology* 118:2188–2194, 1986).

The somatostatin analogue SMS 201-995 effectively decreases growth hormone secretion, but not prolactin secretion, from pituitary adenomas (Lamberts SWJ, et al: *Clin Endocrinol* 25:201–212, 1986).

Laminin in the gonadotrophic cells correlates with their functional state in experimental rats (Holck S, et al: *Lab Invest* 56:481–488, 1987).

In the long-term, 90Y pituitary implantation for acromegaly is highly effective, but hypopituitarism is common (Jadresic A, et al: *Acta Endocrinol (Copenh)* 115:301–306, 1987).

Prolactin and Tumors

Of more then 10,000 screened subjects, 40 with prolactin levels above 75 µg/L were found. Of these, 5 had pituitary prolactinoma, 1 had empty sella, 10 had "big" prolactinemia, 7 were pregnant women, and 13 had drug-induced hyperprolactinemia (Miyai K, et al: *Clin Endocrinol* 25:549–554, 1986).

In a study of 128 histopathologically confirmed pituitary tumors, serum prolactin levels were correlated with histology. If the prolactin level is less than 3,000 milliunits (mU) per liter, surgical removal is necessary for diagnosis and treatment in the absence of a prolactin-secreting adenoma. Prolactin level of 3,000–8,000 mU/L is consistent with any diagnosis, and great care must be taken with dopamine agonist therapy in such patients. A serum prolactin concentration of more than 8,000 mU/L is always attributable to prolactin-secreting adenoma (Bevan JS, et al: *Am J Med* 82:29–32, 1987).

Lymphocytic adenohypophysitis may cause a pituitary mass lesion in the postpartum period. (Meichner RH, et al: *Neurology* 37:158–161, 1987).

Nonfunctioning pituitary adenomas do not regress during bromocriptine therapy but possess membrane-bound dopamine receptors that bind bromocriptine (Bevan JS, Burke CW: *Clin Endocrinol* 25:561–572, 1986).

Prolonged normalization of prolactin level may follow bromocriptine withdrawal (Wang C, et al: *Clin Endocrinol* 27:363–371, 1987).

An injectable form of bromocriptine causes long-lasting suppression of prolactin secretion and shrinkage of prolactinoma (Montini M, et al: *J Clin Endocrinol Metab* 63:266–268, 1986).

On light microscopic quantitative study, bromocriptine causes increase in fibrous tissue content of prolactin-secreting but not nonfunctioning pituitary adenomas (Esiri MM, et al: *J Clin Endocrinol Metab* 63:383–388, 1986).

Preoperative bromocriptine caused marked size reduction in 7 of 7 macroprolactinomas, but if continued beyond 6 weeks, it induced tumor fibrosis, making surgery dangerous and unproductive. Selective transsphenoidal surgery relieved hyperprolactinemia in 70% of patients with mesoprolactinoma or microprolactinoma, usually without loss of pituitary function, with a relapse rate of 1 per 88 patient years follow-up. Invasive prolactinomas and macroprolactinomas showing uneven shrinkage with a short course of bromocriptine should have radiotherapy rather than surgery. Microprolactinomas generally did not benefit from surgery compared with conservative therapy (Bevan JS, et al: *Clin Endocrinol* 26:541–556, 1987).

Of 190 women with prolactinoma, 88 were treated with transsphenoidal resection and 102 with bromocriptine. There were no statistical differences in conception, prolactin levels, and general clinical results (Samaan NA, et al: *Am J Obstet Gynecol* 155:1300–1305, 1986).

Bromocriptine (7.5 mg/d) led to improvement in visual field defects in patients with nonfunctioning pituitary adenomas (D'Emden MC, Harrison LC: *Clin Endocrinol* 25:697–702, 1986).

Sellar lesions may be associated with isolated hyperprolactinemia (Riedel M, et al: *Acta Endocrinol (Copenh)* 113:196–203, 1986).

Dynorphin-A causes increases in plasma prolactin concentration without alteration of other anterior pituitary hormones (Gilbeau PM, et al: *Neuroendocrinology* 45:284–289, 1987).

Preoperative coronal CT scanning had an overall accuracy rate of 92% in 102 patients operated on by Hardy for prolactinoma (Marcovitz S, et al: *AJNR* 9:13–17, 1988).

Treatment of Pituitary Adenomas

In 319 pituitary operations, the transfrontal route was reserved for large adenomas, especially with lateral sellar extension. Postoperative bromocriptine proved useful when prolactin levels failed to normalize. Postoperative radiotherapy was of value in invasive adenomas and in cases where tumor removal was not radical (Guidetti B, et al: *Acta Neurochir (Wien)* 85:117–124, 1987).

Megavoltage radiotherapy effectively decreases prolactin secretion and tumor size in patients with large prolactinomas at the expense of other anterior pituitary functions (Johnston DG, et al: *Clin Endocrinol* 24:675–685, 1986).

Among 78 surgically managed pituitary adenomas, hemorrhage had occurred in 13. Symptoms were headache, drowsiness, diplopia, and visual failure. Correct diagnosis was suggested by skull films and contrast enhanced CT. In some cases without visual abnormality, conservative therapy is reasonable, but in most patients transsphenoidal decompression is the treatment of choice (Tsitopoulos P, et al: *Postgrad Med J* 62:623–626, 1986).

Parasellar Lesions

Among 4 cases of craniopharyngioma (even normal social and work functioning), detailed neuropsychologic testing (Luria-Nebraska battery) disclosed cognitive defects which often correlated with MRI frontal lobe abnormalities (Stelling MW, et al: *Am J Dis Child* 140:710–714, 1986).

Magnetic resonance is superior in demonstrating the differentiation between craniopharyngioma and neighboring normal structures (Baierl P, et al: *Fortschr Rontgenstr* 146:578–583, 1987).

In 9 cases, CT was superior to MR in craniopharyngioma imaging for demonstration of calcification and cyst formation (Freeman MP, et al: *J Comput Assist Tomogr* 11:810–814, 1987).

In 14 patients, transsphenoidal microsurgical removal of metastatic tumors provided decompression of the mass with improvement of presenting symptoms in the majority, and the surgery was free of mortality or serious complications (Branch CL, Jr, Laws ER, Jr: *J Clin Endocrinol Metab* 65:469–474, 1987).

In 31 transcallosal operations, because of the tumor type the final results were considered unsatisfactory in at least 19 (Synowitz HJ: *Zentralbl Neurochir* 48:288–293, 1987).—R.M. Crowell, M.D.

Acoustic Neuromas

MR Detection of Tumor in the Internal Auditory Canal
Daniels DL, Millen SJ, Meyer GA, Pojunas KW, Kilgore DP, Shaffer KA, Williams AL, Haughton VM (Med College of Wisconsin, Milwaukee)
AJR 148:1219–1222, June 1987   19–23

The authors reviewed the magnetic resonance imaging (MRI) findings in 15 patients with tumors within or near the internal auditory canal, who underwent surgery between 1983 and 1986. An initial sagittal scan was obtained to select optimal axial and coronal slice locations for the temporal bones. Spin-echo sequencing was used. Two patients received Gadolinium-DTPA before imaging.

Twelve acoustic neurinomas, 2 facial nerve tumors, and 1 meningioma were evaluated. Short TR and TE images demonstrated a widened canal and tissue displacing cerebrospinal fluid from the auditory canal in cases of intracanalicular tumor. In several cases, the tumor had a homogeneous intensity that was slightly less than that of the brain stem. In some cases, a central thin band of low signal intensity was observed. In one case, intracanalicular disease was not detected by MRI. Gadolinium injection markedly enhanced the intracanalicular and extracanalicular components of an acoustic neurinonoma and a neurofibroma.

Magnetic resonance imaging demonstrated the precise extent of tumors in or near the internal auditory canal in most of these cases. Enhancement with Gadolinium-DTPA will help eliminate uncertainties in MRI of the internal auditory canal, and in distinguishing acoustic neurinoma from extracanalicular meningioma.

▶ Magnetic resonance imaging is superb for the diagnosis of intracanalicular tumors. The single misdiagnosis in this series, a large extracanalicular seventh nerve neurinoma extending into a normal-sized canal, would have been identified with Gadolinium contrast material, which is just now available for widespread use. Note that MR also gives information on the relation of the tumor to vessels in the area, lessening the need for angiography. Magnetic resonance imaging is likely to become the study of choice, because it often is the only study needed for delineation of these lesions.—R.M. Crowell, M.D.

MR Diagnosis of Acoustic Neuromas
Mikhael MA, Ciric IS, Wolff AP (Evanston Hosp-Northwestern Univ)
J Comput Assist Tomogr 11:232–235, March–April 1987   19–24

Until the introduction of magnetic resonance imaging (MRI), computed tomography (CT) combined with intrathecal contrast injection (CT cisternography) was considered the definitive test to rule out lesions in the cerebellopontine angle (CPA) and internal auditory canal (IAC). A total of 243 patients with clinically suspected acoustic neuroma were evaluated radiologically by CT, and in selected cases, by CT cisternography, MRI, or both. Magnetic resonance images were obtained in the axial and coronal planes using slices 5 mm thick or smaller and spin-echo techniques of repetition time (TR) 500–2,000 msec and echo time (TE) 30–90 msec.

Fifty-one acoustic neuromas were diagnosed and removed, including 36 large tumors with extracanalicular extension and 15 intracanalicular small tumors. Among patients studied by routine CT and cisternography, routine CT visualized all 36 large tumors as enhancing lesions but missed the small intracanalicular tumors. The latter were visualized by CT cisternography in 7 patients and by MR in 8. Furthermore, MRI demonstrated 23 (100%) of 23 surgically verified lesions. With the sequence TR 500–820 and TE 30–48 msec, the acoustic neuromas displayed variable intensity: low or isointense with the surrounding brain in 14 tumors, highly intense in 7, and mixed in the presence of necrosis, hemorrhage, or both in 2. With the sequence TR 2,000 and TE 30–90 msec, all acoustic neuromas were shown as high-intensity tumors.

Magnetic resonance, when used with spin-echo technique using both short as well as long sequences for axial and coronal slices 5 mm thick or smaller, allows the diagnosis of acoustic neuromas with accuracy. Moreover, MRI demonstrates the relationship of the lesion to the brain stem, fourth ventricle, and surrounding blood vessels.

▶ Dr. Mikhael and colleagues nicely demonstrate the advantages of MR for the diagnosis of acoustic neuromas. Magnetic resonance actually diagnosed the small intracanalicular tumors as well as the large lesions. Features of importance, including swelling and hemorrhage, were also identified. With present-day technology, CT scanning is occasionally superior for meningiomas in this location. This is likely to change with the increasing experience with gadolinium contrast and MRI imaging. For most cerebellopontine angle tumors, angiography is no longer necessary when satisfactory MR images are available.—R.M. Crowell, M.D.

Preservation of Hearing in Surgical Removal of Acoustic Neuromas of the Internal Auditory Canal and Cerebellar Pontine Angle

Nadol JB, Jr, Levine R, Ojemann RG, Martuza RL, Montgomery WW, Klevens de Sandoval P (Harvard Univ; Massachusetts Eye and Ear Infirmary, Massachusetts General Hospital, Boston)
Laryngoscope 97:1287–1294, November 1987   19–25

Diagnostic modalities such as computed tomography (CT), magnetic resonance imaging (MRI), and auditory-evoked response testing, which allow diagnosis of small tumors of the cerebellopontine angle, and the use of microsurgical techniques have enabled preservation of useful hearing. The treatment of 69 patients with unilateral acoustic neuromas of the internal auditory canal, cerebellar pontine angle, or both was described.

Total tumor removal was accomplished as assessed by microscopic visual inspection in all patients. In all cases, an attempt was made to preserve useful hearing. The success rate of preservation of hearing and facial nerve function was correlated with tumor size (table). Useful hearing, defined as speech reception threshold no worse than 70 dB and a discrimination score of at least 15%, was preserved in 73% of the patients in whom the tumor extension to the posterior fossa was no more than 0.5 cm. Useful hearing was preserved in only 22% of those patients in whom

Preservation of Facial Nerve*

| Status of Facial Nerve / Tumor Size (N) | Postoperative Anatomic Status | | Functional Status | | | | | |
| | | | First Postoperative Day | | | One-Year Postoperative† | | |
	Preserved	Sacrificed	Same as Pre-Op	Paresis	Total Paralysis Due to Surgery	Normal Facial Function	Persistent Paresis	Total Paralysis
IC								
≤0.5 cm (12)	100% (12)	0% (0)	100% (12)	0% (0)	0% (0)	100% (12)	0% (0)	0% (0)
>0.5 cm ≤1.5 cm (35)	100% (35)	0% (0)	66% (23)	29% (10)	6% (2)	97% (34)	3% (1)	0% (0)
>1.5 cm ≤2.5 cm (12)	92% (11)	8% (1)	50% (6)	25% (3)	25% (3)	73% (8)	27% (3)	0% (0)
>2.5 cm (9)	89% (8)	11% (1)	22% (2)	33% (3)	44% (4)	63% (5)	25% (2)	13% (1)
Total (62)	97% (66)	3% (2)	63% (43)	24% (16)	13% (9)	89% (59)	9% (6)	2% (1)

*One patient, with total paralysis preoperatively caused by previous parotid surgery was excluded from analysis.
†Two patients with less than 1 year follow-up were excluded from analysis.
(Courtesy of Nadol JB Jr, Levine R, Ojemann RG, et al: *Laryngoscope* 97:1287–1294, November 1987.)

posterior fossa extension was more than 2.5 cm. No significant correlation was found between preoperative evoked responses and success in hearing preservation.

Useful hearing can be preserved in patients in whom tumors of the internal auditory canal and cerebellopontine angle are completely removed, as judged by microscopic visual inspection. The size of the tumor was correlated with the success rate in hearing preservation.

▶ This report emphasizes that useful hearing can be preserved after suboccipital excision of acoustic neuromas. This is particularly appropriate in patients with small lesions, 0.5 cm or smaller. An effort to save hearing is much less successful when the lesion is larger than 2.5 cm in diameter.—R.M. Crowell, M.D.

Preservation of Hearing by Surgery of Acoustic Neuroma
Frerebeau P, Benezech J, Uziel A, Coubes P, Seignarbieux F, Malonga M (Ctr Médico-Chirurgicol Guy de Chavliac, Montpellier, France)
Neurochirurgie 33:124–128, 1987   19–26

Forty-four patients underwent removal of an acoustic neuroma by a posterior cranial fossa approach between 1981 and 1984, with the goal of preserving hearing. Seven tumors were less than 20 mm in size; 9 exceeded 40 mm. Ten patients had poor hearing preoperatively, 15 had serviceable hearing, and 15 had no hearing. Four others had normal hearing.

Postoperative hearing was preserved in 11 instances, including 8 of the 19 patients who had normal or serviceable hearing preoperatively. Forty-three percent of patients with tumors measuring less than 20 mm—but only 11% of those with large tumors—had hearing preserved.

A suboccipital approach can be useful in preserving hearing when a patient with acoustic neuroma has serviceable hearing preoperatively, and when the tumor is not so large as to preclude this method.

▶ From France comes another report of successful preservation of hearing by suboccipital removal of acoustic neuroma. Data on utility of hearing (speech discrimination scores) are not presented. The ultrasonic aspirator is said to be of use. Hearing and preservation was more common with small tumors (less than 20 mm in diameter).—R.M. Crowell, M.D.

Long-Term Hearing Preservation After Acoustic Neuroma Surgery
Rosenberg RA, Cohen NL, Ransohoff J (New York Univ)
Otolaryngol Head Neck Surg 97:270–274, September 1987   19–27

Advances in instrumentation and better surgical training have led to marked improvement in the treatment of cerebellopontine angle tumors. In some instances, it is technically possible to preserve hearing in treating

Hearing Preserved at or Near Preoperative Level

Patient	Tumor size (cm)	Route	PTA (pre/post)	Speech % (pre/post)	Follow-up (yr)	Symptoms/ signs	CT (cm growth)
BP	1.5	SO	40/43	92/60	1.3	No	—
BA	1.5	SO	23/20	98/100	11.0	No	—
HL*	1.0	SO +	23/48	92/92	7.0	No	0
DW	1.0	MF	25/33	80/72	4.5	No	—
GH	1.5	SO	28/ 8	100/92	6.0	No	—
GS	1.5	SO	68/25	10/88	5.0	No	—
PE	1.5	SO	42/48	64/64	4.0	No	—
FT*	1.5	SO	17/33	94/80	3.0	No	0
JN*	1.0	SO	30/51	96/88	1.5	No	0
					4.81 (mean)		

*Patients without * = group 1A; patients with * = group AB; SO = suboccipital approach; MF = middle fossa approach; + = near-total removal; — = no CT performed; 0 = CT performed, but no tumor seen.
(Courtesy of Rosenberg RA, Cohen NL, Ransohoff J: *Otolaryngol Head Neck Surg* 97:270–274, September 1987.)

tumors of the eighth nerve. However, some studies assert that grossly intact nerves may contain microscopic islands of tumor cells intermingled with nerve fibers. Twenty-one patients who had had acoustic neuroma surgery with attempted preservation of the cochlear nerve were retrospectively studied.

All patients had good functional hearing preoperatively on the involved side or required binaural hearing for safety purposes. Nine patients had surgery with successful anatomical and functional preservation of cochlear nerves and were followed up for an average of 4.8 years. Three of these 9 patients were able to have CT followup. None of the 9 had symptoms or signs of tumor recurrence; no tumor regrowth was seen on CT (table). The remaining 12 patients had anatomical preservation of the cochlear nerve at surgery, but had severe decline or total loss of hearing in the ear undergoing surgery. This group was followed up for an average of 2.9 years. Seven had CT confirmation with followup. Two patients in this group had subtotal removal because of brain stem depression on monitoring while tumor dissection was attempted. At 3 years, 1 patient has shown no recurrence, as confirmed by CT. The second had a recurrence, and underwent surgery again with total removal of the tumor. He has been without signs or symptoms of recurrence for 7 years.

This study demonstrated that functional preservation of the cochlear nerve in patients for whom acceptable hearing results can be attained is technically and biologically possible. Although studies have shown the possibility of microscopic tumor remaining in fibers of the cochlear nerve after dissection, this series demonstrated that clinically the tumor behaves as though it has been totally extirpated.

▶ Total removal of acoustic neuroma with preservation of the cochlear nerve is not associated with significant tumor recurrence. This long-term study of 21 patients provides data that effectively counter the claim that the preserved cochlear nerve harbors islands of tumor cells that may cause recurrence. This report, which will require scientific confirmation by others, firmly supports the effort to preserve hearing, which was achieved in 9 of 21 cases, and thus favors a suboccipital approach to these lesions. A study conducted at the Mayo Clinic found that in 23 patients who underwent operation for residual or recurrent acoustic neuroma over a 10-year period, long-term follow-up for at least 7–8 years was indicated for confirmation that excised tumors do not recur (Ebersold MJ, Harner SG: *Laryngoscope* 97:1168–1171, 1987).—R.M. Crowell, M.D.

Neurofibromatosis 2: Bilateral Acoustic Neurofibromatosis
Martuza RL, Eldridge R (Massachusetts Gen Hosp, Boston; Harvard Univ; Natl Inst of Neurological and Communicative Disorders and Stroke, Bethesda, Md)
N Engl J Med 318:684–688, March 17, 1988   19–28

The neurofibromatoses consist of 2 distinct disorders, the genes for which have recently been located on separate chromosomes. Neurofibromatosis 2, also called bilateral acoustic neurofibromatosis, affects thousands of Americans and has a molecular origin similar to that of some of the common sporadically occurring tumors of the nervous system. The clinical features, diagnostic advances, treatment dilemmas, and basic research findings in neurofibromatosis 2 were reviewed.

The clinical expressions of neurofibromatosis 1 and neurofibromatosis 2 are quite different. The hallmark of neurofibromatosis 2 is bilateral acoustic neuromas. In any child of an affected parent, the risk of such

---

Criteria for Diagnosis of Neurofibromatoses

NEUROFIBROMATOSIS 1

Neurofibromatosis 1 may be diagnosed when two or more of the following are present:

Six or more café au lait macules whose greatest diameter is more than 5 mm in prepubertal patients and more than 15 mm in postpubertal patients

Two or more neurofibromas of any type, or one plexiform neurofibroma

Freckling in the axillary or inguinal region

Optic glioma

Two or more Lisch nodules (iris hamartomas)

A distinctive osseous lesion such as sphenoid dysplasia or thinning of long-bone cortex, with or without pseudarthrosis

A parent, sibling, or child with neurofibromatosis 1 according to the above criteria

NEUROFIBROMATOSIS 2

Neurofibromatosis 2 may be diagnosed when one of the following is present:

Bilateral eighth-nerve masses seen with appropriate imaging techniques (computerized tomography or magnetic resonance imaging)

A parent, sibling, or child with neurofibromatosis 2 and either unilateral eighth-nerve mass or any two of the following: neurofibroma, meningioma, glioma, schwannoma, or juvenile posterior subcapsular lenticular opacity

---

(Courtesy of Martuza RL, Eldridge R: *N Engl J Med* 318:684–688, March 17, 1988.)

tumor development is about 50%. Because its genetic basis and natural history are distinct, it is important to distinguish neurofibromatosis 2 from neurofibromatosis 1 (table). Neurofibromatosis 2 should be suspected in the child, sibling, or parent of a person with known neurofibromatosis 2; in a person with apparent unilateral acoustic neuroma with symptom onset before age 30 years; in a child with meningeal or Schwann-cell tumor; in a person of any age with multiple nervous system tumors not attributable to another disorder; and in a teenager or adult with no family history of neurofibromatosis 1 and 1 or more neurofibromas but only a few cafe au lait spots and no Lisch nodules. Magnetic resonance imaging of the head should be used to search for acoustic neuromas or other intracranial tumors if any findings suggest neurofibromatosis 2. Early diagnosis affords the best opportunity for successful treatment. Complete surgical removal of an acoustic neuroma should be considered in patients with neurofibromatosis 2 who have small tumors when hearing is worsening or when 1 tumor is enlarging and stable hearing still remains in the opposite ear.

▶ Bilateral acoustic neurofibromatosis (neurofibromatosis 2) is a different problem from von Recklinghausen's disease (neurofibromatosis 1). The genetic basis and natural history are different. Martuza and Eldridge present the circumstances for suspicion of neurofibromatosis 2, the method of diagnosis with MR, and the need for complete surgical excision in patients with small tumors and declining hearing or a growing tumor with stable contralateral hearing. Because of the complexity of neurofibromatosis 1 and 2, neurofibromatosis clinics with a variety of specialists appear to be desirable for the management of these patients.—R.M. Crowell, M.D.

Common Pathogenetic Mechanism for Three Tumor Types in Bilateral Acoustic Neurofibromatosis

Seizinger BR, Rouleau G, Ozelius LJ, Lane AH, St George-Hyslop P, Huson S, Gusella JF, Martuza RL (Massachusetts Gen Hosp, Boston; Harvard Univ; Univ of Wales, Heath Park, Cardiff, UK)
Science 236:317–320, Apr 17, 1987   19–29

Bilateral acoustic neurofibromatosis (BANF), also known as central neurofibromatosis, is an autosomal dominant disorder characterized by neoplasia of cells of neural crest origin. Individuals with this gene defect have a predisposition to a variety of tumors of the central and peripheral nervous systems, including meningiomas, gliomas, and spinal neurofibromas. The hallmark of this disorder is the bilateral occurrence of acoustic neuromas, Schwann cell-derived tumors of the vestibular branch of the eighth cranial nerve. The same types of tumors associated with BANF more often occur singly in persons without the inherited tendency. The specific loss of genes on chromosome 22 is a common event in sporadic cases of acoustic neuroma. Tumors of several different histologic types from patients with BANF were investigated.

Genomic DNA was isolated from tumor tissue and lymphocytes from 6 patients with confirmed BANF. Four patients were heterozygous in their normal tissue for at least 1 of the 4 polymorphic DNA markers used. Two patients with acoustic neuroma were constitutionally heterozygous at D22S1, an anonymous DNA locus detected by probe pMS3-18 and mapping to 22q11.2-q13, and D22S9, an anonymous DNA locus detected by probe p22/34 and mapping to 22q11. In DNA from the acoustic neuroma tissue of each patient, heterozygosity was lost for DD22S1 but not for D22S9 (Fig 19–6). In 2 of 3 neurofibromas taken from the upper cervical spinal region of another patient, constitutional heterozygosity for D22S1 was lost. The same allele was lost in both tumors. A meningioma taken from another patient was also found to have lost constitutional heterozygosity for chromosome 22 loci D22S9 and IGLC.

This investigation showed a specific loss of alleles from chromosome 22 in 2 acoustic neuromas, 2 neurofibromas, and 1 meningioma from pa-

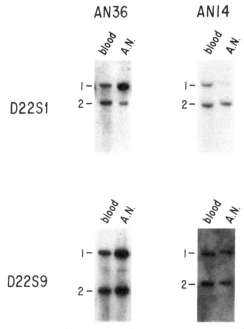

Fig 19–6.—Loss of constitutional heterozygosity for distinct chromosome 22 loci in acoustic neuromas from patients with BANF. Deoxyribonucleic acid was isolated from tumor specimens and corresponding normal tissue (peripheral leukocytes), digested with appropriate restriction enzymes, fractionated by agarose gel electrophoresis, and transferred to nylon membrane. Southern blots were hybridized to 32P-labeled DNA probes pMS3-18 (D22S1) and p22/34 (D22S9), respectively. Patient designations are shown above the autoradiograms. Numbers on the left indicate the observed alleles, with *1* and *2* referring to the larger and smaller allelic restriction fragments, respectively; pMS3-18 reveals an RFLP in Bgl II-digested human DNA with fragments of 9.5 kb ("1" allele) and 6.5 kb ("2" allele); p22/34 detects a RFLP with fragments of 5.8 kb ("1" allele) and 3.2 kb ("2" allele) in Taq I-digested DNA. *Blood*, DNA from peripheral blood leukocytes; *AN*, DNA from acoustic neuroma tissue. (Courtesy of Seizinger BR, Rouleau G, Ozelius LJ, et al: *Science* 236:317–320, Apr 17, 1987.)

tients with BANF. This finding indicates a common pathogenetic mechanism for all 3 tumor types. The 2 neurofibromas, taken from 1 patient, both showed loss of identical alleles, demonstrating that the same chromosome was deleted in both tumors. The third neurofibroma from this patient had no detectable loss of heterozygosity, which suggests the possibility of a more subtle mutational event affecting chromosome 22. Only a portion of chromosome 22 was deleted in the neuromas, narrowing the possible chromosomal location of the gene that causes BANF to the region distal to the D22S9 locus in band 22q11.

▶ Gene probes offer solid evidence of the genetic basis for various inherited CNS tumors. Genetic abnormalities in chromosome 22 have been demonstrated with acoustic neuromas, neurofibromas, and meningiomas in patients with BANF. Specific loss of alleles from chromosome 22 was a common pathogenic mechanism in all 3 tumor types. The identification of progressively smaller deletions on chromosome 22 in these tumor types may well provide a means to clone and characterize the defect. Recently, specific loss of genes on chromosome 22 has been demonstrated in sporadic cases of acoustic neuroma. Application of gene probe techniques offers great promise for understanding pathogenetic mechanisms for the development of CNS tumors and even for the possibility of diagnosis and treatment of these lesions.—R.M. Crowell, M.D.

Brief Notes on Acoustic Neuromas

MRI and Cerebellopontine Tumors

Magnetic resonance detects lesions in the internal auditory canal with great sensitivity. Tumors with small extracanalicular components are seen in the T_1- and T_2-weighted sequences, whereas purely intracanalicular lesions are often visualized only in the T_1-weighted images (Valvassori GE, et al: *AJNR* 9:115–119, 1988).

Of 145 acoustic neurinomas surgically verified, only 2% had normal brain stem auditory evoked potentials. This method remains the least invasive examination providing the earliest diagnosis (Ohoesser M, et al: *Ann Otolaryngol Chir Cervicofac* 103:215–221, 1986).

A small acoustic neuroma may be missed with normal brain stem auditory evoked responses (Leggett JM, Reid A: *J Laryngol Otol* 101:179–183, 1987).

Intracranial and intratemporal facial neuroma generally presents with facial weakness, and the tympanic, vertical, and labyrinthine segments are most commonly involved (Lipkin AF, et al: *Otolaryngol Head Neck Surg* 96:71–87, 1987).

Avascular, contrast enhancing intraosseous petrous apex masses suggest neuroma (Solodnik P, et al: *J Comput Assist Tomogr* 10:1027–1029, 1986).

Direct coronal thin-section CT is the most sensitive means of demonstrating glomus tympanicum chemodectomas. Magnification angiography is also important to avoid aberrant internal carotid artery (Larson TC III, et al: *Radiology* 163:801–806, 1987).

Removal of a large acoustic neuroma eliminated contralateral hemifacial spasm (Nishi T, et al: *Neurology* 37:339–342, 1987).

For cerebellopontine lesions, CT demonstrated the lesions in 95.8%, and MR, in 98.7%. With the exception of metastatic lesions, cholesteatomas, and some meningiomas, MR was usually more helpful. Magnetic resonance is a suitable primary diagnostic modality (Gentry LR, et al: *Radiology* 162:513–520, 1987).

Computed tomography scanning may make the diagnosis of sixth nerve neuroma in the cavernous sinus (Hansman ML, et al: *J Comput Assist Tomogr* 10:1030–1032, 1986).

Facial nerve enhancement with gadolinium in MRI suggests neurofibroma (Daniels DL, et al: *AJNR* 8:605–607, 1987).

Hearing Preservation via Monitoring

Electrophysiologic monitoring is recommended during surgery for acoustic neuroma and other posterior fossa. The best technique is the electrocochleogram, and cochlear nerve action potential is a good backup. In some cases, auditory brain stem response is also helpful. Monopolar constant-voltage intracranial stimulation of the facial nerve is helpful for the identification and preservation of the facial nerve. Audio monitoring of the spontaneous electromyogram provides real-time feedback on facial nerve manipulation (Linden RD, et al: *Can J Neurol Sci* 15:73–81, 1988).

Intraoperative electrocochleography is a reliable intraoperative test for cochlear nerve function in that loss of potentials intraoperatively is always associated with deafness (Sabin HI, et al: *Acta Neurochir (Wien)* 85:110–116, 1987).

In dog experiments, cochlear nerve injuries were found to be caused by cerebellopontine angle manipulations. Retraction of the eighth nerve causes disintegration of the myelin sheath. Hemorrhages within the nerve trunk also can cause loss of function (Sekiya T, Moller AR: *J Neurosurg* 67:244–249, 1987).

Among 16 cases of acoustic neuroma operated via a suboccipital approach, hearing was preserved in 6 of 8 cases with tumors smaller than 1.5 cm. Eighth nerve action potentials were useful in this surgery (Silverstein H, et al: *Otolaryngol Head Neck Surg* 95:285–291, 1986).

One hundred seventy-six operations were performed suboccipitally in 159 patients. One hundred sixty-nine patients had no facial weakness preoperatively, and in 158 of these, the facial nerve was anatomically preserved. Facial results were good in 44%, fair in 43%, and bad or poor in 13%. Anatomical preservation of the cochlear nerve was achieved in 80 patients; of those with a hearing loss below 70 dB, 75% had auditory nerve preserved, and 18% (14 cases) showed preserved hearing postoperatively, with 10 having a speech discrimination over 50% (Fischer G, et al: *Neurochirurgie* 33:169–183, 1987).

Of 44 patients undergoing acoustic neuroma removal, hearing preservation was achieved in 43% of the patients whose lesions were smaller than 20 mm, 25% of those with tumors 20–40 mm, and 11% of those with tumors larger than 4 mm (Frerebeau P, et al: *Neurochirurgie* 33:124–128, 1987).

Hearing preservation in the suboccipital surgery for acoustic neurinoma can be achieved in 43% of tumors smaller than 20 mm, 25% of those 20–40 mm, and 11% of those larger than 40 mm (Frerebeau P, et al: *Neurosurgery* 21:197–200, 1987).

A transtympanic electrode may be used for intraoperative electrocochleographic monitoring (Prass RL, et al: *Otolaryngol Head Neck Surg* 97:343–350, 1987).

In an effort to save hearing in patients with acoustic neuroma, the success rate is higher with suboccipital surgery (Glasscock ME, et al: *Laryngoscope* 97:785–789, 1987).

Experience in 30 patients indicates that preservation of the cochlear nerve action potential correlates well with postoperative preservation of useful hearing in patients with cerebellopontine angle operations (Rowed DW, et al: *Can J Neurol Sci* 15:68–72, 1988).

Successful nerve grafting in iatrogenic intratemporal facial palsy has been reported (Cruz NA, Macha N: *Ann Otolaryngol (Paris)* 104:51–58, 1987).—R.M. Crowell, M.D.

Meningiomas

Cavernous Sinus Meningiomas

Cioffi FA, Bernini FP, Punzo A, Natale M, Muras I (Univ of Naples, Naples, Italy)
Neurochirurgia 30:40–47, 1987   19–30

Less than 1% of all intracranial meningiomas arise from the lateral wall of the cavernous sinus. Although they represent a separate clinical and neuroradiologic entity, in most studies they are included among either the subtemporal or lateral group of parasellar meningiomas. Eleven women and 1 man, aged 36–60 years, were seen in the past 10 years. An interval of 1 month to 12 years elapsed from clinical onset to admission. The most common clinical symptoms were ptosis or diplopia, and deficits of oculomotor nerves were the most common sign on admission.

All operations were performed with the aid of the operating microscope. A frontotemporal craniotomy was performed in 6 patients, and the lesion was reached by temporal craniotomy through a subtemporal approach in 6. Whatever approach used to expose the cavernous sinus region, it was necessary to coagulate the medial group of temporobasal veins near the dura in most patients. Complete piecemeal removal of the tumor could be achieved in only 1 patient without narrowing of the internal carotid artery; a subtotal removal was obtained in 8 patients, and a partial removal was obtained in 3. There were no postoperative deaths. Trigeminal pain as well as proptosis was relieved with no appreciable change in the ophthalmologic disturbances. All patients received prophylactic antiepileptic treatment postoperatively, and their clinical status remained unchanged 14–46 months after operation. Supervoltage x-ray therapy (5,000 rad) was used in 1 patient with an angioblastic meningioma and in 3 patients who had partial excision.

Computed tomographic scanning is the screening procedure of choice in the management of these lesions. However, computed tomography alone does not permit a decision concerning treatment. Angiography may also be used to determine whether the tumor has developed on the lateral wall of the cavernous sinus or originates from the surrounding structures; it can also be used to define features such as intracavernous infiltration.

Improved knowledge about the cavernous sinus now allows for planning a radical operation. In the first cases, the aim was to reduce the tumor mass as much as possible to relieve symptoms without increasing preoperative neurologic deficits. In the later cases, a more aggressive operation was performed, although this is not possible if there is tumoral invasion of the internal carotid artery. In this series, the approach was selected according to tumor size; the frontotemporal approach was used for the largest tumors. Because the dural layer may be indistinguishable from the tumor, only piecemeal removal allows one to recognize when the cavernous lodge has been reached. Although considered ineffective as a primary treatment method, radiotherapy has an established role in treating incompletely excised or malignant meningiomas.

▶ The authors reviewed a 10-year experience with a challenging group of meningiomas. Although CT may detect these lesions, MRI is also quite helpful, depicting the relation to the internal carotid artery and to parenchyma as well. Because only 2-year follow-up is presented, the long-term results of subtotal resection in 11 of the 12 cases cannot be ascertained from this report. It is clear, however, that the surgery was well tolerated, with a minimum of new deficits in these patients. Whether a radical approach with total removal as advocated by Sekhar will produce better results in the long run is unknown, but certainly the perioperative morbidity with this radical approach is much more substantial. For many neurosurgeons, a more conservative subtotal removal will be a reasonable approach. In case of subtotal removal, radiotherapy is probably indicated (Carella et al: *Neurosurgery* 10:332–339, 1982; Petty et al: *J Neurosurg* 62:502–507, 1985).—R.M. Crowell, M.D.

Malignant and Atypical Meningiomas: A Reappraisal of Clinical, Histological, and Computed Tomographic Features
Alvarez F, Roda JM, Pérez Romero M, Morales C, Sarmiento MA Blázquez MG
(Autonomous Univ, Madrid)
Neurosurgery 20:688–694, May 1987   19–31

Meningiomas are considered benign neoplasms, although recurrences and malignancy have been reported. Histologic criteria, such as high cellularity, typical and atypical mitosis, necrosis, infiltration of the underlying brain, poor differentiation, and distant metastasis, were defined as nonbenign meningiomas. Data on a series of 21 patients with atypical and malignant meningiomas were reviewed to correlate the histologic findings with clinical and computed tomographic (CT) features as well as to establish some factors that may predict prognosis. The results were compared with those in 205 patients with benign meningiomas. Malignant meningiomas were defined as those that fulfilled the histologic criteria of malignancy, whereas atypical meningiomas showed high mitotic rate and at least 1 of the histologic criteria.

Twelve male and 9 female patients were studied; this male predominance was significant when compared with that of benign meningiomas.

All tumors were located supratentorially. The most common clinical features were raised intracranial pressure and motor disturbances. On CT, the presence of fringelike extension from smooth and well-defined tumor margins and intratumoral hypodense areas were both significant signs of malignancy of atypia. All patients underwent surgical excision. Of 6 patients with malignant meningiomas, 5 (83.3%) had recurrences, and 4 (66.6%) died during a mean follow-up of 6.9 years (range, 7 months to 17 years). Of 15 patients with atypical meningiomas, 3 (25%) had recurrences and 5 (33.3%) died at a mean follow-up of 3.7 years (range, 1–8 years). Radiotherapy was given to 10 patients, suggesting rapid growth. Of 6 patients with malignant meningiomas, 4 were treated with radiotherapy after the first operation and had tumor intervals of 4–17 years; the remaining 2 were not irradiated; 1 had a vertebral metastases 4 months later, and the other had a recurrence 1 year later. The most striking characteristic on histologic examination was the loss of architectural patterns and increase of cellularity. Eight patients showed clear microscopic cerebral infiltration with digitiform tumoral prolongations that isolated areas of nervous tissue.

Radical surgical excision remains the treatment of choice for malignant and atypical meningiomas. Although these results suggest a beneficial effect of radiotherapy after the first operation for malignant meningiomas, they are not conclusive.

▶ The radiologic and histologic features of meningioma correlate with recurrence rate after surgery. When all of the histologic criteria for malignant meningioma are present and when radiography shows low density in the lesion and fingerlike extensions, there is a very high rate of early recurrence (83%). When a few histologic and radiographic characteristics suggest atypical meningioma, the recurrence rate is substantially less (25%). There is a high preponderance of males in such cases. It is suggested that radiation after the first operation is beneficial. We offer postoperative radiation for atypical and malignant meningiomas.—R.M. Crowell, M.D.

Brief Notes on Meningiomas

Biology of Meningiomas

Of 32 patients suspected of meningioma, MRI demonstrated a positive predictive value of 86%, whereas CT's was only 76% as compared with histology (Mawhinney RR, et al: *Clin Radiol* 37:429–439, 1986).

Meningioma may present with typical migraine attacks (Bouchez B, et al: *Sem Hop Paris* 62:3089–3091, 1986).

Substantial mortality is still reported for posterior fossa tumors (9 of 22 cerebellopontine angle meningiomas = 41%) (Friedrich P, et al: *Zentralbl Neurochir* 47:105–110, 1986).

Careful preoperative venography is important to determine whether the transverse sinus may be ligated in extended supratentorial and infratentorial tumor surgery (Lanzieri CF, et al: *Neuroradiology* 29:360–365, 1987).

Receptor autoradiography and in vitro binding assays demonstrated somatostatin receptors in 13 of 13 human meningiomas (Reubi JC, et al: *J Clin En-docrinol Metab* 63:433–438, 1986).

Computed tomography scans show intraventricular meningiomas to have increased density relative to brain, uniform enhancement, and calcification in virtually all cases (Dolinskas CA, Simeone, FA: *AJNR* 8:1077–1082, 1987).

Fifty meningiomas were stained with monoclonal antibodies to epithelial membrane antigen (50%), keratin (24%), vimentin (18%), and S100 protein (8%) (Meis JM, et al: *Arch Pathol Lab Med* 110:934–937, 1986).

Arachnoid granulations and meningiomas stain positive for vimentin and variably positive for keratin. Hemangiopericytomas and normal pericytes are negative for both vimentin and keratin. This suggests that hemangiopericytoma of the meninges is a variant of meningioma (Holden J, et al: *J Neuropathol Exp Neurol* 46:50–56, 1987).

The authors report 7 cases of papillary meningioma, bringing the reported total to 53 in the literature. Histologic features include necrosis, frequent mitosis, and a rich reticular network. Of the 7 cases, 5 had local recurrences and died 1.4 to 9 years after initial operation. Pulmonary metastases have been demonstrated. This is an aggressive lesion with poor prognosis (Pasquier B, et al: *Cancer* 58:299–305, 1986).

To diagnose cerebellar hemangioblastoma, screening is advisable in individuals at risk for Von Hippel-Lindau disease, with annual retinal examination from 5 years and biennial CT of the head and abdomen from 15 and 20 years, respectively (Huson SM, et al: *Brain* 109:1297–1310, 1986).

In 14 cases of solid hemangioblastoma, lesions were often mistaken for meningioma, and death or poor result occurred in 50% of the cases. Vertebral angiography is helpful in diagnosis (Young S, Richardson AE: *J Neurol Neurosurg Psychiatry* 50:155–158, 1987).—R.M. Crowell, M.D.

20 Ischemia

Introduction

In the area of *anterior circulation,* a number of landmark studies have appeared. As regards diagnosis, computed tomographic scanning can now provide in a noninvasive fashion information on carotid occlusion, pseudoocclusion, dissection, and stenosis (Abstract 21–1). The gold standard of carotid artery diagnosis, neuroangiography, has been studied regarding complications (Abstract 21–2). The authors document a 0.4% permanent ischemic complication rate, with the interesting finding that such complications are 3 times as common between 24 and 72 hours as between 0 and 24 hours. The group at Wake Forest University documents a declining morbidity and mortality of carotid endarterectomy, with stroke morbidity of 2.1% and operative mortality of 2.6% for symptomatic patients (Abstract 21–4). Traumatic dissections of the extracranial internal carotid artery are recognized with increasing frequency, are usually best treated with anticoagulants, and only occasionally require surgical repair (Abstract 21–3). There is a place for emergency carotid endarterectomy, with some patients improving remarkably following restoration of carotid flow (Abstract 21–5). A controlled study from the University of Washington suggests an advantage for endarterectomy in the management of asymptomatic high-grade internal carotid artery stenosis (Abstract 21–6). Radiation-induced carotid atherosclerosis is readily identified on angiography, but the surgical management is quite difficult, often involving special patch graft techniques (Abstract 21–7). A randomized study has indicated the benefits of patching in routine carotid endarterectomy (Abstract 21–8).

In the area of *posterior circulation*, vertebral artery injury cases seldom develop neurologic deficits and may best be treated by percutaneous endovascular techniques (Abstract 21–10). Vertebrobasilar insufficiency may be treated by a host of ingenious surgical revascularization techniques outside the skull, but the indications remain speculative (Abstract 21–11).

In *medical management* of cerebrovascular disease, the prognosis of patients with retinal embolism has been studied (Abstract 21–12). Patients with cholesterol retinal emboli have high risk of stroke. In a randomized, controlled trial of hemodilution in acute ischemic stroke, the results did not bear out a beneficial effect for this treatment method (Abstract 21–13).

Robert M. Crowell, M.D.

Anterior Circulation

Computed Tomographic Evaluation of Extracranial Carotid Artery Disease
Hodge CJ Jr, Leeson M, Cacayorin E, Petro G, Culebras A, Iliya A, (SUNY Health Sciences Ctr, Syracuse)
Neurosurgery 21:167–176, August 1987

20–1

The techniques currently used to assess the pathologic abnormalities of the carotid artery, such as digital subtraction angiography (DSA) and standard transfemoral angiography (TFA), generally emphasize the luminal consequences of the abnormality instead of the pathologic condition itself. To investigate the efficacy of axial CT in imaging pathologic processes of the carotid artery, CT scanning was used to assess the cervical carotid arteries at the bifurcation and above in a series of patients believed to have ischemic cerebral dysfunction secondary to abnormalities of the cervical carotid arteries.

A General Electric 8800 or 9800 scanner was used to obtain high-resolution images during and after intravenous Conray-60 infusion. The contrast agent, 100 ml, was injected during the dynamic portion of the scan. A slow infusion of 150 ml of the contrast agent followed for about 15 minutes. During the dynamic portion of the scan, 5-mm overlapping CT slices were taken in the axial plane at intervals of 2.5 mm for a maximum of 16 slices. When the dynamic scan was completed, a series of 24 to 43 contiguous high-resolution 1.5-mm slices was obtained through the same cervical area. Planar reconstructions of the axial data were generally of little value. Standard transfemoral cervical carotid and cerebral angiographic results were compared to the CT images. The CT scan was useful for determining the presence of degenerative atheromatous changes such as carotid artery calcification, subintimal hemorrhage, carotid occlusion, carotid segmental occlusion, carotid pseudoocclusion, and carotid artery dissection. Computed tomography scans were found particularly useful for identifying atheromatous carotid artery disease when the carotid angiogram appeared nearly normal and for identifying the cause of postoperative carotid stenosis.

Computed tomography imaging of the carotid artery permits extension of the information gained by conventional angiography. The CT scan views not only the lumen of the vessel, but also the arterial wall, allowing definition of the thickness and composition of the wall. This technique improves the diagnostic radiologic evaluation of carotid disease when combined with angiography.

▶ This is a landmark paper in cerebrovascular diagnosis. Hodge and colleagues present data that establish the importance of CT evaluation of extracranial carotid artery disease. They show that carotid occlusion, pseudoocclusion, dissection, and stenosis can be identified with CT. Further studies are needed to confirm these findings and especially to determine the sensitivity and reliability of CT diagnosis as compared with angiography and pathologic data. Most importantly, the authors present CT images of intimal thickening, atheromatous debris, and other details of plaque anatomy that are not provided by other studies. Correlation of such data with clinical course may help identify dangerous plaques, particularly in asymptomatic patients. Such correlations could assist in establishing indications for endarterectomy.— R.M. Crowell, M.D.

Clinical Events Following Neuroangiography: A Prospective Study
Dion JE, Gates PC, Fox AJ, Barnett HJM, Blom RJ (Univ Hosp, Univ of Western Ontario, London, Ont)
Stroke 18:997–1004, November–December 1987   20–2

Studies assessing the risks of cerebral angiography have traditionally been retrospective, and none included events occurring more than 24 hours after angiography. To identify predictable risk factors and to compare these risk factors with those previously identified, the authors prospectively evaluated clinical events occurring up to 72 hours after cerebral angiography in 1,002 consecutive procedures in 724 patients.

The procedures were performed from 1983 to 1984. The ischemic event rate between 0 and 24 hours was 1.3% (0.1% permanent) (table). This incidence was higher (2.5%) in patients examined for cerebrovascular disease, but the difference was not significant. Between 24 and 72 hours after angiography, an additional 1.8% of patients became ischemic (0.3% permanent). Cerebral ischemic events occurred as either recurrences or worsening of preexisting conditions twice as often as de novo. All permanent ischemia was a worsening of a preexisting phenomenon. A significant increase in the incidence of neurologic events between 0 and 24 hours was noted when the procedure lasted longer than 60 minutes and when there was systolic hypertension. Trends toward higher incidence were observed with the use of increased volume of contrast, increased serum creatinine, when transient ischemic attacks or stroke were indications, and when at least 3 catheters were used. The incidence of neurologic events between 24 and 72 hours increased significantly with increased amounts of contrast used, age, and diabetes. The incidence of nonneurologic events, mostly hematomas, was significantly raised by multiple factors.

This prospective study demonstrated that clinical events do occur beyond the usual observation period of 24 hours but confirms the low risk of cerebral angiography when performed judiciously.

▶ This important prospective study confirms the safety of neuroangiography in experienced hands. The authors document a 0.4% permanent ischemic complication rate. It is documented by prospective examination by a neurologist. Importantly, significant ischemic complications between 24 and 72 hours were 3 times as common as those between 0 and 24 hours after the examination. This serves as a warning, therefore, to those who favor outpatient angiography. Note also that complications were common when the procedure lasted longer than 60 minutes. In order to achieve these low complication rates, obviously

Neurologic Events According to Indication and Angiographic Technical Data*

Indication	% of procedures (N=1,002)	Mean age (years)	No. catheters	Duration (min)	Neurologic				Non-neurologic
					Transient		Permanent		
					0–24 hrs	24–72 hrs	0–24 hrs	24–72 hrs	
TIA/stroke	28.4	57.7	1.9	60.4	2.5% (7)	1.4% (4)	—	0.7% (2)	14.0%
Known aneurysm and AVM	21.8	43.1	1.2	53.4	0	0.9% (2)	—	—	3.7%
Postoperative aneurysm	22.6	47.9	1.3	37.6	1.3% (3)	0.9% (2)	—	0.4% (1)	6.6%
SAH (recent)	12.0	43.9	1.3	51.7	0.8% (1)	2.5% (3)	0.9% (1)	—	5.0%
Postoperative AVM	8.8	33.7	1.1	44.4	0	3.4% (3)	—	—	2.3%
Others	6.4	46.1	1.3	50.3	1.6% (1)	1.6% (1)	—	—	0.2%
Total	100	47.6	1.4	50.2	1.2% (12)	1.5% (15)	0.1% (1)	0.3% (3)	7.2%

*TIA, transient ischemic attack; AVM, arteriovenous malformation; and SAH, subarachnoid hemorrhage.
(Courtesy of Dion JE, Gates PC, Fox AJ: Stroke 18:997–1004, November–December 1987.)

the angiographer must be well-trained and maintain a high-volume experience (Dion JE, et al: *Stroke* 18:997–1004, 1987).

Theodotou et al (*Surg Neurol* 28:90–92, 1987) report that in 159 transfemoral cerebral angiograms for patients with carotid stenosis, no patient asymptomatic prior to study developed complications, whereas patients with transient ischemic attacks (TIAs) had a 4.5% incidence and patients with stroke in evolution had a 7.7% incidence of complications. Patients with completed strokes did not have angiographic complications. Stroke in progress has too high an angiographic risk, whereas TIAs and completed strokes do not. McIvor et al. conclude that the neurologic morbidity of cerebral angiography is clearly influenced by the experience of the vascular radiologist (McIvor J, et al: *Br J Radiol* 60:117–122, 1987).—R.M. Crowell, M.D.

Traumatic Dissections of the Extracranial Internal Carotid Artery
Mokri B, Piepgras DG, Houser OW (Mayo Clinic and Found, Rochester, Minn)
J Neurosurg 68:189–197, February 1988   20–3

Extracranial internal carotid artery (ICA) dissections, although uncommon, are not rare. As clinicians become more familiar with the clinical and angiographic features of this entity, the number of patients reported increases. The management of 18 patients with traumatic extracranial ICA dissections was described.

The patients, aged 19–55 years, had sustained blunt head or neck injury of marked or moderate severity. Motor vehicle accidents were the main cause of injury. The most common presenting symptoms were delayed focal cerebral ischemic symptoms. Focal unilateral headache associated with oculosympathetic paresis or bruit was noted less commonly. After head injury, the abrupt onset of focal cerebral symptoms after a lucid interval should raise the suspicion of arterial injury, especially when computed tomography does not show abnormalities that would explain the evolving neurologic deficits on the basis of direct trauma to the brain. Unilateral headaches, oculosympathetic palsy, and bruits also aid in making the diagnosis. Focal cerebral ischemic symptoms can appear months or years after trauma. Such delayed symptoms are caused by embolization from a thrombus in a residual dissecting aneurysm. Commonly seen angiographic findings in decreasing order of frequency were aneurysm, stenosis of the lumen, occlusion, intimal flap, distal branch occlusion, and slow ICA-to-middle cerebral artery flow (Fig 20–1). Two patients in this series died of massive cerebral infarction and edema. Some patients were left with severe neurologic deficits, but most had a good recovery.

▶ Internal carotid artery dissections are not uncommon after head and neck trauma. A Horner's syndrome and unilateral headache may also suggest the diagnosis. Focal neurologic deficit may occur even years after dissection, presumably on an embolic basis. The treatment is usually with anticoagulants. Only occasionally will surgical repair of the dissected artery be required. Angio-

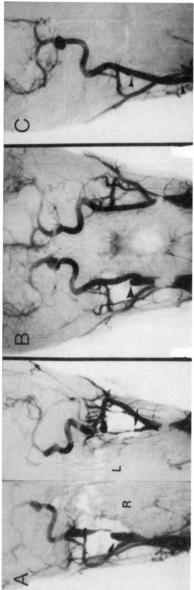

Fig 20–1.—Angiograms showing traumatic bilateral dissection of the internal carotid artery (ICA). **A**, initial angiograms on July 23, 1981, showing tapered stenosis of the left ICA with abrupt reconstitution of the lumen at the carotid canal and a tiny aneurysm proximally (*arrows*). An aneurysm is visualized in the midsegment of the extracranial portion of the right ICA with distal stenosis of the lumen. **B**, angiogram on February 24, 1983, showing resolution of the stenosis and aneurysm of the left ICA after superficial temporal artery-middle cerebral artery anastomosis. Stenosis of the right ICA has resolved, but a residual dissecting aneurysm persists (*arrowhead*). The patient then underwent resection of the right ICA aneurysm with interposition of a vein graft. **C**, angiogram on March 7, 1983, showing the vein graft, with its proximal and distal points identified by *arrowheads*. (Courtesy of Mokri B, Piepgras DG, Houser OW: *J Neurosurg* 68:189–197, February 1988.)

graphic follow-up is recommended, although many of these lesions improve substantially over the course of time. Kline et al. (*Ophthalmology* 94:227–230, 1987) suggest that painful Horner's syndrome may result from spontaneous internal carotid artery dissection.—R.M. Crowell, M.D.

Declining Morbidity and Mortality of Carotid Endarterectomy: The Wake Forest University Medical Center Experience

Till JS, Toole JF, Howard VJ, Ford CS, Williams D (Lewis-Gale Clinic, Salem, Va; Wake Forest Univ, the Quaker Med and Neurological Group, High Point, NC)
Stroke 18:823–829, September–October 1987   20–4

Because of unacceptable mortality and stroke morbidity rates after carotid endarterectomy for patients with transient ischemic attacks (TIAs), the Wake Forest University Medical Center undertook measures to reduce them. These measures included a TIA and stroke registry with continuing audit of patient management and outcome, more rigorous case selection, use of superficial cervical plexus block so that the patient acts as his own monitor of brain function, the use of a shunt only for patients who could not tolerate carotid clamping, meticulous removal of plaque and all detritus, and patient ambulation within 72 hours postoperatively. To determine whether these measures have contributed to a decline in morbidity and mortality, the records of 356 patients who underwent 389 carotid endarterectomies from 1979 through 1983 were reviewed. The 30-day mortality and morbidity for stroke and myocardial infarction were recorded.

Of the 155 asymptomatic patients who underwent endarterectomy, major morbidity included 2 myocardial infarctions and 1 stroke (1.9%). There were 3 deaths, 2 myocardial infarctions and 1 stroke, for a perioperative mortality rate of 1.9%. For the 234 symptomatic patients, stroke morbidity was 2.1% and operative mortality was 2.6%. Stroke morbidity for both groups combined was 1.5% and operative mortality was 2.3%, compared with a stroke morbidity of 16% and mortality of 6% reported in 1978 in patients treated before implementation of quality control measures. The perioperative stroke rate (morbidity plus mortality) was 2.6%, including 9 that were ipsilateral to the carotid endarterectomy, suggesting distal embolism as the probable cause.

The dramatic improvement in operative mortality and morbidity is attributed to the quality control measures implemented to correct unacceptable rates reported in 1978.

▶ Till and his group present encouraging data on the results of carotid endarterectomy at Wake Forest University. They attribute this improved postoperative profile to increased attention to detail in the matter of selection, to improved technique, and to performance of the operation only by experienced operators. Nonetheless, the serious morbidity and mortality for the asymptomatic group was 3.8%, and for the symptomatic group it was 4.7%. It remains to be proved that this outcome is an improvement over the natural history of the condition, particularly in the asymptomatic patient. One can only await the results of the North American Symptomatic Carotid Endarterectomy Trial with regard to scientific validation of the procedure.— R.M. Crowell, M.D.

Emergency Carotid Endarterectomy

Walters BB, Ojemann RG, Heros RC (Massachusetts Gen Hosp, Boston; Harvard Univ)
J Neurosurg 66:817–823, June 1987   20–5

The indications for emergency carotid endarterectomy are not well defined. A retrospective review was undertaken of the 64 emergency carotid endarterectomies performed by the Neurological Service at Massachusetts General Hospital from July 1976 to December 1985. Patients included 40 men and 24 women, with a mean age of 64 years (range, 32–87 years).

Preoperative angiographic findings were correlated with outcome. Of the 27 patients with severe stenosis and marked delay in blood flow, 25 (93%) were the same or improved postoperatively; no patient in this group died. Eleven patients had stenosis and an intraluminal filling defect, 6 of whom had an intraluminal clot; 8 (73%) were the same or improved after surgery, and 2 (18%) died. Of the 16 patients with presumed complete occlusion, 14 (88%) were the same or improved and 1 (18%) died. Of 10 patients who had moderate to severe stenosis, severe ulceration, or both, 8 (80%) were the same or improved after surgery and 1 (10%) died. Based on the preoperative and postoperative clinical status, the final clinical condition was closely correlated with the presenting status. No patient died who was intact (with history of transient ischemic attack or had only mild deficits preoperatively; 92% were improved or the same after surgery. Of 15 (7%) patients with moderate deficits preoperatively, 80% were the same or improved after surgery and 1 (7%) died. Of the 13 patients with severe deficits, 10 (77%) were the same or improved and 3 (23%) died. Of the 4 deaths in the total series, 2 were attributable to cardiac causes and 2 to unrelated disease processes.

Indications for emergency carotid endarterectomy include the following: (1) the sudden onset of a neurologic deficit with loss of a previously noted carotid artery bruit; (2) sudden onset of deficit from proven carotid artery occlusion during angiography; and (3) presence of transient ischemic attacks or acute, spontaneous mild, moderate, or severe neurologic deficit in the presence of 1 or more of these angiographic findings: severe stenosis in the proximal internal carotid artery (ICA) with a marked delay in flow, stenosis in the proximal ICA and the presence of an intraluminal filling defect, or complete occlusion of the ICA. Emergency surgery may be of benefit in patients with severe deficit who are alert and without evidence of significant infarction.

▶ The MGH group presents encouraging data for the utilization of emergency carotid endarterectomy in selected groups. A new point emerging from the study was that even cases with severe deficits at the time of surgery may improve following carotid endarterectomy. The question of how late one may operate after the onset of the deficit was not clarified. In the current medicolegal climate, it is prudent for such surgery to be practiced by surgeons already well experienced with endarterectomy in the setting of stable neurologic status. In a related study, of 7 patients with emergency carotid endarterectomy for hemiplegia, 2 of 3 patients with rapid downhill course despite medical therapy became neurologically intact after surgery (Benes, V, Jr: *Zentralbl Neurochir* 48:1–8, 1987). Prompt surgical relief of thrombosis appears to be the preferred approach (Painter TA, et al: *J Vasc Surg* 5:445–451, 1987). Of 2,651 patients with carotid endarterectomy at the Cleveland Clinic, 11 (0.4%) had symptomatic thrombosis of the internal carotid artery and underwent urgent reoperations. Eight (73%) recovered substantially and 1 died of a fatal hemorrhagic cerebral infarction.—R.M. Crowell, M.D.

Operative Versus Nonoperative Management of Asymptomatic High-Grade Internal Carotid Artery Stenosis: Improved Results With Endarterectomy
Moneta GL, Taylor DC, Nicholls SC, Bergelin RO, Zierler RE, Kazmers A, Clowes AW, Strandness DE Jr, (Univ of Washington, Seattle)
Stroke 18:1005–1010, November–December 1987   20–6

Developments in ultrasonic duplex scanning have improved the diagnosis of carotid artery disease, making it possible to accurately classify the degree of stenosis. Because high-grade carotid artery stenosis is an important predictor of a neurologic event, endarterectomy was recommended at 1 center to patients with asymptomatic internal carotid stenosis of 80% to 99%.

From 1983 to 1986, 129 high-grade internal carotid artery stenoses were identified in 115 patients. Fifty-six carotid endarterectomies were performed, and 73 lesions were followed without surgery. Surgical and nonsurgical groups were comparable in age, prevalence of hypertension, cardiac disease, diabetes, and aspirin use. Life table analyses to 24 months showed a higher rate of stroke—19% versus 4% —in the nonsurgical group (Fig 20–2). Transient focal neurologic deficits occurred in 28% of the nonsurgical group and 5% of the surgical group, and carotid

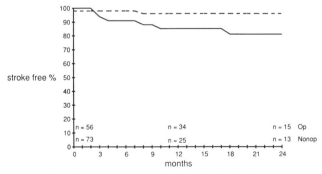

Fig 20–2.—Life-table analysis for occurrence of stroke in the distribution of nonoperated *(solid line)* vs. operated *(broken line)* sides after carotid endarterectomy (includes perioperative events) *(P = .08)*. (Courtesy of Moneta GL, Taylor DC, Nicholls SC, et al: *Stroke* 18:1005–1010, November–December 1987.)

occlusion occurred in 29% and 0%, respectively. Eight of the 9 strokes that occurred among the nonsurgically treated patients did so within 9 months of the diagnosis of high-grade lesions, and none was preceded by a transient ischemic attack. One perioperative stroke occurred, for an incidence of 1.8%, but there were no in-hospital operative deaths and no difference in the late death rates of the 2 groups.

The preservation of neurologic status in patients with asymptomatic high-grade internal carotid artery stenosis can be improved with carotid endarterectomy.

▶ Strandness's group presents controlled data that suggest a benefit for carotid endarterectomy in asymptomatic high-grade internal carotid stenosis. However, the control mechanism was not a randomized one in that patients were selected for surgery on the basis of their referring physician's preferences. In addition, with regard to the crucial endpoints of stroke and death, there was no statistically significant difference between the operated and unoperated groups. The crucial question of efficacy and safety of this treatment must await a properly controlled clinical trial. In follow-up of 135 patients with asymptomatic carotid stenosis, Schroeder et al. found an annual stroke rate of 1.1%. This is not considered high enough to warrant prophylactic endarterectomy, with the possible exception of a patient with greater than 90% stenosis (Schroeder T, et al: *Arch Surg* 122:795–801, 1987). A multicenter cooperative study is being undertaken to evaluate the incidence of TIAs, stroke, and death in previously asymptomatic patients with arteriographically confirmed internal carotid stenosis (50% or more) randomly allocated to carotid endarterectomy plus aspirin therapy versus aspirin therapy alone (A Veterans Administration Cooperative Study: *Stroke* 17:534–539, 1986).—R.M. Crowell, M.D.

Management of Radiation-Induced Accelerated Carotid Atherosclerosis
Loftus CM, Biller J, Hart MN, Cornell SH, Hiratzka LF (Univ of Iowa, Iowa City)
Arch Neurol 44:711–714, July 1987   20–7

Improved therapeutic regimens for systemic and head and neck malignancies have prolonged survival times. However, long-term survivors who were treated with cervical irradiation are at risk for radiation-induced acceleration of carotid arteriosclerosis. The neurologic presentation of such patients mimics naturally occurring atheromatous disease, but the patients are often younger and have less concurrent coronary or systemic vascular disease. Treatment in 2 patients with radiation-induced-accelerated atherosclerosis was described.

Case 1.—Man, 50, who had hypertension, received 60 Gy to the cervical area to treat a neck mass. The malignancy did not recur, but 8 years later, arteriography revealed more than 95% stenosis of the distal right common carotid artery, marked ulceration at the carotid bifurcation, and irregularity at the proximal portion of the right internal carotid artery. With aspirin and antihypertensive therapy, the patient remained asymptomatic for 1½ years until left inferior quadrantanopia developed in 1 eye. Angiography showed occlusion of the internal artery, with an irregular internal carotid stump. At endarterectomy, a thick, fibrotic, friable occlusive lesion in the common carotid was found. The patient recovered and was without neurologic symptoms while taking aspirin.

Case 2.—Man, 41, was treated at age 18 years with extensive cervical and mediastinal irradiation for Hodgkin's disease. While the disease was in remission, he experienced fluent aphasia and numbness on 1 side of the face and in 1 arm. Angiography revealed severe bilateral carotid disease. For 1½ months, he did well with warfarin sodium therapy until he experienced several short episodes of tingling and numbness in 1 hand. Bilateral aortointernal carotid arterial bypass with saphenous vein interposition grafts was done. Five months later, a second left aorta-to-internal carotid artery bypass was needed because the left bypass graft was occluded. The patient has done well with maintenance aspirin therapy.

These patients with radiation-induced accelerated carotid atherosclerosis typify the presentation and characteristics of this disease. Angiographic findings included disproportionate involvement of the distal common carotid artery and unusually long carotid lesions, and pathologic findings included internal elastic lamina destruction and replacement of the normal intima and media with fibrous tissue.

▶ This report emphasizes the severe fibrosis associated with radiation-induced accelerated carotid atherosclerosis. As in the 2 reported cases, medical therapy usually fails. Most authors have emphasized direct carotid exploration, as in case #1. Sometimes endarterectomy can be performed. An alternative is an on-lay patch graft of saphenous vein or Gortex (Marty AT, Logan JA: *Indiana Med* 77:90–91, 1984). As in case #2 reported here, the more complex bypass techniques may result in complications. Jones and Frusha (*South Med J* 79:1517–1520, 1986) conclude that carotid occlusive disease after irradiation may require special approaches, such as saphenous vein bypass.—R.M. Crowell, M.D.

Benefits of Carotid Patching: A Randomized Study
Eikelboom BC, Ackerstaff RGA, Hoeneveld H, Ludwig JW, Teeuwen C, Vermeulen FEE, Welten RJT (St Antonius Hosp, Nieuwegein-Utrecht, the Netherlands)
J. Vasc Surg 7:240–247, February 1988   20–8

Some researchers claim that carotid artery patching results in a decreased incidence of recurrent stenosis after endarterectomy. A prospective study was done to determine the value of carotid artery patching with random selection between primary closure and saphenous vein patching.

One hundred twenty-nine consecutive endarterectomies were assessed by duplex scanning at 3, 6, and 12 months after surgery. Intravenous digital subtraction angiography (DSA) was performed in the first postopera-

One-Year Duplex Restenosis Rates in Men and Women
With Primary Closure and Patch

	No.	*1 yr duplex restenosis (No.)*
Women, primary closure	11	6 (55%)
Men, primary closure	37	4 (11%)
Men, patch	43	2 (5%)
Women, patch	14	0 (0%)
Total	105	12 (11%)

(Courtesy of Eikelboom BC, Ackerstaff RGA, Hoenveld H, et al: *J Vasc Surg* 7:240–247, February 1988.)

tive days for control of the surgical technique and after 1 year to provide a reference for duplex scanning. Sixty-two patients had primary closure and 67 had the patching technique. Risk factors in each group were comparable: the mean patient age was 63 years, 74% were men, 57% had hypertension, 41% had coronary disease, 37% had peripheral arterial disease, and 9% had diabetes mellitus. In each group, the left side was operated on in 55% of patients; 18% were asymptomatic. Postoperative DSA was normal in 81% of patients; 17% had residual lesions, 2% had occlusions. A complete 1-year follow-up was possible in 81% of the patients. Duplex scanning showed recurrent stenosis of more than 50% in 11% of patients (table). This was significantly higher after primary closure (21%) than with patch closure (3.5%), and was significantly higher in women than in men. Recurrent stenosis occurred in 6 of 11 women with primary closure, 4 of 37 men with primary closure, 2 of 43 men with patching, and none of 14 women with patch closure. Duplex scanning at 1 year also showed that recurrent stenosis occurred more frequently when residual lesions were seen on postoperative DSA compared with normal DSA. Most recurrent stenoses occurred within 6 months of surgery. Duplex scanning graded these as more severe than did DSA.

This study demonstrated that the rate of recurrent carotid stenosis is decreased by patching, particularly in women, and may be further reduced by intraoperative detection and correction of technical imperfections.

▶ This randomized controlled study demonstrates a low rate of early occlusion and late restenosis for carotid vein patch grafting. Rupture occurs with saphenous vein graft taken from the ankle, and therefore harvesting from the groin is rational. This study adds substantial weight to the existing literature favoring patch grafting (Sundt, Imparato, Cleveland Clinic). In experimental studies, venous patch grafting did not influence carotid artery patency, endothelial regeneration, or wall healing. On the other hand, vein-patch angioplasty does increase vessel diameter and prevents the development of circumferential intimal thickening (Stewart GW, et al: *Arch Surg* 122:364–371, 1987). In a controlled series of carotid endarterectomies, no difference was found in restenosis frequencies between those performed with simple closure and those with vein patch graft (Curley S, et al: *J Vasc Surg* 6:350–354, 1987).—R.M. Crowell, M.D.

Carotid Body Tumours: A Review of 52 Cases
Gaylis H, Davidge-Pitts K, Pantanowitz D (Univ of the Witwatersrand, Johannesburg, South Africa)
S Afr Med J 72:493–496, Oct 3, 1987   20–9

During a 22-year period (1962–1984), 52 carotid body tumors were seen in 50 patients. Two patients had bilateral carotid body tumors and unilateral paragangliomas of the glomus intravagale, for a total of 54 paragangliomas. The patients' ages ranged from 23 to 80 years; the female/male ratio was 2:1, and the right side was affected twice as often as the left. The clinical course was slow in most patients, and almost all presented with a mass in the neck, which had been present for periods ranging from 2 weeks to 20 years. The tumors ranged in diameter from 1.5 to 8.5 cm and were characteristically mobile from side to side, but not vertically.

One patient had a recurrent carotid body tumor, the first one having been removed 23 years earlier. In all of the 38 patients who underwent carotid arteriography, the characteristic features of a tumor blush with splaying of the carotid bifurcation were seen, occasionally displaced anteriorly. The tumor was confirmed either by biopsy or excision in 48 patients. A biopsy specimen of an enlarged cervical lymph node before excision of the tumor revealed paraganglioma in 2 patients. Computed tomography demonstrated an enhancing mass in 13 patients. Circumferential spread of the tumor around the internal and external carotid arteries was also seen. No patient had significant hypertension and the results of endocrine studies, when undertaken, were normal.

Of the 50 patients, 4 were treated nonsurgically; 3 were too frail and elderly to undergo surgery and 1 had an extensively fixed tumor previously subjected to radiotherapy. The 46 remaining patients underwent surgery, although the operation was abandoned after a trial dissection in 2 patients because of inability to separate the tumor from the internal carotid artery and insufficient length of accessible internal carotid artery distal to the tumor for insertion of a graft. In the remaining 44 patients, 46 tumors were excised. In 6 patients, it was necessary to insert a graft. One patient died of a pulmonary embolus and 1 died of respiratory failure after hemiplegia. Eight patients were left with cranial nerve palsy, which had been present preoperatively in 5 patients. Seven tumors were malignant.

The slow growth of these tumors and the morbidity and mortality resulting from surgical complications were reasons often given for a conservative approach. With the introduction of modern techniques in vascular surgery and the unpredictable biologic behavior of these tumors, these reasons are no longer valid. Although the morbidity in this series was not inconsiderable, complications occurred almost exclusively in patients with larger tumors.

Most carotid body tumors grow slowly, but if not removed in time they also kill slowly. Since malignancy cannot be ruled out on the histologic features of the primary tumor, a conservative approach is not warranted unless there are medical contraindications to surgery.

▶ The authors advocate an aggressive approach toward carotid body tumors. This is also the recommendation of another recent publication on the subject from Sundt and colleagues (*J Neurosurg* 64:169–182, 1986). In the latter study, vascular grafting was not required in any case, nor were there any hemispheral symptoms. Both studies indicate that cranial nerve deficits are difficult to avoid, particularly in the larger tumors. A substantial percentage of these tumors may be malignant, and thus careful follow-up is recommended.— R.M. Crowell, M.D.

Brief Notes on Anterior Circulation

Other Noninvasive Studies

Intravenous digital subtraction angiography has a sensitivity of only 79% for stenosis and 23% in the diagnosis of ulcerated plaques (Friedrich JM, et al: *J Radiol* 68:275–283, 1987).

Agreement between DSA and duplex scanning is about 90% regarding restenosis after carotid artery surgery (Zbornikova V, et al: *Stroke* 17:1137–1142, 1986).

In 149 patients studied with intravenous DSA compared with surgical findings, there was good correlation in 79% with regard to degree of stenosis (Freidrich JM, et al: *VASA* 16:16–24, 1987).

A 6-year follow-up indicates that intravenous digital subtraction angiography has a place in the clinical arena, but it is relatively limited. Intra-arterial DSA, however, has increasing utility because it provides the opportunity of using less contrast, which leads to greater safety (Carmody RF, et al: *Invest Radiol* 21:899–905, 1986).

Prediction of carotid bifurcation ulceration was poor with B-mode ultrasound (O'Leary DH, et al: *Radiology* 162:523–525, 1987).

Complications and Long-Term Results of Carotid Endarterectomy

Of 100 carotid endarterectomies, angiography showed complete occlusion of the operated carotid artery in 16 cases, of which 13 were asymptomatic. Perioperative findings suggest that embolism, rather than hemodynamic ischemia, was the important cause of persistent symptoms (Van Alphen HAM, Polman CH: *Stroke* 17:1251–1253, 1986).

Ten cases are described with cerebral hyperfusion after carotid endarterectomy. Intraoperatively there was a dramatic increase in cerebral blood flow, and postoperative headaches and seizures were common. (Reigel MM, et al: *J Vasc Surg* 5:628–634, 1987).

Massive intracerebral hemorrhage may occur following carotid endarterectomy, particularly in the setting of extreme arterial stenosis, involvement of multiple extracranial vessels, presence of postoperative hypertension, and use of anticoagulant or antiplatelet medications (Haffner DH, et al: *Arch Surg* 122:305–307, 1987).

Glossopharyngeal nerve injury may complicate carotid endarterectomy (Rosenbloom M, et al: *J Vasc Surg* 5:469–471, 1987).

Forty-six of 47 patients survived combined coronary and carotid artery surgery without neurologic or cardiac complications, but there was one death (Minami K, et al: *J Thorac Cardiovasc Surg* 95:303–309, 1988).

When bilateral vocal cord paresis complicates a second operation for carotid endarterectomy, temporary tracheostomy may be utilized until 1 vocal cord resumes function (Tyers MR, Cronin K: *Anaesth Intensive Care* 14:314–316, 1986).

Isoflurane, when compared to enflurane and halothane, decreases the frequency of cerebral ischemia during carotid endarterectomy (Michenfelder JD, et al: *Anesthesiology* 67:336–340, 1987).

A review of results from carotid endarterectomy throughout Cincinnati did not show influence by type of surgical specialty or operative caseload (Kempczinski RF, et al: *J Vasc Surg* 3:911–916, 1986).

In a military hospital experience of 201 consecutive carotid endarterectomies, complications were present in 35.8% of the patients, with 8.9% being major complications (Oller DW, Welch H: *Am Surg* 52:479–484, 1986).

After carotid endarterectomy for amaurosis fugax, 2 strokes in 448 patient years of follow-up were reported (Bernstein EF, Dilley RB: *J Vasc Surg* 6:333–340, 1987).

Of 214 patients with 248 carotid endarterectomies, hemodynamically restenosis occurred in 15% at 6–12 months on noninvasive testing (DeGroote RD, et al: *Stroke* 18:1031–1036, 1987).

Carotid endarterectomy often fails to ameliorate nonhemispheric symptoms, especially in patients with hemodynamically insignificant lesions. When ocular pneumoplethysmography (OPG) suggests a hemodynamically significant lesion, 72% were relieved. With normal OPG only 32% were asymptomatic (Ouriel K, et al: *J Vasc Surg* 4:115–118, 1986).

In 33 carotid endarterectomies for recurrent carotid stenosis, pathologic lesions included recurrent atherosclerosis, neointimal fibromuscular hyperplasia, and lesions with elements of both. Embolic events rather than reduced blood flow appeared to be more common than previously reported. (Hunter GC, et al: *Arch Surg* 122:311–315, 1987).

Follow-up of 292 carotid endarterectomy operations over the long term showed restenosis of 15% in 5 years. The late neurological symptom rate was 14% in 5 years and was associated with widespread vascular disease rather than restenosis (Ackroyd N, et al: *J Cardiovasc Surg* 27:418–425, 1986).

Ocular pneumoplethysmographic testing (OPG-Gee) is said to indicate improvement in ocular blood flow on the side opposite the carotid repair only in patients with totally occluded contralateral vessels (Gee W, et al: *J Vasc Surg* 4:129–135, 1986).

External Carotid Surgery

Of 10 patients with bilateral internal carotid artery occlusion undergoing external carotid artery revascularization, only 1 transient ischemic attack and no strokes occurred in follow-up (Friedman SG, et al: *J Vasc Surg* 5:715–718, 1987).

External carotid artery reconstruction can be performed with little risk in symptomatic patients with occlusion of the internal carotid artery and ECA stenosis or cul-de-sac formation (Santiani B, et al: *Surg Gynecol Obstet* 164:105–110, 1987).

Experience with 14 external carotid endarterectomies leads to the conclusion that this is a safe and durable procedure, but periodic follow-up with noninvasive testing is needed to detect distal developing stenoses (Fisher DF, et al: *Am J Surg* 152:700–703, 1986).

Other Technical Considerations

A controlled, randomized study of local anesthetic injection of the carotid sinus nerve during carotid endarterectomy revealed no difference except for intraoperative hypertension in a greater number of those patients subjected to such local injection (Elliott BM, et al: *Am J Surg* 152:695–699, 1986).

Among 1,935 cases undergoing carotid endarterectomy, statistics were analyzed regarding the influence of shunt. The risk was 0.5%. The benefit based on likelihood of cerebral infarction estimated from CBF studies was 12% major deficits, 15% minor or transient deficits (Sundt TM, Jr, et al: *Ann Surg* 203:196–204, 1986).

In dog experiments, endarterectomy led to depression of fibrinolytic activator activity at the endarterectomy site for 24 hours, a period of increased thrombogenicity for which anticoagulation therapy would be justifiable (Hiatt JR, et al: *Arch Surg* 122:712–714, 1987).

Other Topics

Decision analysis suggests that, for patients with a risk of less than 3% per year, carotid endarterectomy is not indicated. For risk between 3% and 5% per year, low-risk surgery can be expected to provide benefit. For stroke risk between 5% and 10%, even high-risk surgery is favored (Matchar DB, Pauker SG: *JAMA* 258:793–798, 1987).

In a review of 157 carotid endarterectomies performed in 1 year by the same surgeon at a community hospital and a university hospital, neurologic results were the same but costs were 56% higher per patient at the university institution (Green RM, McNamara JA: *Surgery* 102:743–748, 1987).

Posterior Circulation

Vertebral Artery Injury: Diagnosis and Management
Golueke P, Sclafani S, Phillips T, Goldstein A, Scalea T, Duncan A (Kings County Hosp, Downstate Med Ctr, SUNY Health Sciences Center, Brooklyn, NY)
J Trauma 27:856–865, August 1987   20–10

Little information is available on the management of vertebral artery injuries. The authors review their experience with 23 patients with vertebral artery injuries caused by 19 gunshot wounds, 2 stab wounds, 1 shotgun wound, and 1 blunt injury.

Twelve patients had unilateral vertebral artery thrombosis, 7 had vertebral arteriovenous (AV) fistulae, and 4 had mural injury without thrombosis. Six (26%) patients developed major neurologic deficits, of which 5 could be directly attributed to central nervous system missile injury. One patient had transient vertebrobasilar ischemia on the basis of a vertebral AV fistula. Four vertebral AV fistulas were managed by therapeutic embolization alone; 2 patients underwent surgical management alone. One patient had therapeutic embolization of the proximal vertebral artery and surgical distal vertebral artery ligation for an AV fistula. Four (17.4%) patients died as a result of a direct central nervous system missile injury.

The authors concluded that unilateral vertebral artery occlusion seldom results in a neurologic deficit if there is a normal contralateral vertebral artery and posterior inferior cerebellar artery blood supply is preserved. Accurate assessment of a vertebral artery injury requires contralateral vertebral arteriography. Management of vertebral artery injury is simplified by proximal and distal therapeutic embolization. An anterior approach to the C1–2 vertebral artery is a satisfactory method of obtaining distal surgical control, obviating the need to unroof the bony canal of the vertebral artery. Angiography is needed to identify occult vascular injuries in patients with penetrating neck trauma.

▶ This communication illustrates that patients with vertebral artery injury seldom develop neurologic deficits in the absence of contralateral vertebral artery pathology and preservation of posterior-inferior cerebellar artery blood supply. Obviously, contralateral vertebral artery angiography is needed for full demonstration of arterial pathology and collateral circulation in these cases. As amplified by the UCSF group, percutaneous endovascular embolization and occlusion of fistulas usually obviate a need for surgery. On a related topic, Leys et al. describe a case of bilateral spontaneous dissection of the extracranial vertebral arteries. Anticoagulation appears to be the best treatment (Leys D, et al: *J Neurol* 234:237–240, 1987).—R.M. Crowell, M.D.

Vertebrobasilar Insufficiency: I. Microsurgical Treatment of Extracranial Vertebrobasilar Disease
Spetzler RF, Hadley MN, Martin NA, Hopkins LN, Carter LP, Budny J (Barrow Neurological Inst, Phoenix, and SUNY Buffalo)
J Neurosurg 66:648–661, May 1987   20–11

Both transient ischemic attacks and brain-stem or cerebellar infarction may result from thromboocclusive disease of the extracranial vertebrobasilar circulation. Forty patients with such disease, causing repeated ischemic symptoms despite maximum medical treatment, were treated surgically. The 24 men and 16 women had a mean age of 59 years. Two thirds of the patients were hypertensive. Focal symptoms of posterior circulatory ischemia were present in all patients. Patients were significantly disabled but had no fixed brain-stem or cerebellar deficits.

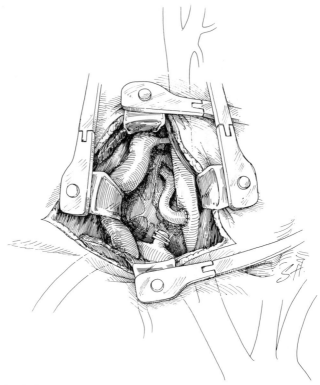

Fig 20–3.—Artist's representation of the operative exposure and completed vertebral artery to common carotid artery transposition. The use of dual Cloward retractors maintains the deep exposure. (Courtesy of Spetzler RF, Hadley MN, Martin NA, et al: *J Neurosurg* 66:648–661, May 1987.)

Ten patients had occlusion of the proximal subclavian artery and angiographic "steal" from the vertebrobasilar circulation; in these patients, vertebral-to-common carotid transposition was performed (Fig 20–3). Symptoms were relieved in all cases, and no patient had symptoms of upper limb ischemia. Eighteen patients had severe stenosis of the vertebral artery origin. Four of 18 proximal vertebral artery operations were complicated. Six patients were treated for proximal vertebral artery occlusion; 4 underwent lateral external carotid-to-vertebral artery anastomosis.

▶ Clear-cut indications for posterior circulation revascularization have not been established, but this report shows that a variety of ingenious procedures can be performed by experienced surgeons to correct vascular anatomical lesions with low morbidity. It is to be emphasized that the rate of stroke after a TIA from extracranial unilateral vertebral obstruction is quite low, and the associated death rate from coronary disease is markedly elevated (Moufarrij NA, et al: *Stroke* 15:260–263, 1984). Even patients with bilateral intracranial vertebral occlusive disease may have surprisingly good outcomes when treated with anticoagulants (Barnett HJM, et al: *Surg Neurol* 26:227–235, 1986). We need more data, especially controlled data, to establish the efficacy of surgical revascularization. In the meantime, careful studies should be confined to a few experienced centers, adequately funded and critically monitored.—R.M. Crowell, M.D.

General Topics

Prognosis of Patients With Retinal Embolism
Howard RS, Ross Russell RW (St Thomas' Hosp, London)
J Neurol Neurosurg Psychiatr 50:1142–1147, September 1987   20–12

Retinal emboli—calcific and cholesterol—can occur without any loss of vision, during or after temporary loss of vision, and in patients with uniocular field defects. These emboli can be of fibrin platelet aggregates, cholesterol fragments, pieces of calcified cardiac valve, or mixed or infected thrombus, neoplasm, fat, air, or foreign material.

Cases of cholesterol and calcific retinal emboli in 61 men and 24 women, 35–84 years of age, were studied retroactively. Loss of vision was temporary (< 4 hours) in 17 and permanent in 68. Four to 5 years was the average period of follow-up. Group A included 69 patients with cholesterol retinal emboli; 11 were treated with carotid endarterectomy. The other 58 were told to quit smoking and lose weight. Some were on high blood pressure medication, aspirin and/or dipyridamol. Group B included 15 patients with calcific emboli. Two of group B patients were

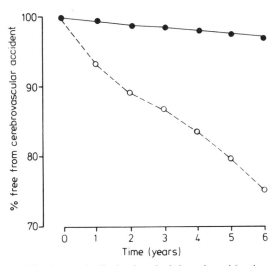

Fig 20–4.—Survival free from stroke (fatal and nonfatal) for males and females combined after presentation with visual loss caused by cholesterol emboli, compared with the expected stroke rate for the equivalent age and sex in Oxfordshire, 1981–1983. (Courtesy of Howard RS, Ross Russell RW: *J Neurol Neurosurg Psychiatr* 50:1142–1147, 1987.)

treated with carotid endarterectomy. Group C had 1 patient with a fibrin-platelet embolus, who was treated with carotid endarterectomy and did not have permanent loss of vision.

After 6 years' follow-up, group A patients who did not have surgery showed a significantly higher mortality from fatal stroke than was expected ($P < .001$), and all cerebrovascular incidence was also significant ($P < .001$). The prognosis of patients with retinal embolism is seen in Figure 20–4. Calcific emboli in 11 of the 15 group B patients had a cardiac source. The mortality in group B indicates that patients with calcific retinal emboli be referred for cardiac evaluation.

Permanent loss of vision caused by cholesterol emboli—group A— indicates occlusion of a branch or central retinal artery. The mortality after such visual loss can result from extensive and ulcerating atheroma. In this study, the higher group A mortality was mainly due to stroke. Thus, cholesterol retinal emboli suggest carotid atheroma and can be a significant predictor of cerebrovascular disease.

▶ This careful study indicates that patients with cholesterol retinal emboli have a high risk of stroke and should be treated with carotid endarterectomy for appropriate carotid occlusive lesions. Patients with calcific retinal emboli should be referred for cardiac evaluation in that many of these emboli have a cardiogenic source. This contribution does not shed light on what to do for patients with fibrin platelet emboli or central retinal artery occlusion by emboli of carotid or cardiac source.—R.M. Crowell, M.D.

Multicenter Trial of Hemodilution in Acute Ischemic Stroke: I. Results in the Total Patient Population

Scandinavian Stroke Study Group
Stroke 18:691–699, July–August 1987   20–13

In a single-center, randomized controlled trial, the combination of venesection and infusion of plasma expanders was used to achieve rapid hemodilution in an attempt to enhance neurologic recovery in acute ischemic stroke. Treated patients had better early neurologic recovery and fewer functional impairments. Encouraged by these results, a stratified and randomized multicenter trial involving 15 large and small hospitals was undertaken to explore the beneficial effects of hemodilution in acute ischemic stroke in its natural habitat. Patients with acute ischemic stroke of less than 48 hours' duration and with hematocrits of 38%–50% on admission were randomized to a hemodilution (n = 183) or a control (n = 190) group. The groups did not differ in sex distribution, medical history, age, neurologic deficits, hematocrit, and blood pressure at entry. Hemodilution involved graded venesection of 250–1,000 ml during the first 2 days, with the same amount of dextran 40 infused during the 2–4 hours after venesection, and 500 ml of dextran 40 daily to maintain hemodilution.

The mean hematocrit was reduced from 44.2% to 37.1% in the hemodilution group. Three-month survival expressed as life table product was 0.84 in the hemodilution group and 0.88 in control patients. Among survivors, neurologic score and activities of daily living performance did not differ between groups during the 3-month follow-up period. The length of hospital stay in an acute-care hospital and need for long-term institutional care were not reduced in the hemodilution group. There was a tendency for more patients to die and more cardiovascular events to occur during the first 5 days of treatment in the hemodilution group.

Contrary to the previous single-center study, this study fails to demonstrate any beneficial effects of a simple standardized hemodilution regimen in a general stroke population with acute ischemic stroke. Neither mortality nor clinical outcome in survivors is improved by hemodilution.

▶ Although the pilot study was positive, the larger multicenter trial is negative for hemodilution in acute ischemic stroke. Of course, it remains possible that patients with fresher stroke, specific subgroups of arterial pathology, or treatment with more vigorous hemodilution might still benefit. Only further carefully designed, prospective controlled studies will be able to demonstrate any utility in these subgroups. In a related report, Lyden et al. found that hemodilution with low–molecular-weight hydroxyethyl starch improves outcome in focal cerebral ischemia in rabbits (Lyden PD, et al: *Stroke* 19:223–227, 1988).—R.M. Crowell, M.D.

Treatment of Acute Cerebral Infarction With a Choline Precursor in a Multicenter Double-Blind Placebo-Controlled Study
Tazaki Y, Sakai F, Otomo E, Kutsuzawa T, Kameyama M, Omae T, Fujishima M, Sakuma A (Kitasato Univ, Sagamihara; Yokufukai Geriatric Hosp, Tokyo; Research Inst for Brain and Blood Vessels, Akita; Natl Cardiovascular Ctr, Osaka, Kyoto Univ, Kyoto; Japan, et al)
Stroke 19:211–216, February 1988   20–14

Cytidine 5'-diphosphocholine (CDP-choline) is an essential precursor for phosphatidylcholine synthesis, 1 of the main structural components of cell membranes that are degraded to highly toxic substances. Based on pharmacologic observations in animals, the authors conducted a multicenter, double-blind, placebo-controlled trial to assess the efficacy and safety of CDP-choline treatment for well-established acute cerebral infarction.

In all, a total of 272 patients, aged 20–90 years, were entered in the study. All had acute cerebral infarction and suffered from moderate to mild disturbances in consciousness. All were admitted within 14 days of ictus. By random assignment, 133 patients received CDP-choline treatment, 1,000 mg per day administered intravenously once a day for 14 days, and 139 patients received placebo. Complete neurologic and medical evaluations were done just before treatment, and on days 1, 2, 3, 7, and 14 of treatment. Improvements in levels of consciousness did not differ between the 2 groups on days 1, 2, or 3, but were significantly improved on days 7 and 14 for those receiving CDP-choline. At final assessment, the rates of improvement were 51% for the CDP-choline group and 33% for the placebo group. Differences in global improvement ratings increased as treatment progressed.

This study demonstrated that CDP-choline produced significant improvements in level of consciousness in patients with well-established acute cerebral infarction compared with placebo. Cytidine 5'-diphosphocholine was also found to be entirely safe.

▶ This study suggests that CDP-choline is beneficial for treatment of acute cerebral infarction. Although significant improvement was demonstrated in this controlled study, the results of this study suggest that Cytidine 5'-diphosphocholine benefits patients with acute cerebral infarction. This controlled double-blind study produced a specifically significant beneficial result. However, patients were most frequently admitted to this study several days after the onset of symptoms, and many were affected by disturbance of consciousness. Since patients with less severe and earlier ischemia would be more likely to benefit, further studies in this group appear warranted.—R.M. Crowell, M.D.

Brief Notes on General Topics

Stroke

In a review of 61 cases of angiographically proved internal carotid artery occlusion, the presence of cerebral infarction on CT scan was well correlated with a persisting neurologic deficit. Patients without CT evidence of infarction frequently had transient ischemic attacks. In the few cases with cerebral infarction despite good collateral, a mechanism of embolus was suggested (Harrison MJG, Marshall J: *J Neurol Neurosurg Psychiatry* 51:269–272, 1988).

Gadolinium leads to enhancement of cerebral infarction (Imakita S, et al: *Neuroradiology* 29:422–429, 1987).

Occlusion of the posterior-inferior cerebellar artery including the branch to the pontomedullary region produces the lateral medullary infarction extending to the lower pons (Fisher CN, Tapia J: *J Neurol Neurosurg Psychiatry* 50:620–624, 1987).

Evans and Hayes reported 83 patients with transient ischemic attacks and essentially normal angiography. In follow-up from 3 to 132 months, 6 patients suffered cerebral infarction and 5 had further TIAs (*J Vasc Surg* 6:548–552, 1987).

Hemiataxia and ipsilateral hemisensory defect may be found in anterior choroidal artery territory infarct (Bogousslavsky J, et al: *Rev Neurol (Paris)* 142:671–676, 1986).

Sixteen documented cases of anterior choroidal artery syndrome are reported with hemiplegia, hemianesthesia, and homonymous hemianopia. Computed tomography scan confirmed the diagnosis (Decroix JP, et al: *Brain* 109:1071–1085, 1986).

Of 515 first-ever strokes in a community-based study, lacunar infarct was confirmed in 34 CT scans for crude annual incidence of 0.33 per 1,000. The case fatality rate was 9.8% at 1 year, with 11.8% of patients having recurrent strokes and 66% being capable of independent existence (Bamford J, et al: *Stroke* 18:545–551, 1987).

Transient focal cerebral ischemia can result from digital palpation of the carotid artery in the neck (Martin MA, Bernstein M: *Can J Surg* 30:136–138, 1987).

Of 6 patients with isolated supraclinoid occlusive disease of the internal carotid artery, 5 had 1 or more risk factors for atherosclerosis (Lagreze HL, et al: *Eur Neurol* 26:40–45, 1987).

Venous Occlusion

Increased intracranial pressure can result from bilateral thrombosis of the transverse sinus. A gortex graft was used as a venous bypass in a patient reported by Saiki and co-workers (*Neurol Med Chir Tokyo* 26:634–638, 1986). The right transverse sinus was linked to the right internal jugular vein, with a good postoperative result.

Superior sagittal sinus thrombosis may occur with sickle cell trait, causing cerebral infarction and requiring aggressive management including intracranial pressure monitoring, cerebrospinal fluid drainage, and even barbiturate coma (Feldenzer JA, et al: *Stroke* 18:656–660, 1987).

Computed tomography may permit evaluation of deep cerebral vein thrombosis (Gupta KL, et al: *Ala J Med Sci* 24:40–45, 1987).

Bypass Surgery

A few patients with symptoms from hemodynamic compromise may still benefit from extracranial-intracranial arterial bypass (Mehdorn HM, Grote W: *Neurochirurgia* 30:72–81, 1987).

Of 300 patients undergoing stable xenon cerebral blood flow studies, 9 were selected with global low flow and nonhemispheric symptoms for flow-augmenting procedures. In each case, disabling transient symptoms were relieved without postoperative death, and there was but a single stroke, probably related to postoperative hypertension (Yonas H, et al: *J Vasc Surg* 5:289–297, 1987).

Diamox may lead to a paradoxical decrease in focal cerebral blood flow, and this is correlated with an improved focal cerebral blood flow after extracranial-intracranial bypass grafting (Vostrup S, et al: *Stroke* 17:1291–1298, 1986).

In the EC-IC Bypass Study, patients with higher hemoglobin concentration suffered no more ischemic strokes than those with lower values (Wade JPH, et al: *Stroke* 18:68–71, 1987).

Experiments show that satisfactory results are obtained with rapid nonsuture arterial anastomosis using a stent and clip methodology (Gentili F, et al: *Can J Neurol Sci* 14:92–95, 1987).

Experiments in rat vascular anastomoses demonstrate that fibrin adhesive may be helpful (Hamm KD, et al: Zentralbl Neurochir 47:322–333, 1986).

Emboli

Among 25 patients undergoing carotid angiography for central retinal artery occlusion, 14 (56%) were found to have ipsilateral extracranial carotid disease. Ten underwent endarterectomy with removal of either ulcerated plaque or tight stenosis. Eleven patients had no abnormalities on angiography (Sheng FC, et al: *Am J Surg* 152:175–178, 1986).

Among 47 cases of posterior cerebral artery occlusion, 43 were consistent with embolism. Prodromes include photopsias, hemianopic blackout, headache, transient numbness, episodic lightheadedness, spells of bewilderment, and rarely, tinnitus. Photopsias did not closely resemble scintillating displays of migraine. When stroke occurred, visual complaints predominated. Sensory deficit occurred in one third of cases. In 25 cases of memory impairment, the dominant hemisphere was involved in 24. Mechanisms included local embolism, vertebral distal stump embolism, embolus in transit, and hemorrhagic infarction (Fisher CM: *Can J Neurol Sci* 13:232–239, 1986).

Serial CT scanning can disclose evolution of hemorrhagic infarction, suggesting an embolic mechanism (Laureno R, et al: *Brain* 110:93–105, 1987).

Pretreatment with perfluorocarbons protects against cerebral air emboli in rabbits (Spiess BD, et al: *Stroke* 17:1146–1149, 1986).

Between 1951 and 1984, 7 adult patients at the Mayo Clinic had cerebral infarction as a result of nonmyxomatous tumor emboli (O'Neill BP, et al: *Cancer* 60:90–95, 1987).

Treatment of Cerebral Infarction

Mannitol improves postischemic recovery of focal cerebral blood flow after experimental middle cerebral artery occlusion (Tanaka A, Tomonaga M: *Surg Neurol* 28:189–195, 1987).

Barbiturates may be protective, but isoflurane is not, during temporary focal ischemia in primates (Nehls DG, et al: *Anesthesiology* 66:453–464, 1987).

Modification of experimental cerebral infarction by new pharmacologic agents or restoration of blood flow to areas of focal cerebral ischemia suggests that a more aggressive approach may be considered in selected patients with acute stroke (Meyer FB, et al: *Mayo Clin Proc* 62:35–55, 1987).

In a rat middle cerebral artery occlusion model, nimodipine-treated rats 1 hour after occlusion had improved neurologic outcome and less infarction as compared with controls, suggesting a mechanism of action on the penumbra of the ischemic area (Germano IM, et al: *J Neurosurg* 67:81–87, 1987).

Hyperglycemia reduces the extent of cerebral infarction in rats (Ginsberg MD, et al: *Stroke* 18:570–574, 1987).

Administration of MK-801, a noncompetitive antagonist of N-methyl-d-aspartate receptors, protects against ischemia injury in the gerbil (Gill et al: *J Neurosci* 7:3343–3349, 1987).

Other Topics

Immunohistochemical techniques provide early detection of cerebral ischemia damage and repair in the gerbil (Matsumoto M, et al: *Mayo Clin Proc* 62:460–472, 1987).

Serotonin levels are decreased in the acute period of cerebral infarction. Serotonin levels appear to vary with the type and stage of cerebral infarction (Ishizaki F: *J Neural Transm* 69:123–129, 1987).

Celiac disease may present with isolated vasculitis of the central nervous system (Rush PJ, et al: *Am J Med* 81:1092–1094, 1986).

Giant cell arteritis may be associated with peripheral neuropathy (Golbus J, McCune J: *J Rheumatol* 14:129–134, 1987).

Cerebral astrocytes secrete plasminogen activator, with modulation by drugs and pathologic processes (Toshniwal PK, et al: *J Neurol Sci* 80:307–321, 1987).—R.M. Crowell, M.D. Autoprocessing Division

21 Hemorrhage

Introduction

Intracranial aneurysms were the subject of many interesting contributions in the past year. Intraoperative digital subtraction angiography has now reached the point where an intraoperative angiogram can indicate to the surgeon whether the aneurysm clip is properly placed or needs to be adjusted (Abstract 21–1). Unruptured familial intracranial aneurysms have been detected by intravenous digital subtraction angiography (Abstract 21–2). Intravascular volume expansion may not increase cerebral blood flow in patients with ruptured cerebral aneurysms (Abstract 21–3). In patients at high risk for vasospasm after subarachnoid hemorrhage, high-dose methylprednisolone appears to have beneficial results (Abstract 21–4). In another study of clinical vasospasm after subarachnoid hemorrhage, hypovolemic hemodilution and arterial hypertension appear to have a beneficial effect, although ongoing controls were not provided (Abstract 21–5). Common carotid occlusion is touted as an effective operation for unclippable carotid aneurysms (Abstract 21–8). In a study with historical controls, a deliberate policy of early operation on supratentorial aneurysms is reported to have a beneficial effect on mortality (Abstract 21–6). For large and giant cerebral aneurysms, etomidate therapy, temporary arterial occlusion, and intraoperative angiography are advocated as beneficial (Abstract 21–7). A collagen type III deficiency has been discovered in patients with ruptured intracranial saccular aneurysm (Abstract 21–9). Circulating immune complexes and complement activation have been noted following rupture of intracranial aneurysms (Abstract 21–10). Two interesting studies have appeared documenting the natural history and pathologic features of fusiform aneurysms of the basilar artery (Abstracts 21–11 and 21–12).

Arteriovenous malformations were the subject of a number of studies. According to a Mayo Clinic study, unruptured arteriovenous malformations carry a substantial rate of deterioration, with a 2.2% rupture rate per year and a risk of death of 29% (Abstract 21–13). By contrast, M.J. Aminoff calculates that conservative management of unruptured cerebral arteriovenous malformations is warranted (Abstract 21–14). Sugita and colleagues have described successful results in the surgical management of sylvian fissure arteriovenous malformations (Abstract 21–15). Deep-seated trigonal arteriovenous malformations are best attacked through an interhemispheric approach when mesially placed but through a middle temporal gyrus approach when they extend laterally beyond the P_2-P_3 junction (Abstract 21–16). Staged treatment of arteriovenous malformations of the brain has been recommended for deep-seated and giant lesions (Abstracts 21–17 and 21–18). Cavernous angiomas have a characteristic MRI appearance with a central zone of high signal and periphery of low signal (Abstract 21–19). Occasionally, a hemorrhagic neo-plasm may mimic such an occult vascular malformation (Abstract 21–20).

Robert M. Crowell, M.D.

Aneurysms

Intraoperative Digital Subtraction Neuroangiography: A Diagnostic and Therapeutic Tool

Hieshima GB, Reicher MA, Higashida RT, Halbach VV, Cahan LD, Martin NA, Frazee JG, Rand RW, Bentson JR (Univ of California, San Francisco, Los Angeles, Irvine)

AJNR 8:759–767 September–October 1987   21–1

Intraoperative digital subtraction angiography (DSA) offers the advantages of immediate image processing, a lower dose of contrast material required, and the depiction of blood vessels unobscured by extraneous bony structures or partially radiopaque surgical hardware. A review was made of experience with intraoperative digital subtraction neuroangiographic procedures in 43 patients.

A portable imaging system was used to perform intraoperative neuroangiography on 53 occasions. Thirty-two procedures were done for diagnostic purposes after resection of arteriovenous malformations (AVMs) in 12 patients, single aneurysm clipping in 9, multiple feeding-artery aneurysm clipping and resecting of an AVM in 2, multiple aneurysm clipping without associated AVM in 2, and endarterectomy in 2. In 7 patients, unexpected problems were discovered and were immediately treated surgically in 4. Angiography was used therapeutically in 21 other patients. In 5, intraoperative angiography was used with embolization therapy of direct carotid cavernous fistulas. In 2 patients, 5 intraoperative angiographic procedures were done to treat pseudoaneurysms of the petrous or cavernous internal carotid artery. Five AVMs were embolized together with intraoperative angiographic monitoring. A dural arteriovenous fistula of the transverse sinus was totally obliterated by intraoperative embolization in 1 patient. In another patient, direct surgical exposure and catheterization of the common carotid artery facilitated balloon occlusion of the cavernous carotid artery above the level of a giant cavernous carotid aneurysm.

Intraoperative DSA is a valuable diagnostic and therapeutic tool. With a combined interventional neuroangiographic and neurosurgical approach, intraoperative angiography opens new avenues for treatment of intracranial vascular abnormalities.

▶ Intraoperative DSA appears to offer great promise. According to this report from the University of California, Los Angeles, the method is practical and carries minimal risk. The demonstrated images are of sufficient resolution and quality to permit surgical decision making, as in clip reposition for aneurysms or further resection of residual AVM. Further experience will be needed to find the precise indications for such studies and the limits of DSA's sensitivity. However, intraoperative angiography has for some time been desirable, and this general technical approach appears to have solved the major problems. It is expected that such an approach will be used in major neurovascular operating theaters.—R.M. Crowell, M.D.

Detection of Unruptured Familial Intracranial Aneurysms by Intravenous Digital Subtraction Angiography: Screening of Two Affected Families
ter Berg JWM, Overtoom TMD, Ludwig JW, Bijlsma JB, Tulleken CAF, Willemse J (Univ Hosp, Utrecht; St. Antonius Hosp, Nieuwegein; Univ of Utrecht; Regional Hosp Almelo, Almelo, the Netherlands)
Neuroradiology 29:272–276, 1987   21–2

Asymptomatic members of families in which intracranial aneurysms occur have a greater chance of harboring such lesions. Elective screening by intravenous digital angiography (ivDSA) was done of the asymptomatic members of 2 families affected by IA.

In the first family, 7 members were known to have intracranial aneurysms. In the second family, 1 member had proved ruptured intracranial aneurysm, and another member had subarachnoid hemorrhage. The standard projections used in the screening procedure were right off-lateral, 15–20 degrees out of the horizontal plane; left off-lateral; Towne-Twining projection; and posteroanterior projection. In the first family, 36 asymptomatic members were tested. In 1 person, a 6×15-mm aneurysm was found at the left posterior communicating artery. Of the 4 members tested in the second family, 1 aneurysm with a diameter of 6 mm was

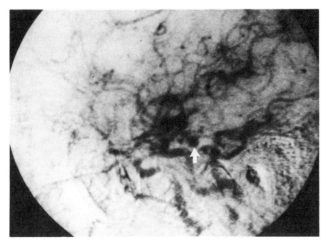

Fig 21–1.—Right off-lateral projection with the ivDSA method in patient that shows the aneurysm at the left posterior communicating artery *(arrow)*. (Courtesy of ter Berg JWM, Overtoom TMD, Ludwig JW, et al: *Neuroradiology* 29:272–276, 1987.)

found at the left posterior communicating artery (Fig 21–1). Conventional cerebral angiography confirmed both intracranial aneurysms, and the patients underwent neurosurgical treatment.

Two intracranial aneurysms among 40 asymptomatic members of 2 families known to be affected by these lesions were detected by screening with ivDSA. Screening of first-degree relatives of persons with familial intracranial aneurysm by ivDSA is strongly advocated.

▶ This communication describes detection of familial intracranial aneurysms by screening with intravenous digital subtraction angiography. Two intracranial aneurysms among 40 asymptomatic patients were detected. However, in 2 patients ivDSA failed to detect a lesion demonstrated on cerebral angiography, indicating a potential false-negative defect in this method of screening. It may be that MRI will be as sensitive for the detection of these lesions as ivDSA, which after all has some inherent risks. Another approach would involve the identification of individuals on the basis of a blood test by biochemical or genetic survey. In a related study, Jaksche and Zent report 4 cases of familial intracranial aneurysm among 10 family members (Jaksche H: *Zentralbl Neurochir* 47:351– 353, 1986).—R.M. Crowell, M.D.

Effects of Intravascular Volume Expansion on Cerebral Blood Flow in Patients With Ruptured Cerebral Aneurysms

Yamakami I, Isobe K, Yamaura A (Kimitsu Gen Hosp, Chiba Univ, Chiba, Japan)
Neurosurgery 21:303–309, September 1987   21–3

Ischemic neurologic deficits from vasospasm may be caused by severe luminal narrowing of the extraparenchymal conducting arteries, lowered cerebral perfusion pressure, and decreased cerebral blood flow (CBF). Intravascular volume expansion with or without induced arterial hypertension improves symptomatic vasospasm. To clarify the effect of intravascular volume expansion on CBF in patients after subarachnoid hemorrhage (SAH), 55 pairs of regional CBF measurements using the xenon-133 inhalation method were performed before and after volume expansion in 35 patients with ruptured cerebral aneurysms. All patients underwent aneurysmal clipping. Volume expansion was achieved with a half-hour intravenous infusion of 500 ml of 5% human serum albumin, and CBF was calculated as the hemispheric mean value of the initial slope index.

Hemoglobin levels were significantly decreased after volume expansion, suggesting adequate volume expansion. Mean arterial blood pressure remained unchanged after volume expansion. Cerebral blood flow was significantly decreased after volume expansion during the first 2 weeks after SAH, but it remained unchanged after volume expansion during the third through the fourth weeks after SAH. After volume expansion, CBF decreased significantly among the 18 patients with symptomatic vasospasm, but remained unchanged among the 37 patients with asymptomatic vasospasm.

These data show that volume expansion after SAH and intracranial operation fails to increase CBF or reverse symptomatic vasospasm. It appears that correction of systemic hypovolemia into normovolemia prevents the development of symptomatic vasospasm, but increasing the intravascular volume above normal by volume expansion in normovolemic patients does not increase CBF, nor does it reverse symptomatic vasospasm. Volume expansion in patients with symptomatic vasospasm may even prove harmful to these patients. Further reduction of cerebrovascular resistance by hemodilutional volume expansion in these patients, who may already have damage in the blood-brain barrier and increased cerebral blood volume, may further increase cerebral blood volume and raise intracranial pressure. It appears that volume expansion with albumin has 2 effects on patients after SAH; the beneficial effect is the augmentation of CBF, mainly by improvement of hemorrheologic characteristics, and the detrimental effect is the reduction of CBF, possibly by increasing cerebral blood volume and increasing intracranial pressure.

▶ The data indicate that volume expansion after SAH and intracranial operation fails to increase CBF or to reverse symptomatic vasospasm. The data did not, however, discount the utility of normal or increased intravascular volume as a guard against insidious drops in systemic arterial blood pressure, which could be deleterious in such patients. In addition, the study did not repeat the treatment of volume administration, as is commonly used in many centers for the treatment of delayed ischemia. In addition, angiographic and CT data would have been useful in focusing on patients most likely to benefit from volume expansion therapy.

In short, one cannot generalize from this single study to dismiss the potential value of volume expansion in patients with cerebral vascular vasospasm.— R.M. Crowell, M.D.

Preliminary Report: Effects of High Dose Methylprednisolone on Delayed Cerebral Ischemia in Patients at High Risk for Vasospasm After Aneurysmal Subarachnoid Hemorrhage

Chyatte D, Fode NC, Nichols DA, Sundt TM, Jr (Yale Univ; Mayo Clinic, Rochester, Minn)

Neurosurgery 21:157–160, August 1987   21–4

The overall management of aneurysm repair after subarachnoid hemorrhage remains disappointing, partly because of delayed cerebral ischemia resulting from vasospasm. Increasing evidence suggests that chronic cerebral vasospasm may be linked to the inflammatory response that follows subarachnoid hemorrhage, and experimental studies suggest that massive doses of methylprednisolone can prevent or markedly reduce posthemorrhagic chronic vasospasm. High-dose methylprednisolone was administered within 72 hours of aneurysmal subarachnoid hemorrhage in 21 patients judged to be at high risk for vasospasm because of either poor admitting grade or a large amount of subarachnoid blood as shown by computed tomography. Management results were compared with those of 21 contemporary patients matched for grade, number of hemorrhages, time from hemorrhage to admission, time from hemorrhage to operation, aneurysm location, age, and sex.

Patients treated with high-dose methylprednisolone were twice as likely to have excellent results and half as likely to die than those who were not. The incidence and severity of delayed cerebral ischemia were reduced in patients treated with methylprednisolone compared with controls. No major side effects were associated with steroid treatment, although in 4 patients hyperglycemia developed that required insulin therapy.

These results support the hypothesis that chronic posthemorrhagic cerebral vasospasm is an inflammatory vasculopathy. Early treatment with high-dose methylprednisolone is a safe and effective method of lessening the incidence and severity of chronic cerebral vasospasm and improving the outcome in patients at risk after subarachnoid hemorrhage.

▶ This report presents encouraging results in the treatment of patients with subarachnoid hemorrhage using high-dose methylprednisolone. Although this is only a preliminary report, the treated group clearly fared better than the controls. We must await further results before these approaches may be advocated for general use, however. Steroid therapy certainly has significant hazards of its own, and only a large, appropriately controlled study will establish the utility of this method of treatment.—R.M. Crowell, M.D.

Clinical Vasospasm After Subarachnoid Hemorrhage: Response to Hypervolemic Hemodilution and Arterial Hypertension

Awad IA, Carter LP, Spetzler RF, Medina M, Williams FW, Jr (Barrow Neurological Inst, Phoenix)
Stroke 18:365–372, March–April 1987   21–5

The greatest cause of morbidity and mortality after subarachnoid hemorrhage is delayed neurologic deterioration from vasospasm. The incidence and 24-month clinical course of symptomatic vasospasm subarachnoid hemorrhage were investigated in 118 patients admitted within 2 weeks of subarachnoid hemorrhage not attributed to trauma, tumor, or vascular malformation.

Of these, 113 had aneurysms. Early surgery was performed when possible. Hypertensive hypervolemic hemodilution therapy was begun at the first sign of clinical vasospasm. Forty-two patients (35.6%) had signs and symptoms of clinical vasospasm; spasm was confirmed by angiographic assessment in 39. All patients with clinical vasospasm received hypervolemic hemodilution therapy to achieve a hematocrit of 33% to 38%, a central venous pressure of 10 to 12 mm Hg or a pulmonary wedge pressure of 15 to 18 mm Hg, and a systolic arterial pressure of 160 to 200 mm Hg, or 120 to 150 mm Hg for unclipped aneurysms, for the duration of clinical vasospasm.

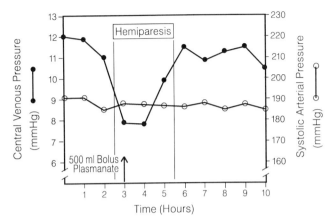

Fig 21–2.—Hemodynamic parameters in 1 patient. Hemiparesis appeared whenever the central venous pressure dropped below 10 mm Hg despite elevated systolic arterial pressure and optimal hematocrit. (Courtesy of Awad IA, Carter LP, Spetzler RF, et al: *Stroke* 18:365–372, March–April 1987.)

In some patients, neurologic deficits fluctuated markedly with changes in arterial pressure despite optimal volume status; in others, neurologic deficits fluctuated markedly with changes in volume status, despite maximal hypertension (Fig 21–2). During the course of treatment, 60% of patients with clinical vasospasm had improved by at least 1 grade, in 24% a stable neurologic status was maintained, and 16% continued to worsen. At the end of therapy, 47.6% had become neurologically normal, 33.3% had a minor neurologic deficit, and 19% had a major deficit or had died. Cardiopulmonary deterioration occurred in 3 patients without Swan-Ganz catheters; all resolved with appropriate diuresis. One patient rebled and subsequently died despite hypervolemic hemodilution therapy. Less than 7% of all patients with subarachnoid hemorrhage died or sustained a major neurologic deficit from clinical vasospasm.

Early surgery and aggressive management of clinical vasospasm with hypervolemic hemodilution therapy can be carried out with minimal morbidity. This strategy may lower the incidence of mortality and morbidity from vasospasm after subarachnoid hemorrhage.

▶ Hypertension and hemodilution may improve, with low risk of worsening, the condition of some patients with symptomatic vasospasm. Sustained improvement was observed in 60% of the patients; 14% worsened or died. The temporal profile suggested that therapy was the likely cause of improvement. Early surgery did not seem to lead to an increase in the frequency of vasospasm. Controlled studies will be needed to validate this approach, but a host of uncontrolled reports buttress the contention.—R.M. Crowell, M.D.

Effect on Management Mortality of a Deliberate Policy of Early Operation on Supratentorial Aneurysms
Disney L, Weir B, Petruk K (Univ of Alberta)
Neurosurgery 20:695–701, May 1987

The optimal timing of operation for acutely ruptured intracranial aneurysms is controversial. In 1978 the University of Alberta adopted a policy of early definitive aneurysm operation as a result of the favorable outcome of such treatment, as opposed to delayed operation, in a retrospective analysis of earlier treatment protocols. In all, 736 patients with intracranial aneurysms seen from 1968 to 1975 were admitted on the day of or the day after subarachnoid hemorrhage (SAH) from a supratentorial aneurysm. Of these patients, 205 were managed from 1968 through 1977, when the interval between SAH and operation for ruptured aneurysm was random, and 232 were managed from 1978 through early 1985, when the policy of early aneurysm operation was implemented. Postoperative and management mortality and morbidity rates were related to the grade of the patient at the time of admission and the time interval before operation.

Overall, there was a significant reduction of 8% in postoperative mortality and of 9% in management mortality for all grades after the institution of the policy of early operation. Management mortality and postoperative mortality rates for patients treated before 1978 were 47% and 19%, respectively, for all grades, and these were reduced to 38% and 11%, respectively, for patients treated after 1978. Management mortality for patients operated on on days 0 to 3 was lower than for those operated on later after SAH in both treatment periods. Postoperative mortality was reduced in all patients operated on from 1978 to 1985, regardless of the interval from SAH to operation; management mortality was reduced overall, as well as for patients operated on on days 0 to 3, in those treated from 1978 to 1985. In addition, morbidity decreased across all grades and on days 0 to 3 with early operation. A policy of early definitive aneurysm operation has contributed to a reduction of both postoperative and management mortality.

▶ Dr. Weir and his group provide data with historical controls suggesting that early operation on supratentorial aneurysms improves mortality and morbidity. Furthermore, the recent results of the International Cooperative Study on the Timing of Aneurysm Surgery demonstrate that the overall outcome from early operation is equivalent or better (particularly in the case of alert patients) to that of delayed operation in a large number of neurosurgical centers throughout the world. For experienced groups such as the Edmonton unit, early surgery appears to offer substantial advantages. Whether this will also be the case for less experienced surgeons remains an area of significant concern.—R.M. Crowell, M.D.

Use of Etomidate, Temporary Arterial Occlusion, and Intraoperative Angiography in Surgical Treatment of Large and Giant Cerebral Aneurysms
Batjer HH, Frankfurt AI, Purdy PD, Smith SS, Samson DS (Univ of Texas, Dallas)
J Neurosurg 68:234–240, February 1988   21–7

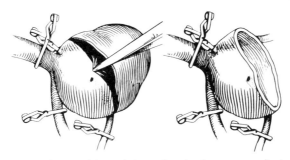

Fig 21–3.—Schematic drawing of the surgical procedure showing temporary clipping and opening of the aneurysm *(left)*, followed by evacuation of the aneurysmal contents and resection, leaving a clippable cuff of tissue *(right)*. (Courtesy of Batjer HH, Frankfurt AI, Purdy PD, et al: *J Neurosurg* 68:234–240, February 1988.)

The surgical treatment of large and giant aneurysms is complicated by their typically atheromatous and thick walls, frequent thrombosis with calcification, and broad-based necks that often incorporate perforating arteries and other vital vessels. Sometimes it is necessary to arrest at least focally the intracranial circulation and open or excise these aneurysms to facilitate vascular reconstruction. In patients whose disease has destroyed autoregulatory function or who have inadequate sources of anatomical collateral supply, such a maneuver may cause permanent ischemic injury. Experience with 14 patients who had large and giant intracranial aneurysms was reviewed.

The patients were treated at 1 center in a 13-month period. They were treated while under electroencephalographic monitoring to document electric burst suppression induced by administration of etomidate, followed by temporary clipping to allow vascular repair and intraoperative angiography to document parent artery patency (Fig 21–3). Up to 60 minutes of internal carotid artery occlusion, 35 minutes of middle cerebral artery occlusion, 19 minutes of upper basilar artery occlusion, and 4.5 minutes of lower basilar artery occlusion were well tolerated. Ten patients had a good outcome. Three patients had a poor outcome 3–7 months after surgery and 1 patient died.

This early experience with etomidate suggests that it has significant potential value as a protective agent during iatrogenic cerebral ischemia. Its administration can be safely and systemically titrated with intraoperative electroencephalographic monitoring.

▶ This study indicates that 14 patients were treated with temporary intracranial arterial clipping for obliteration of intracranial aneurysms under etomidate cerebral protection, with good results in 10. These results suggest, but do not prove, that etomidate may be helpful as a cerebral protection agent. Alternative approaches, such as mannitol or hypertension therapy, interruption of temporary clipping, and evoked potential monitoring, may produce results as good or better. Further data will be required to decide which of these approaches is superior.

In a related study, middle cerebral artery (MCA) occlusion up to 19 minutes with moderate hypothermia was carried out for treatment of 5 MCA aneurysms. Monitoring of somatosensory evoked potentials was done, and no occlusion was maintained for longer than 3 minutes in the presence of a severely disturbed SEP. There was good recovery of neurologic function in all cases (Mooij JJA, et al: *Neurosurgery* 21:492–496, 1987).— R.M. Crowell, M.D.

Common Carotid Occlusion for Unclippable Carotid Aneurysms: An Old But Still Effective Operation

Swearingen B, Heros RC (Massachusetts Gen Hosp, Boston; Harvard Univ)
Neurosurgery 21:288–295, September 1987   21–8

An intracranial aneurysm is optimally treated by a direct surgical approach with clipping of the neck of the aneurysm and preservation of the parent vessel. However, this is often impossible with giant aneurysms and rarely advised for intracavernous aneurysms. Eight women and 1 man aged 38–68 years with unclippable internal carotid artery (ICA) aneurysms underwent a 1-treatment procedure.

All had headache, visual loss, cranial nerve palsy, or complex partial seizures. Radiologic findings included giant cavernous aneurysm, giant ICA bifurcation aneurysm, fusiform giant ICA aneurysm, giant paraclinoid aneurysm, and in 1 patient, bilateral carotid giant aneurysm. Eight patients underwent common carotid ligation after angiographic assessment (Fig 21–4). Tolerance to carotid occlusion was judged intraoperatively by awake examination, electroencephalogram (EEG) monitoring, and carotid stump pressure measurements. In none of the patients did a permanent deficit develop. Seven of 8 treated aneurysms thrombosed.

Carotid ligation has a clear role in the treatment of unclippable carotid aneurysms. Prophylactic revascularization procedures may be needed in only a minority of patients, as most ischemic complications from carotid ligation appear to be thromboembolic. Screening procedures such as cerebral blood flow recordings, intraoperative examination with the patient awake, intraoperative EEG monitoring, and preoperative determination of angiographic cross flow during temporary carotid occlusion are useful in selecting patients who cannot tolerate carotid occlusion because of insufficient collateral circulation. After common carotid ligation, patients must be followed with periodic CT to ascertain whether aneurysmal thrombosis has occurred. If it has not occurred within 3 to 6 months, these patients may be considered for additional procedures. Carotid occlusion alone is inadequate for patients with rapidly progressing visual loss or signs of brain stem compression.

▶ This report suggests that common carotid occlusion may be safer and more effective than ICA occlusion. However, the experience in London, Ontario, which is substantially more extensive, suggests that ICA occlusion with a balloon catheter with the patient awake is probably more effective and safer than common carotid artery occlusion (Peerless et al: *Neurosurgery* 21:295, 1987).

Matsuoka et al. report excellent results with direct attack on intracavernous

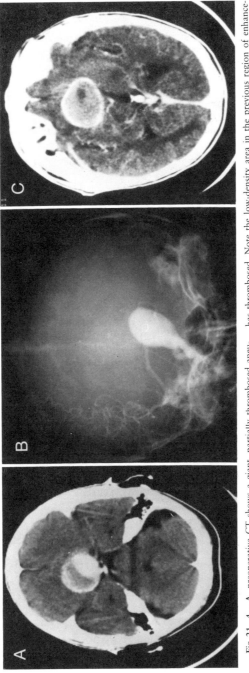

Fig 21–4.—A, preoperative CT shows a giant, partially thrombosed aneurysm. **B,** angiography demonstrates a giant paraclinoid aneurysm. **C,** postoperative CT shows that the lumen no longer enhances, suggesting that the aneurysm has thrombosed. Note the low-density area in the previous region of enhancement. (Courtesy of Swearingen B, Heros RC: *Neurosurgery* 21:288–295, September 1987.)

carotid aneurysms in 4 cases. Technical adjuncts include elevation of the head, removal of the anterior clinoid process, and wide mobilization of the distal optic nerve. Also helpful were incision of the cavernous sinus on its superior aspect to avoid injury to cranial nerves, control of bleeding with Oxycel soaked in Biobond, and repair of paranasal sinus with fascia (Matsuoka Y, et al: *Surg Neurol* 26:360–364, 1986).—R.M. Crowell, M.D.

Collagen Type III Deficiency in Patients With Rupture of Intracranial Saccular Aneurysms

Østergaard JR, Oxlund H (Aarhus Kommunehospital, Univ of Aarhus, Aarhus, Denmark)
J Neurosurg 67:690–696, November 1987   21–9

The pathogenesis of intracranial saccular aneurysms is complex. The fibrous structure of collagen and elastin plays an important role in the load-bearing capacity of arteries. Because the major collagen structures of arteries are type I and type III collagen fibers, studies were made of the mechanical properties and relative amounts of these collagen types in intracranial and extracranial arteries of patients with ruptured aneurysms.

Samples of the middle cerebral artery (MCA) and the brachial artery were obtained from 14 patients who had died after rupture of intracranial saccular aneurysms. Samples were also taken from a control group of 14 age- and sex-matched patients who had died of other causes. The biomechanical properties of ring-shaped arterial specimens were investigated by loading the specimens at a constant deformation rate until they ruptured. Collagen amounts were determined by sodium dodecyl sulfate-polyacrylamide gel electrophoresis studies of cyanogen bromide peptides of collagen prepared from the samples.

A deficiency of type III was demonstrated in specimens of the MCA in 6 of 14 patients with ruptured aneurysms. The deficiency of collagen type

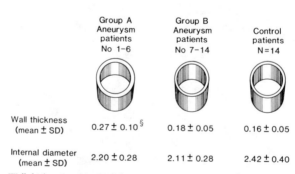

	Group A Aneurysm patients No 1–6	Group B Aneurysm patients No 7–14	Control patients N = 14
Wall thickness (mean ± SD)	0.27 ± 0.10 §	0.18 ± 0.05	0.16 ± 0.05
Internal diameter (mean ± SD)	2.20 ± 0.28	2.11 ± 0.28	2.42 ± 0.40

Fig 21–5.—Wall thickness and internal diameter (mm) of the middle cerebral artery of patients with aneurysm and controls. Group A comprised aneurysm patients with a collagen type I;type III ratio exceeding the mean value + 2 SD of the control group. In group B, the collagen type I:type III ratios were all below the mean value + 2 SD of the control group. § = P < .05 when compared with controls. No, case number; N, number of patients. (Courtesy of Østergaard JR, Oxlund H: *J Neurosurg* 67:690–696, November 1987.)

III was accompanied by a significant increase in the arterial wall thickness, although no difference was found in the internal diameter (Fig 21–5). Also, this deficiency was not accompanied by changes in the mechanical arterial strength, but it resulted in a significant increase in the extensibility at stress values corresponding to blood pressures between 100 and 200 mm Hg. No difference was found between aneurysm patients and the control group in biochemical properties of the brachial artery, despite the significant deficiency of collagen type III in patients with aneurysms.

Increases in vascular extensibility of the MCA may represent changes in the fibrous structure and functional integrity of the cerebral arteries of patients with aneurysm and collagen type III deficiency. Along with aggravating hemodynamic stresses, this deficiency may be an important factor in the pathogenesis of saccular aneurysms.

▶ This paper helps to put cerebral aneurysm on a biochemical basis, by demonstrating a collagen type III deficiency in some patients with aneurysms. It would be of interest to find out whether patients with familial saccular aneurysm show this lesion in a molecular fashion. The tools to uncover the molecular basis and even the genetic basis of cerebral aneurysm are already at hand. It may be that the fruits of such efforts may uncover a blood test for the identification of patients with aneurysm.—R.M. Crowell, M.D.

Immune Complexes and Complement Activation Following Rupture of Intracranial Saccular Aneurysms
Østergaard JR, Kristensen BØ, Svehag S-E, Teisner B, Miletic T (Aarhus Kommunehospital, Aarhus; Odense Univ, Odense, Denmark)
J Neurosurg 66:891–897, June 1987   21–10

Previous studies suggest that immunologic reactions are involved in cerebral vasospasm. To investigate further, circulating immune complexes (CIC) and complement activation were monitored during a 2-week period in 18 patients with ruptured cerebral aneurysms and in 7 patients with cerebral hematoma unrelated to saccular aneurysms. The findings were correlated with outcome and development of angiographic vasospasm.

On admission, CIC was detected in 13 (72%) of patients with ruptured aneurysms compared with 3 of 21 healthy blood donors. Eight of the 13 aneurysm patients positive for CIC were in Hunt and Hess grade III or IV at admission, and only 2 recovered fully at 3-months' follow-up. In contrast, of the 5 patients with negative CIC on admission, 1 was in grade III and the rest were in grades I and II. Five patients with positive CIC died, whereas none of the CIC-negative patients died. Eight of 9 patients who had angiographically observed vasospasm had CIC on admission, compared with only 1 of 4 without vasospasm. Patients with vasospasm, in contrast to those who did not have vasospasm and patients with hematoma unrelated to aneurysm rupture, had a twofold increase in plasma

C3d levels at the time when the spasm occurred. The increase in plasma C3d concentration was positively associated with the presence of CIC.

Most patients with ruptured cerebral aneurysms have CIC on admission to the hospital. The presence of CIC on admission is associated with the development of angiographic vasospasm, poor prognosis, and complement activation.

These data suggest that immunologic processes involving complement-activating immune complexes are involved in the pathogenesis of cerebral vasospasm following rupture of saccular aneurysms. The early occurrence of CIC in these patients may be explained by the repeated leakage of small amounts of blood into the subarachnoid space with concomitant release of damaged tissue, which may act as an autoantigen.

▶ This creative study extends observations regarding immune reactions in cerebrovascular vasospasm. Further studies along this line may help to define further the importance of circulating immune complexes in the process of vasospasm.

In a related study, Seifert et al. (*Surg Neurol* 27:243–52, 1987) found that high levels of thromboxane B^2 in the cerebrospinal fluid are associated with ischemic complications in patients with subarachnoid hemorrhage.—R.M. Crowell, M.D.

Fusiform Aneurysms of the Basilar Artery: A Review of 15 Cases
Milandre L, Bonnefoi B, Pellissier JF, Ali Cherif A, Khalil R (Centre Hospitalier Universitaire de La Timone, Marseille, France)
Sem Hôp Paris 63:365–370, Feb 5, 1987   21–11

In contrast to sacculated aneurysms, which arise from arterial dilatation of a weakened area in the artery and have a high risk of rupture, fusiform aneurysms of the basilar trunk (FABT) are fairly common congenital arterial malformations that usually remain asymptomatic and rarely rupture. However, FABTs may be associated with a wide range of symptoms. The true incidence of FABT is unknown. Findings were reviewed in 13 men and 2 women aged 59–78 years treated during a 10-year period; FABT was diagnosed either at autopsy or at radiographic examination.

The lesion was first diagnosed at autopsy in 6 patients, after conventional arteriography and confirmed at autopsy in 2 patients, and after computed tomography and confirmed by angiography in 7 patients. Ten patients had arterial hypertension, 6 patients had coronary insufficiency, ischemic vascular accidents, or both, and 1 patient had facial hemiparesis several years before having a stroke. Thirteen patients had several FABT-associated abnormalities: In 10 patients, basilar trunk ectasia also involved 1 or 2 vertebral arteries (Fig 21–6). Additional involvement of the posterior cerebral arteries was observed in 1 patient, and of 1 or 2 internal carotid arteries in 8. Two patients also had aortic aneurysms. Only 2 patients with trigeminal neuralgia improved and remained stabi-

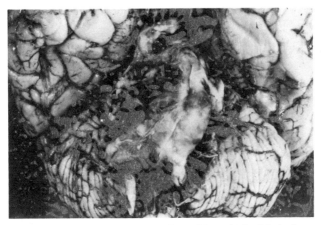

Fig 21–6.—Fusiform aneurysm in situ involving the caudal two thirds of the basilar artery and extending to the distal portion of the vertebral arteries. (Courtesy of Milandre L, Bonnefoi B, Pellissier JF, et al: *Sem Hôp Paris* 63:365–370, February 1987.)

lized after undergoing removal of the gasserian ganglion by balloon angioplasty. In all cases, FABT had caused deformity of the cerebral trunk, and all patients had severe and diffuse atherosclerosis.

When FABTs are found, other arterial aneurysms at other sites, especially along the aorta, can be expected and should be looked for.

▶ These lesions are now picked up with some regularity through the use of CT and MR. This study may delineate the relationship of the lesion to adjacent parenchyma. The course is unpredictable, but in case of progressive symptomatology, intervention may be warranted. With a balloon catheter, we promoted thrombosis of a distal vertebral giant aneurysm of this type with resolution of clinical symptoms of brain stem compression. In 2 other cases, shunting of hydrocephalus was helpful. In 2 other cases, decompression of the posterior fossa with dural patch graft led to clinical improvement. Occlusion of the aneurysm with distal bypass grafting has not been rewarded with success in the Mayo Clinic experience.—R.M. Crowell, M.D.

Fusiform Intracranial Aneurysms: Clinicopathologic Features
Shokunbi MT, Vinters HV, Kaufmann JCE (Univ Hosp, London, Ont)
Surg Neurol 29:263–270, April 1988   21–12

Fusiform intracranial aneurysms are uncommon vascular lesions and their pathology has not been well documented. In particular, their microscopic features have not been studied systematically. Autopsy records from 1972 to 1985 were reviewed, and 7 fusiform aneurysms were reported in 5 patients aged 56–65 years. The basilar trunk was the most common site of the aneurysm (Fig 21–7).

Four aneurysms were of giant proportions and contained laminated

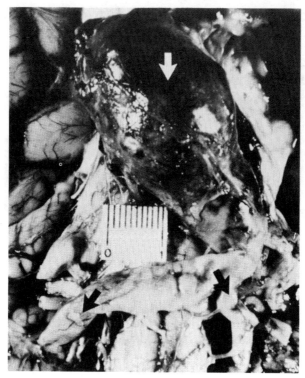

Fig 21–7.—Basal view of the brain: giant fusiform aneurysm of the basilar trunk *(white arrow)* and ectatic atherosclerotic vertebral arteries *(black arrows)* are shown. (Courtesy of Shokunbi MT, Vinters HV, Kaufmann JCE: *Surg Neurol* 29:263–270, April 1988.)

thrombi. Microscopic assessment of the aneurysm walls demonstrated atheromatous degeneration, focal wall attenuation, mural hemorrhage, rupture, and acute and chronic inflammatory cell infiltration.

Rupture is not rare, and atherosclerosis is only 1 mechanism in the pathogenesis of these lesions.

▶ This careful pathologic study indicates that atherosclerosis, as well as infiltration and hemorrhage, may be present in fusiform intracranial aneurysms. Rupture is not uncommon and may lead to subarachnoid hemorrhage with potentially lethal outcome.—R.M. Crowell, M.D.

Brief Notes on Aneurysms

Fifty asymptomatic aneurysms were surgically treated. Two patients died, 5 were unchanged with neurologic deficit, and 43 were cured (Jomin M, et al: *Presse Med* 16:375–377, 1987).

Aneurysms are reported in association with glioma, meningioma, and pituitary adenoma (Plangger CA, et al: *Nervenarzt* 58:279–286, 1987).

The authors add 4 cases of traumatic aneurysm after penetrating brain wound to 24 they find in the literature. They emphasize the need for routine angiography in this situation (Rahimizadeh A, et al: *Acta Neurochir (Wien)* 84:93–98, 1987).

Among 1,076 patients with intracranial aneurysm, the maximum risk of rebleeding was observed between day 4 and day 9, with fewer rebleeds in patients whose condition was graded as good (Rosenorn J, et al: *J Neurosurg* 67:329–332, 1987).

Of 150 patients with subarachnoid hemorrhage admitted within 6 hours, 33 rebled, with 29 rebleeds occurring within the first 24 hours. Moreover, the rebleeding rate was highest of all within 6 hours, this rebleeding was more severe than the initial, and the chance of rebleeding was higher with the higher clinical grades (Inagawa T, et al: *Surg Neurol* 28:93–99, 1987).

Holter monitoring showed arrhythmia in 96 of 107 patients monitored within 24 hours after subarachnoid hemorrhage. Life-threatening ventricular arrhythmia occurred in 4, and changes suggesting myocardial ischemia were found in 8 (Di Pasquale et al: *Am J Cardiol* 59:596–600, 1987).

At the Beijing Neurosurgical Institute, 520 patients with intracranial aneurysm were operated upon. Spasm was common, as was recurrent hemorrhage. Microsurgery is used routinely at this time. Carotid ligation is uncommonly utilized. Extra-intracranial bypass is utilized prior to direct attack on giant aneurysms. Operative results are not available (Zhong-cheng W, et al: *Chin Med J* 99:263–267, 1986).

Although no difference was found in subarachnoid hemorrhage patients with and without subsequent ischemic complications with regard to white blood cell count on admission, WBC count rose significantly at the time of clinical manifestation of ischemia, suggesting a possible role for WBCs in the pathogenesis of cerebral ischemia (Spallone A, et al: *Surg Neurol* 27:253–258, 1987).

In a comparison of needles, catheters, and techniques, it was concluded that the Cordis CSF catheters are more effective than other methods for the intraoperative removal of CSF (Artru AA, Katz RA: *Neurosurgery* 22:101–104, 1988).

Giant Aneurysms

Computed tomography and MR imaging have demonstrated in giant intracranial aneurysms hyperdensity representing fresh clot in the wall of a thrombosed mass. It is suggested that the giant aneurysm grows by recurrent hemorrhage into its wall (Schubiger O, et al: *Neuroradiology* 29:266–271, 1987).

Partially thrombosed giant aneurysm can simulate an arteriovenous malformation on MR imaging (Camras et al: *J Comput Assist Tomogr* 11:326–328, 1987).

Other Vasospasm Treatments

In a study of 70 patients with subarachnoid hemorrhage, nimodipine did not prevent vasospasm but significantly reduced the severity of vasoconstriction and the incidence of delayed neurologic deficit, probably by increasing tolerance to focal cerebral ischemia (Seiler RW, et al: *Acta Neurochir (Wien)* 85:7–16, 1987).

Oral nimodipine reduces prostaglandin and thromboxane production by arteries chronically exposed to periarterial hematoma and tranexamic acid (Pickard JD, et al: *J Neurol Neurosurg Psychiatry* 50:727–731, 1987).

Pharmacokinetic studies of nimodipine indicate that IV administration leads to mean plasma concentrations of 26.6 ng/ml. Oral nimodipine led to mean plasma concentration of 13.2 ng/ml. In patients with delayed ischemic dysfunction, plasma concentration fell within the range of patients who did not have such deficits, suggesting that therapeutic failure cannot be attributed to individual deviations in the pharmacokinetics (Vinge, E, et al: *Eur J Clin Pharmacol* 30:421–425, 1986).

In an experimental model of delayed cerebral vasospasm, 5-lipoxygenase inhibitor had a beneficial effect (Yokota M, et al: *Stroke* 18:512–518, 1987).

Systemic heparinization in the early management of ruptured intracranial aneurysms led to improved results in 104 cases with concurrent controls (Kapp J, et al: *Neurosurgery* 20:564–570, 1987).

Early Surgery

One hundred fifty patients were operated on within 72 hours of subarachnoid hemorrhage over a 7-year period in Freiburg. Seventy-nine percent of the 23 patients were in grades I to III; 21% were in grades IV and V. Seventy-one percent had a severe hemorrhage. Thirteen percent of the patients suffered permanent or fatal postoperative deterioration, and 11% developed delayed deficits. Patients in good preoperative condition had a good early outcome in 69%, a fair outcome in 21%, and a poor outcome in 4%, with 6% fatality (Gilsbach JM, et al: *Acta Neurochir Wien* 90:91–102, 1988).

A prospective, multicenter study was carried out in 120 patients with subarachnoid hemorrhage treated with early surgery and nimodipine. During surgery, the drug was placed on the exposed arteries, and postoperatively it was given intravenously for 1 to 2 weeks. At 6 months, 93% of patients were completely recovered, 16% minimally disabled, 5% moderately disabled, and 3% severely disabled, with 3 deaths. The study supports the concept that early surgery and nimodipine can reduce delayed ischemic deficit. Delayed ischemic deficit with permanent disability occurred in only 2 patients (Auer LM, et al: *Acta Neurochir (Wien)* 82:7–13, 1986).

In a controlled study involving 30 patients, patients with acute intracerebral hematoma caused by rupture of an aneurysm who had surgery did better than those treated conservatively. The mortality was 80% in the conservatively treated group and 27% in the surgical group. It is suggested that the aneurysm should be clipped at the same operation (Heiskanen O, et al: *Acta Neurochir (Wien)* 90:81–83, 1988).

In 57 cases of patients with significant intracranial hematoma from ruptured aneurysm, a significant mortality (10% at a minimum) was noted (Freger P, et al: *Neurochirurgie* 33:1–11, 1987).

Two hundred forty cases were entered by the University of Toronto into the International Cooperative Study on Timing of Aneurysm Surgery. Comparing surgery at less than 3 days and after 4 or more days, no significant differences were found in the incidence of technical complications between these 2 groups (Tucker WS: *Can J Neurol Sci* 14:84–87, 1987).—R.M. Crowell, M.D.

Arteriovenous Malformations

The Natural History of Unruptured Intracranial Arteriovenous Malformations

Brown RD, Jr, Wiebers DO, Forbes G, O'Fallon WM, Piepgras DG, Marsh WR, Maciunas RJ (Mayo Clinic and Found, Rochester, Minn)
J Neurosurg 68:352–357, March 1988   21–13

Whether an arteriovenous malformation (AVM) of the brain should be managed conservatively or interventionally is controversial. A long-term follow-up study of 70 female and 98 male patients aged 6 to 74 years was carried out to define the natural history of clinically unruptured intracranial AVMs. All were seen at 1 center between 1974 and 1985. Four patients had 2 angiographically distinct lesions.

Follow-up information was obtained on 166 patients until death, surgery, or other intervention or for at least 4 years after diagnosis was made. The mean follow-up was 8.2 years. Cerebral arteriograms and computerized tomography scans of the head were reviewed.

Thirty-one patients (18%) had intracranial hemorrhage, 29 from rupture of an AVM. In 2 cases the hemorrhage was secondary to rupture of an AVM or aneurysm. Mean risk of hemorrhage was thus found to be 2.2% per year. The observed annual rates of hemorrhage increased with time. The risk of death from rupture was 29%. Twenty-three percent of survivors had significant long-term morbidity. The size of the AVM and the presence of hypertension, whether or not treated, were no value in predicting rupture. A significant risk of hemorrhage among survivors persisted for 20 years. The 29% mortality from hemorrhage noted is higher than previously reported.

▶ This 11-year follow-up of 168 patients with unruptured AVM indicates a 2.2% rupture rate per year. The risk of death from rupture was 29%. The risk of significant morbidity was 23%. This study supports a recommendation of surgical therapy for patients with unruptured intracranial AVMs.— R.M. Crowell, M.D.

Treatment of Unruptured Cerebral Arteriovenous Malformations
Aminoff MJ (Univ of California, San Francisco)
Neurology 37:815–819, May 1987   21–14

A conservative approach to unruptured arteriovenous malformations (AVMs) usually appears to be most appropriate. Although a cerebral AVM is a potential risk to life or the quality of life, pharmacologic measures or partial obliteration by nonoperative means counter most nonhemorrhagic manifestations. The benefit of removing an AVM, in eliminating the risk of intracranial bleeding, is countered by the risks of operative treatment.

The reported risk of bleeding in patients with an unruptured AVM is about 1% to 3% yearly, and mortality from a first hemorrhage ranges from 6% to 14%. From 4% to 23% of survivors may remain severely disabled after hemorrhage. Some workers have reported low operative risk for malformations that appear small angiographically. Even with the best mortality and morbidity rates for surgery (table) and poor rates for conservative management, there is no clear advantage to operat-

Results of Surgical Treatment of Cerebral
Arteriovenous Malformations*

Source	Total no. of pts	No. of operated pts	Operative results Percent mortality	Percent morbidity
Wilson et al	83	65	6	28
Parkinson & Bachers	100	90	11	20
Stein & Wolpert	81	55	2	5
Pellettieri et al	166	119	5	15§
Guidetti & Delitala	145	95	6	6
Fults & Kelly	131	48	11†	
Luessenhop & Rosa	450	90	2	11
Davis & Symon	129	69‡	2	9§
Adelt et al		43	7	7§
Heros & Tu		103	1	16

*Data shown are from several different series published since 1979. Percentages
are expressed to nearest whole number.
†Perioperative mortality was 11%; total mortality, 19%.
‡Patients underwent elective surgery only.
§"Moderate," "severe," or "significant" disability.
(Courtesy of Aminoff MJ: *Neurology* 37:815–819, May 1987.)

ing on unruptured cerebral AVMs, at least during a 20-year period.

Realistic estimates of the outcome of surgery in patients of unruptured cerebral AVM do not warrant surgical excision. With a single rupture, however, the risk of hemorrhage is increased, and excision may be more appropriately considered.

▶ Dr. Aminoff convincingly marshals data against surgery for unruptured AVMS. He carefully compares rates of hemorrhage (1%–3% per year) with published surgical results (1% to 11% mortality; 5% to 28% morbidity). Assuming a 20-year follow-up, he finds an advantage to conservative therapy over even the best surgical results (1% mortality, 16% morbidity reported by Heros RC, Tu Y-K; *Clin Neurosurg* 33:187–236, 1986). Decision analysis supports this conclusion unless the operative morbidity was less than 18% with an operative mortality of 1% (Iansek R, et al: *Lancet* 1:1132–1135, 1983; Aminoff MJ: *Clin Neurosurg* 33:177–185, 1986).

There are concerns with this argument; for example, many younger patients can be expected to survive beyond 20 years' follow-up. Also, 0% mortality and 4% morbidity can be achieved with small lesions, according to Luessenhop and Rosa (*J Neurosurg* 60:14–22, 1984). For a counter view, see Heros RC, Tu YK: *Neurology* 37:279–286, 1987.—R.M. Crowell, M.D.

Sylvian Fissure Arteriovenous Malformations
Sugita K, Takemae T, Kobayashi S (Shinshu Univ, Matsumoto, Japan)
Neurosurgery 21:7–14, July 1987   21–15

Arteriovenous malformations in or adjacent to the sylvian fissure are relatively difficult to remove, because they involve the middle cerebral ar-

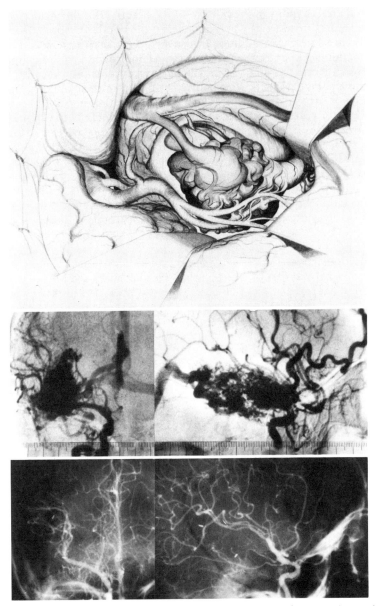

Fig 21–8.—Drawing *(top)* and preoperative *(center)* and postoperative *(bottom)* angiograms in patient with right pure and lateral sylvian fissure arteriovenous malformation. (Courtesy of Sugita K, Takemae T, Kobayashi S: *Neurosurgery* 21:7–14, July 1987.)

tery and are surrounded by critical structures such as the basal ganglia and the internal capsule. The surgical experience with 16 sylvian fissure arteriovenous malformations was reviewed. Pure sylvian fissure malformations were distinguished from lateral and medial malformations, depending on the site of the nidus, and from deep sylvian fissure lesions, in which there is a nidus in the bottom of the fissure or in the insular cortex.

The feeders in all cases were branches of the middle cerebral artery (Fig 21–8). In some cases, additional feeders from the choroidal and posterior communicating arteries were present. Nine patients with hemiparesis or hemiplegia at the time of surgery had remarkable improvement postoperatively. Five patients who had recovered from their initial deficits at the time of surgery did not have new deficits. Seizures persisted postoperatively in 1 patient without subarachnoid bleeding, but responded to drug treatment. The surgical outcome was rated as excellent in 10 cases, good in 3, and fair in 2. One patient died of infection and rebleeding from a residual nidus; staged surgery had been planned in this case.

Satisfactory operative results were obtained in all surviving patients with sylvian fissure arteriovenous malformation in this study. A large malformation extending deeply remains difficult to remove, because the nidus involves the basal ganglia; the 1 patient in this series with such a lesion died.

▶ These are difficult AVMS to excise because of their relation to critical MCA branches and basal ganglia. Stereoscopic angiography CT and MRI can help to determine the relationship of the nidus to the MCA and its branches. The sylvian fissure is split widely to permit individual dissection of MCA branches, which are divided only after assurance that they do not pass on to crucial frontal structures. Ventriculo-striate branches may be dissected from the nidus. Staging may be useful. Sugita achieved 10 excellent, 3 good, and 2 fair results; there was 1 fatality (the latter from rehemorrhage in a comatose patient with planned second-stage surgery). Modern microsurgery by an experienced master can procure good results with sylvian AVMs.—R.M. Crowell, M.D.

Surgical Approaches to Trigonal Arteriovenous Malformations
Batjer H, Samson D (Univ of Texas Health Science Ctr, Dallas)
J Neurosurg 67:511–517, October 1987   21–16

Most intracranial arteriovenous malformations (AVMs) have some ependymal representation, but lesions in which the nidus of the malformation is mostly in the ventricular system are rare. Only about 5% of AVMs fall into this anatomical category. These AVMs are often deemed inoperable because of their deep location and sometimes intimidating vascular patterns. Fifteen patients with AVMs in the ventricular trigone were seen between July 1981 and February 1986. The mean age was 24 years, and 10 were females. The most common presenting symptom was intracranial hemorrhage; intraventricular hemorrhage occurred in 11 patients, with multiple episodes documented in 5.

Three relationships were noted between the nidus of the AVM and the trigone. In the first, seen in 9 patients, the bulk of the AVM extended laterally from the lateral wall of the trigone. In the second type, seen in 5 patients, the malformation involved the trigone and projected from the medial ependymal surface into the splenium of the corpus callosum. One

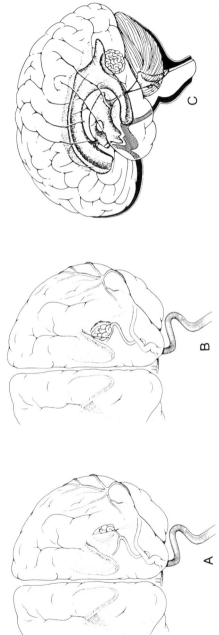

Fig 21-9.—A, artist's depiction of a laterally projecting AVM, antero-posterior view. The AVM lies lateral to the P2–P3 junction of the posterior cerebral artery. This pattern was seen in 9 patients. B, medially projecting AVM extending medial to the P2–P3 junction. This pattern was seen in 5 patients. C, this pattern of AVM projecting inferiorly from the floor of the trigone was seen in 1 patient. (Courtesy of Batjer H, Samson D: *J Neurosurg* 67:511–517, October 1987.)

patient had an AVM projecting inferiorly from the floor of the trigone, demonstrating cortical representation on the parahippocampal gyrus (Fig 21–9).

An interhemispheric surgical approach was used in 8 patients, a middle or inferior temporal gyrus incision in 6, and a subtemporal route in 1. After a mean follow-up of 15 months, 8 patients were neurologically normal. Four patients had homonymous hemianopsia, 1 of whom had this deficit before surgery. One patient awakened normally but a delayed thalamic syndrome developed on the fourth postoperative day, probably because of retrograde thrombosis in the posterior cerebral artery. Another patient, a 5-year-old boy, had progressive right-sided dystonia from documented moyamoya disease that involved the left basal ganglia. He later sustained an intraventricular hemorrhage from a trigonal AVM. Although the AVM was resected uneventfully, the dystonia worsened perioperatively and a 1-cm hemorrhage was found in the left basal ganglia. Another patient awakened densely hemiparetic and aphasic with a homonymous hemianopsia, a catastrophe believed to be related to proximal occlusion of the patient's fetal-type posterior cerebral artery.

In this series, 13 of the 15 patients returned to their previous form of work or educational level after removal of trigonal AVMs. An interhemispheric approach is recommended if the nidus projects medially from the trigone and is observed medial to the P_2–P_3 junction of the posterior cerebral artery on angiography. A middle temporal gyrus approach should be considered if the nidus is lateral to the P_2–P_3 junction, even when the lesion is in the dominant hemisphere. A subtemporal approach should be reserved for inferiorly projecting AVMs with cortical representation on the fusiform or parahippocampal gyrus in the nondominant hemisphere.

▶ Batjer and Samson report good results for excision of trigonal AVMs. Among 15 cases, there was 1 devastating deficit, 2 moderate, and 4 visual field defects only. Middle temporal gyrus incision led to only mild neurologic disturbance while providing excellent exposure. This type of approach seems preferable whenever the lesion extends more than 3 cm lateral to the midline.—R.M. Crowell, M.D.

Staged Treatment of Arteriovenous Malformations of the Brain

Andrews BT, Wilson CB (Univ of California, San Francisco)
Neurosurgery 21:314–323, September 1987   21–17

The treatment of large complex arteriovenous malformations (AVMs) of the brain remains challenging. In 28 patients aged 15–60 years with AVMs, therapy consisted of multiple surgical procedures, or endovascular embolization followed by surgery. Clinical symptoms in 13 patients were associated with intracranial hemorrhage; progressive neurologic deficit not caused by hemorrhage was present in 6, intractable headache in 5, and seizures in 4 patients.

Thirteen patients with large high-flow AVMs comprised group A; these

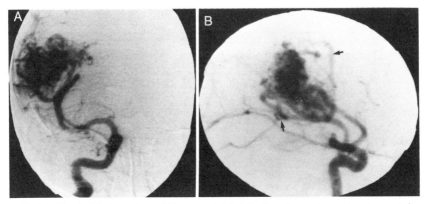

Fig 21–10.—A right internal carotid intra-arterial digital subtraction angiogram in anteroposterior (**A**) and lateral (**B**) views shows that the AVM is supplied by branches of the middle cerebral artery. Note poor filling of the adjacent cortical blood vessels and the anterior cerebral artery. Branches supplying the AVM also supply adjacent cortex at the periphery of the AVM *(arrows)*. (Courtesy of Andrews BT, Wilson CB: *Neurosurgery* 21:314–323, September 1987.)

patients had staged treatment because of the risk of normal perfusion pressure breakthrough (Fig 21–10). The initial afferent artery occlusion was done surgically in 9 patients and by endovascular embolization in 4. No patient had malignant cerebral edema or intracranial hemorrhage suggestive of normal perfusion breakthrough after surgery, although 1 patient had an intraventricular hemorrhage after initial embolization.

In the 9 patients comprising group B, the AVM had a complex multiple arterial supply that precluded resection from a single operative exposure. Seven of these patients had supratentorial AVMs; 2 had AVMs of the posterior fossa. In 6, the AVM was in the midline and received bilateral arterial input. Six patients underwent staged surgical procedures, and 3 had endovascular embolization followed by surgery. Two had intracerebral hemorrhages — 1 after an initial surgical procedure and 1 after embolization.

In the 4 patients in group C, the AVM had a major dural component treated separately from the parenchymal component. Embolization through the external carotid artery obliterated the dural component in 3 patients. In the fourth patient, a persistent internal carotid supply necessitated dural malformation resection. The parenchymal component was surgically excised in 2 cases. The 2 patients in group D had separate surgical procedures for an aneurysm associated with a parenchymal AVM.

Overall, 19 of the 28 patients had complete excision, and 9 had partial obliteration of AVMs. Of 27 patients followed for a mean of 18.6 months, 16 were in excellent condition, 8 were in good condition, and 3 in poor condition with serious neurologic deficits. One patient had an intracranial hemorrhage 22 months after incomplete AVM obliteration.

Staged treatment of selected patients with AVMs of the brain may avoid normal perfusion pressure breakthrough. This approach allows satisfactory obliteration of selected malformations that have multiple complex arterial supplies or a dural component and those associated with an aneurysm.

▶ Andrews and Wilson report good results for staged treatment of large AVMs and those fed by disparate arterial supplies. The problem of normal perfusion pressure breakthrough, a terrifying situation with malignant edema and uncontrolled hemorrhage, appears to be effectively countered by this approach. Apparently, the cerebrovascular tree, given time to gradually adjust, can avoid this devastating complication.

It is not clear whether endovascular obliteration of feeders or open surgical occlusion of feeders is preferable. Nor is the best embolic material established. It is to be expected with progress in percutaneous catheter technique that further advances in this area will make it even more attractive. It may be that especially difficult portions of the AVM might be obliterated by radiosurgical techniques after elimination of much of the lesion by embolic or direct surgical obliteration.

It is clear that risk of hemorrhage continues to exist as long as there is angiographic evidence of AVM. The recurrent hemorrhage in the partially obliterated lesion and the 3 hemorrhages between staged procedures in the current presentation bear witness to this fact.— R.M. Crowell, M.D.

Surgical Management of Large AVM's by Staged Embolization and Operative Excision

Spetzler RF, Martin NA, Carter LP, Flom RA, Raudzens PA, Wilkinson E (Barrow Neurological Inst, Phoenix)
J Neurosurg 67:17–28, July 1987   21–18

The surgical treatment of giant arteriovenous malformations (AVMs) —lesions more than 6 cm adjacent to or in eloquent areas of the brain and that have deep drainage—is complicated and risky. The results of treatment of 20 such patients with a stepwise reduction of flow through preoperative and intraoperative embolization followed by final excision were presented.

The 10 male and 10 female patients were aged 17–56 years. Initial treatment consisted of transfemoral embolization with Ivalon particles and sometimes a mix of Gelfoam. Usually, 1 major group of feeding vessels was embolized during each stage of management. Most commonly, the AVM was fed by the middle cerebral artery, the anterior communicating artery, and the posterior cerebral artery, thus requiring 3 separate surgical approaches for embolization. Complete excision of the AVM was achieved in 18 patients. No related deaths occurred, and only 4 complications occurred. In 1 patient normal perfusion pressure breakthrough occurred hours after surgery. This patient had extensive hemorrhagic infarction resulting in right hemiplegia and aphasia and was left with a major neurologic deficit. Another patient had a postoperative intracerebral and intraventricular hemorrhage; her recovery was protracted but complete, except for a residual homonymous hemianopsia. In another patient, a preoperative speech difficulty increased and never completely re-solved. The fourth patient developed contralateral upper extremity weakness that did not completely resolve.

This staged approach to giant AVM treatment is proposed to render previously inoperable or marginally operable AVMs to totally excisable lesions. The level of morbidity and mortality in this series was considered acceptable.

▶ The Barrow group reports good results by complex embolization and exci-sion. It is important to note that the embolizations, including intraoperative em-bolizations, have been staged, whereas the actual dissection of the lesion is carried out in a single operation, not several. A partial dissection of the lesion would be expected to have a substantial risk of hemorrhage before total exci-sion. This approach as described may be refined yet further with the introduc-tion of newer catheter techniques and embolization methods (such as Vinuela's cocktail of avitene, alcohol, and PVA).— R.M. Crowell, M.D.

The MRI Appearance of Cavernous Malformations (Angiomas)
Rigamonti D, Drayer BP, Johnson PC, Hadley MN, Zabramski J, Spetzler RF
(Barrow Neurological Inst, Phoenix)
J Neurosurg 67:518–524, October 1987   21–19

Magnetic resonance imaging (MRI) is emerging as the most effective diagnostic method in most disorders affecting the CNS. The importance of MRI is apparent when a high-field strength system is used to assess brain hemorrhage. A study was done to define the MRI characteristics of pathologically verified cavernous angiomas and to compare the merits of computed tomography (CT) with those of MRI in delineating these ab-normalities.

Angiographic, CT, and MRI findings were compared in 10 patients with 16 verified cavernous angiomas. Findings on angiography were neg-ative in 4 cases. In 2 studies an avascular area was demonstrated, and the remaining 4 angiograms depicted a mass lesion with displacement of ad-jacent vessels. A subtle vascular anomaly was seen in 3 of the latter 4 pa-tients in the form of focal capillary blush or venous pooling. Multiple le-sions were shown in only 1 case. Dilated arteries, rapid arteriovenous shunting with enlarged drainage veins, or abnormal draining veins sug-gesting arteriovenous or venous malformations were not shown by an-giography in any case. Results on CT were negative before and after con-trast media administration in 3 cases. In the remaining 7, CT depicted a hyperdense lesion in the precontrast study (Fig 21-11). Faint contrast en-hancement was observed in 5 of the 7 patients. Computed tomography confirmed a mass lesion suggested by vessel displacement on angiography in 4 cases. Multiple lesions were seen in only 3 patients. Fourteen lesions total were seen on CT. Magnetic resonance imaging demonstrated the le-sions in every case, with 27 separate lesions seen on T_2-weighted images. Eighteen larger lesions appeared as areas of mixed signal intensity (SI)

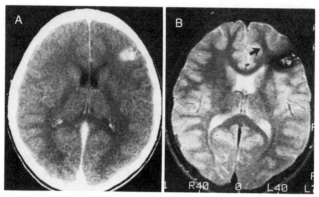

Fig 21–11.—**A,** CT scan with contrast enhancement showing a calcified, minimally enhancing lesion. **B,** MRI (TR 2,500 msec, TE 80 msec) showing the same lesion as a central core of mixed increased and decreased signal intensity (SI) surrounded by a dense black rim of decreased SI caused by hemosiderin-laden macrophages. The *arrow* points to a smaller lesion characterized by a core of predominantly decreased SI "black dots"). (Courtesy of Rigamonti D, Drayer BP, Johnson PC, et al: *J Neurosurg* 67:518–524, October 1987.)

with a reticulated appearance and a prominent surrounding rim of decreased SI. Eight smaller lesions were seen as punctate areas of reduced SI. Multiple lesions were seen in 5 patients, and mass effect was seen in 4. T_1-weighted studies were less sensitive than T_2-weighted studies, detecting 23 of the 27 lesions.

High-field strength MRI yielded positive findings in all verified cavernous angiomas, whereas CT findings were positive in only 7 of 10. On T_2-weighted images, the combination of a reticulated core of mixed SI with a surrounding rim of decreased SI strongly suggests a cavernous malformation.

▶ This timely essay confirms that lesions shown on MR with a high signal and peripheral rim of low-intensity signal on T_2 are pathologically cavernous angiomas. The ease and specificity of MRI diagnosis gives rise to a substantial patient population hitherto missed with negative angiography. It is known that these lesions can occasionally rebleed, but the precise natural history is unknown, and thus the vigor and risk of appropriate management remain uncertain. Moreover, it is difficult to gauge the efficacy of treatment in that there is no convenient endpoint as in angiographic obliteration.— R.M. Crowell, M.D.

Hemorrhagic Neoplasms: MR Mimics of Occult Vascular Malformations
Sze G, Krol G, Olsen WL, Harper PS, Galicich JH, Heier LA, Zimmerman RD, Deck MDF (Mem Sloan-Kettering Cancer Ctr, New York Hosp, New York; Univ of California, San Francisco)
AJNR 8:795–802, September–October 1987   21–20

Angiographically occult vascular malformations of the brain typically appear on magnetic resonance (MR) imaging as central foci of

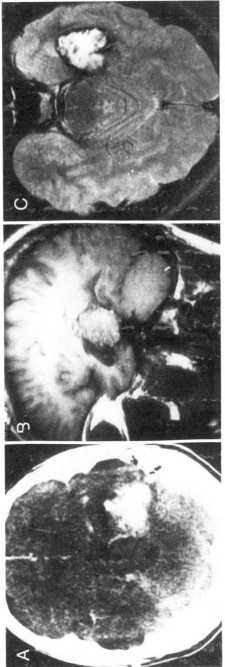

Fig 21–12.—A 34-year-old man with seizure disorder. Surgical pathology: cryptic vascular malformation. **A,** contrast-enhanced CT scan shows large enhancing mass with primarily intraventricular location and trapping of distal temporal horn. **B,** T1-weighted sagittal MR images (TR 600 msec, TE 25 msec) confirm intraventricular location of mass. In addition, the mass is primarily isointense, with a few foci of increased signals. **C,** T2-weighted MR images (TR 2,000) msec, TE 70 msec) now show lesion to be of high signal, with scattered areas of lesser signal. In addition, a prominent hypointense rim surrounds lesion, creating an appearance most consistent with the paramagnetic effect of hemosiderin. (Courtesy of Sze G, Krol G, Olsen WL, et al: *AJNR* 8:795–802, September–October 1987.)

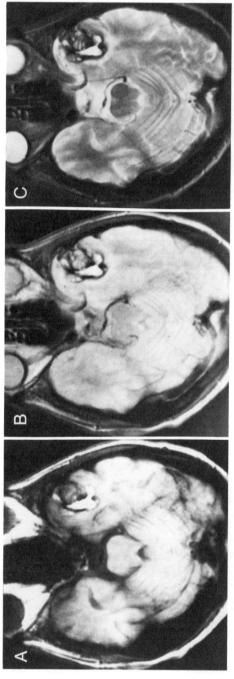

Fig 21–13.—A 66-year-old man with melanoma. Surgical pathology: metastatic melanoma. The metastasis was hemorrhagic and virtually amelanotic. **A,** T1-weighted images (TR 600 msec, TE 20 msec) show a lesion of mixed isointensity and hyperintensity, with surrounding hypointensity. The lesion has an appearance similar to that described as typical for cryptic vascular malformations. **B** and **C,** proton density and T2-weighted MR images (TR 2,000 msec, TE 35/70 msec). Central core remains either isointense or hyperintense, and peripheral hypointensity has increased. Although there is a minimal amount of surrounding edema and mass effect, these features can also be seen in cryptic vascular malformations. (Courtesy of Sze G, Krol G, Olsen WL: *AJNR* 8:795–802, September–October 1987.)

high-intensity signal surrounded by a peripheral zone of low intensity. These findings are also similar to the MR appearance of many primary or secondary hemorrhagic neoplasms. The MR appearances were reviewed in 24 patients.

Six of the 24 patients had occult vascular malformations, 5 of which were documented surgically. In 2 of these patients, a central focus of isointensity was present on T_1-weighted images (Fig 21–12). In 3 others, the central focus was hyperintense. The remaining 18 patients had hemorrhagic neoplasms. Three were primary lesions that closely resembled occult vascular malformations. In 15 patients with hemorrhagic metastasis, the average number of lesions was 3. In 2 patients computed tomography (CT) missed multiple punctate metastases that were clearly visible on MR. The usual MR finding was of areas of high central signal.

Although foci of adjacent nonhemorragic tumor may be seen in larger neoplasms, nodular areas without the high signal of subacute blood are also present in occult vascular malformations. The peripheral dark rim becomes more prominent and hypointense on the second echo of the long TR sequence (Fig 21–13).

Magnetic resonance findings considered typical of occult vascular malformation may actually represent hemorrhagic tumor. Neoplasm must be considered even if a small, single lesion is present. In questionable cases, CT may provide further information. Certainly, further patient evaluation or follow-up is required.

▶ This report extends previous investigations of MR imaging of angiographically occult vascular malformations (Lemme-Plaghos L, et al: *AJNR* 7:217–222; 1986; New P, et al: *AJNR* 7:771–779, 1986). The authors point out that central foci of high intensity signal with peripheral low intensity may also be seen with hemorrhagic neoplasms. In most of their cases, however, multiplicity of lesions led to the diagnosis of multiple metastases. In all 3 cases of primary brain neoplasm, the CT suggested the correct diagnosis. However, I have personally observed 2 cases of brain stem solitary lesions in which the MR suggested occult malformation or tumor, and the CT scan was inconclusive. For such lesions, careful follow-up evaluation or biopsy is indicated. The distinction becomes particularly important as one considers the possibility of stereotactic radiosurgical treatment.—R.M. Crowell, M.D.

Brief Notes on AVMs

Cerebral angiography may confirm complete spontaneous regression of the cerebral arteriovenous malformation (Leramo OB, Clarke WFB: *South Med J* 80:529–532, 1987).

A case of spontaneous disappearance of a brain arteriovenous malformation is reported (Besel VR, et al: *Zentral bl Neurochir* 48:43–49, 1987).

In a study of vascular malformations of the posterior fossa, Silber et al. and colleagues found clinical presentation as hemorrhage, progressive deficit, disequilibrium, or trigeminal neuralgia in patients with typical arteriovenous lesions as well as venous angiomas. Computed tomography with infusion was abnormal in 95%. Angiography established or confirmed the diagnosis in most of the patients (*Arch Neurol* 44:965–969, 1987).

Careful follow-up demonstrated spontaneous enlargement of 0.2% to 2.8% per year among 6 patients with arteriovenous malformations (Mendelow AD, et al: *J Neurol, Neurosurg, Psychiatry* 50:980–987, 1987).

Of 18 patients with cerebral circulation studied during removal of arteriovenous malformation, 2 cases developed perfusion breakthrough syndrome and had low cerebral blood flow and disturbed CO_2 reactivity before excision and marked increase in local blood flow after excision (Barnett GH, et al: *Neurosurgery* 20:836–842, 1987).

Embolization

Glutaraldehyde cross link collagen (GAX) is recommended as a new material for therapeutic embolization (Strother CM, et al: *AJNR* 8:509–515, 1987).

A Tracker catheter system may redirect a symptomatic errant intracranial silastic sphere embolus with recovery (Russell EJ, Levy JM: *Radiology* 165:631–633, 1987).

Venous Angioma

Cerebral varix has been associated with a venous angioma on CT and angiographic study (Dross P, et al: *AJNR* 8:373–374, 1987).

Asymptomatic cerebellar venous angioma can be suspected on CT scan and confirmed by angiography. Data indicate that conservative management is appropriate (Hankey GJ, et al: *Aust N Z J Med* 17:441–443, 1987).

Value of MRI

Magnetic resonance imaging in 15 patients with AVM demonstrated the AVM in all cases with good delineation of feeding arteries and draining veins without bony artifact. The relationship of the AVM to surrounding parenchyma was well appreciated. Often, the MRI appearance can lead to a judgment of operability, making angiography unnecessary. Magnetic resonance imaging is more useful than CT for the management of specific cases (Leblanc R, et al: *Neurosurgery* 21:15–20, 1987).

In 20 cases of AVMs studied with MR, CT, and angiography, the size of malformations looked smaller on MR because draining veins can be separated out by MR. Magnetic resonance was also better in detecting hemorrhage, which could be mistaken for old infarction on CT. It is more accurate in the definition of the AVM nidus (Noorbehesht B, et al: *Neuroradiology* 29:512–518, 1987).

Slow flow vascular malformations of the brain stem on MR are characterized by isointense to hyperintense central signal surrounded by well-defined thin band of low signal intensity suggesting subacute or chronic hematoma (Griffin C, et al: *Neuroradiology* 29:506–511, 1987).

Fifteen malignant lesions with hemorrhage were diagnosed on MRI (Atlas SW, et al: *Radiology* 164:71–77, 1987).

Intracerebral Hemorrhage

A review of 112 patients with intracerebral hemorrhage confirmed etiologic distinction between lobar and thalamic/basal ganglionic hemorrhage but not reported differences in clinical presentation and outcome (Lipton RB, et al: *J Neurol* 234:86–90, 1987).

An intracerebral hematoma developing during MR examination showed heterogeneous density on CT study immediately following the MR examination (Nose T, et al: *J Comput Assist Tomogr* 11:184–187, 1987).—R.M. Crowell, M.D.

22 Spine

Introduction

In the *cervical spine,* a prospective evaluation indicated that surface coil MR imaging was as good as myelography in the evaluation of cervical radiculopathy (Abstract 22–1). Cervical spine involvement in rheumatoid arthritis is beautifully imaged by MR techniques (Abstract 22–2). Cervical spine stenosis secondary to ossification of the posterior longitudinal ligament is more common in American populations than was originally thought, is well demonstrated by CT, and is best treated by an anterior approach (Abstract 22–3). An anterior retropharyngeal approach may be effectively utilized to reach deep lesions at C1, C2, and C3 (Abstract 22–4). Anterior plate fixation is advocated for traumatic lesions of the lower cervical spine (Abstract 22–5).

In the field of *lumbar disease,* MR can diagnosis lumbar arachnoiditis in all but the mildest cases (Abstract 22–6). Postoperative assessment is also significantly advanced with surface coil MRI (Abstract 22–7). In a controlled study, posterior fusion offered superior results for grades III and IV spondylolisthesis (Abstract 22–9). Posterior lumbar interbody fusion may be effectively accomplished with plates (Abstract 22–10). A long-term prospective study of lumbosacral diskectomy finds good results for patients with neurologic signs and confirmatory radiology (Abstract 22–11).

Regarding *spinal tumors,* intra-axial tumors of the cervical medullary junction may now be removed with modern technical adjuncts, yielding good results (Abstract 22–12). Magnetic resonance imaging is currently the method of choice for evaluating metastatic spinal disease (Abstract 22–13). Radical excision is advocated for the treatment of spinal chordomas (Abstract 22–15). Luque rod stabilization appears to have a place in the treatment of metastatic disease of the spine (Abstract 22–14). Congenital intraspinal lipomas produce progressive neurologic disability and should be removed even when asymptomatic (Lhowe D, et al: *J Pediatr Orthop* 7:531–537, 1987). Modern radiographic techniques permit subdivision of spinal arteriovenous fistulas and AVMs for appropriate management (Abstract 22–16). Magnetic resonance is very helpful in the follow-up of syringomyelia after surgery (Abstract 22–17).

In *basic studies,* it has been demonstrated that measurement of epidural blood flow is useful in the serial evaluation of spinal cord blood flow (Abstract 22–18).

Robert M. Crowell, M.D.

Cervical

Cervical Radiculopathy: Prospective Evaluation With Surface Coil MR Imaging, CT With Metrizamide, and Metrizamide Myelography

Modic MT, Masaryk TJ, Mulopulos GP, Bundschuh C, Han JS, Bohlman H (Univ Hosp of Cleveland, Case Western Reserve Univ, Cleveland)
Radiology 161:753–759, December 1986   22–1

Theoretically, surface coil magnetic resonance (SCMR) imaging could provide an examination in assessment of cervical radiculopathy that is competitive in quality with computed tomography with metrizamide (CTM) and metrizamide myelography (MM). A prospective study was done to compare the accuracy of these 3 methods in determining cervical radiculopathy.

All imaging studies were performed on 52 patients, and the studies were evaluated for disease location and type. Surgical findings were used as the objective measure of accuracy. Twenty-eight patients had subsequent cervical surgery at 39 levels from an anterior interbody approach. Predictions made with SCMR imaging were confirmed surgically in 74% of the patients. The CTM predictions were confirmed in 85% of the patients, and the MM, in 67%. When SCMR imaging and CTM were used jointly, there was a 90% agreement with surgical findings. When CTM and MM were used together, the agreement with surgical findings was 92%. Generally, SCMR was as sensitive as CTM for identifying disease level, but was not as specific for disease type. The MM was least specific for disease type. The CTM's major advantage was its ability to distinguish bone from soft tissue, for which contrast material is not necessary.

Imaging with SCMR is a viable alternative to MM. Together with CT, if needed, SCMR imaging provides a thorough examination of the cervical region.

▶ Modic and colleagues suggest that cervical roots are nicely imaged by magnetic resonance imaging without resorting to myelography. These methods present attractive images. On the other hand, images available in many clinical settings are not so refined. In many institutions, for the time being myelography will remain an important adjunct in the evaluation of cervical root disease.

In another study, Modic and his colleagues found that oblique MR imaging permitted an 82% concurrence of MR findings with surgical findings relative to cervical radiculopathy, only slightly lower than findings on CT metrizamide myelography (Modic MT, et al: *Radiology* 163:227–231, 1987).—R.M. Crowell, M.D.

Cervical Spine Involvement in Rheumatoid Arthritis: MR Imaging

Aisen AM, Martel W, Ellis JH, McCune WJ (Univ of Michigan)
Radiology 165:159–163, October 1987   22–2

The cervical spine is often involved in patients with long-standing rheumatoid arthritis. Magnetic resonance (MR) imaging was used to

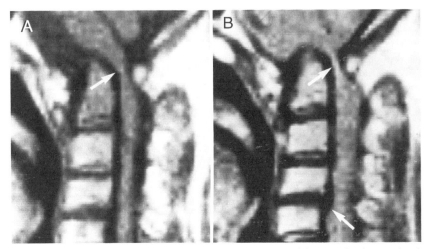

Fig 22–1.—Images of a 54-year-old man with a 26-year history of rheumatoid arthritis and with weakness that later progressed to quadriparesis. **A,** T1-weighted MR image (SE 500/28) demonstrates erosion of the dens with absence of the superior portion, craniovertebral setting, and marked constriction of the neuraxis (*arrow*) at the cervicomedullary junction. **B,** T2-weighted image (SE 1,500/56) reveals a subtle zone of increased signal intensity at the site of constriction (*upper arrow*) and diminished signal in the C4–C5 disk, with an indentation on the dura at this level (*lower arrow*). (Courtesy of Aisen AM, Martel W, Ellis JH, et al: *Radiology* 165:159–163, October 1987.)

evaluate 18 rheumatoid patients who had neck pain, reduced neck motion, or neurologic deficit referable to the cervical spine. Most had classic adult-type rheumatoid arthritis. Imaging used relatively T_1-, T_2-, and intermediately weighted pulse sequences.

All patients but 1 had plain x-ray evidence of rheumatoid involvement of the cervical spine. The odontoid process was better appreciated on MR images than on plain radiographs. The dens was eroded in 14 patients (Fig 22–1). In 6 patients the skull was settled on the upper cervical spine because of occipitoatlantoaxial joint erosion. A focal zone of increased signal intensity in the cord adjacent to a site of constriction may have represented cord edema. Minor cervical subluxations were not visualized by MR imaging in several instances. All patients with indentation or distortion of the caudal brain stem or cervical cord had neck pain or reduced motion, and most had related neurologic abnormalities.

Magnetic resonance imaging makes it possible to follow the progression of rheumatoid disease in the cervical spine. Findings of progressive destructive change might prompt more aggressive drug therapy. Asymptomatic patients with significant abnormalities might be advised to limit their activity or use a cervical brace.

▶ As demonstrated in this report, MR beautifully depicts pathology around the cervico-vertebral junction in rheumatoid arthritis. In some cases MR studies may be the only ones required, although myelography is still frequently used in symptomatic cases requiring surgical intervention. Yulish et al. report that juvenile rheumatoid arthritis may also be assessed by MR imaging (Yulish BS, et al: *Radiology* 165:149–152, 1987).—R.M. Crowell, M.D.

Cervical Spine Stenosis Secondary to Ossification of the Posterior Longitudinal Ligament

Harsh GR IV, Sypert GW, Weinstein PR, Ross DA, Wilson CB (Univ of California, San Francisco; Univ of Florida, Gainesville)
J Neurosurg 67:349–357, September 1987   22–3

Ossification of the posterior longitudinal ligament (OPLL) is a cause of cervical spine stenosis and myelopathy among Japanese patients. Ossification of the posterior longitudinal ligament in North Americans is thought to be rare. Diagnostic and treatment methods for this entity remain controversial. Twenty patients were seen with symptomatic OPLL of the cervical spine, representing 10% to 20% of those undergoing surgery in the past 3 years for myelopathy secondary to structural spinal compression at the present institutions. Sixty percent were Caucasian. The median patient age was 47.5 years, and men outnumbered women by 4:1. Six patients had previously undergone laminectomy or diskectomy. Cervical radiographs and standard myelography sometimes suggested the diagnosis; axial CT metrizamide myelography with small interslice intervals was invaluable in diagnosing and in operative planning (Fig 22–2). Magnetic resonance imaging was not needed for the diagnosis.

Retrovertebral calcification extended over 1 to 5 bodies. The size of the mass ranged from 5 to 16 mm in anteroposterior diameter, reducing the residual canal diameter to a mean caliber of 9.42 ± 2.41 mm. Anterior cervical decompression by medial corpectomy and diskectomy with fusion was done, and uniformly reduced preoperative myelopathy. Complications included transient neurologic deterioration in 2 patients, recurrent laryngeal nerve palsy in 1, and halo device pin site infections in 2. At

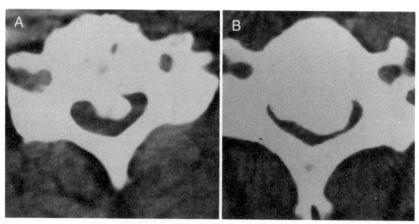

Fig 22–2.—Preoperative axial CT scans without metrizamide. These scans of 2 different patients demonstrate the variability in shape of the ossified mass. A, the calcified ligament extends from the medial aspect of the vertebral body and the mass appears pedunculated. B, the calcified mass is seen as an irregularly shaped osteoma protruding from the entire posterior surface of the vertebral body. (Courtesy of Harsh GR IV, Sypert GW, Weinstein PR, et al: J Neurosurg 67:349–357, September 1987).

a mean follow-up period of 15 months, improvement was noted in each category: extremity weakness, hypesthesia, hypertonia, and urinary dysfunction. In addition, all fusions produced solid unions.

These data indicate that OPLL of the cervical spine is an unexpectedly prevalent cause of myelopathy among patients treated in the United States. Thin-section axial CT metrizamide myelography with small inter-slice intervals is invaluable for diagnosing OPLL. Anterior decompression and stabilization by medial corpectomy, diskectomy, removal of the cal-cified mass, and fusion comprise a safe and effective method of treatment.

▶ Ossification of the posterior longitudinal ligament is more common in Caucasians than was previously thought. An anterior decompression is safe and effective treatment. Computed tomography scanning readily makes the diagnosis. Microsurgical anterior corpectomy and fusion provide the best anatomical relief of compression with superior clinical results. Posterior decompression by laminectomy does not eliminate the progressive encroachment.—R.M. Crowell, M.D.

The Anterior Retropharyngeal Approach to the Upper Part of the Cervical Spine
McAfee PC, Bohlman HH, Riley LH, Jr, Robinson RA, Southwick WO, Nachlas NE (Johns Hopkins Univ)
J Bone Joint Surg [Am] 69A:1371–1383, December 1987   22–4

An anterior approach to decompress the cervical spinal cord may be indicated for disease above the level of the third disk. An anterior retro-pharyngeal approach provides adequate exposure for removing lesions of the atlas and axis and stabilizing the upper cervical spine. It is a cranial extension of the anterior cervical approach described by others, and it is entirely extramucosal. A modified transverse submandibular incision is used. The retropharyngeal space is dissected after preserving the hypoglossal nerve (Fig 22–3). Anterior decompression usually begins by removing the disk between the second and third vertebrae or the first normal disk at the caudad edge of the lesion.

Seventeen patients had this operation, most for tumor of the upper cervical spine. Intralesional excision of a malignancy was the most frequent procedure. No postoperative infections occurred, and there were no acute respiratory problems. The anterior bone graft shifted in 2 cases. Three patients had transient hypoglossal or facial paresis postoperatively. All 12 patients followed for 2 years or longer had solid anterior fusion without later loss of spinal stability.

The anterior retropharyngeal approach to the upper cervical spine provides better exposure than the lateral approach. Tracheostomy is avoided in most patients. In some cases, posterior stabilization and arthrodesis may be done at the same session.

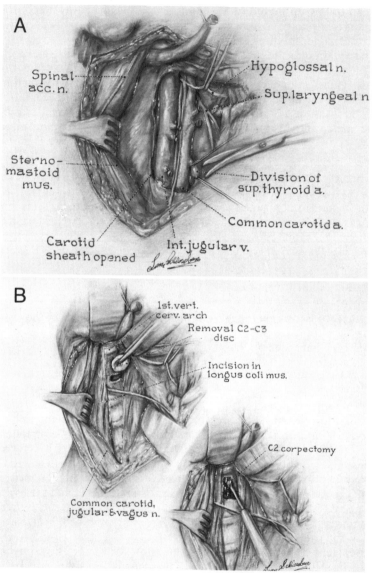

Fig 22–3.—A, after the superficial layer of the deep cervical fascia is incised along the anterior border of the sternocleidomastoid muscle, the superior thyroid artery and vein are divided. The hypoglossal and superior laryneal nerves are mobilized. Additional branches of the carotid artery and internal jugular vein are ligated to allow mobilization of the contents of the carotid sheath laterally as the hypopharynx is mobilized medially. **B,** the first step of the anterior spinal decompression is meticulous removal of the disk between the second and third cervical vertebrae. The longus colli muscle is dissected in a lateral direction, exposing the second cervical vertebral body and anterior arch of the atlas. Removal of the body of the second cervical vertebra can then be performed with a high-speed burr. (Courtesy of McAfee PC, Bohlman HH, Riley LH Jr, et al: *J Bone Joint Surg* [Am] 69-A:1371–1383, December 1987.)

▶ This report describes a promising approach to the "no man's land" of the upper cervical spine. The standard anterior cervical exposure of this area is difficult, and the transoral approach to the dens, although effective in some hands, has sometimes been associated with infections and a need for tracheostomy. Therefore this report, without incidence of postoperative infection or major neurologic deficit and no tracheostomies, suggests that this logical extension of the anterior cervical approach may well be useful right up to the clivus. Obviously, careful anatomical experience with this type of method (as in the autopsy dissecting room) is necessary before its appropriate clinical application.— R.M. Crowell, M.D.

Anterior Plate Fixation of Traumatic Lesions of the Lower Cervical Spine
de Oliveira JC (Oporto Med School, Oporto, Portugal)
Spine 12:324–329, 1987   22–5

Since 1979, an H-shaped plate, with 2 screws for each vertebra, has been used to fuse the cervical spine in patients with traumatic lesions. Steel plates, 18–30 mm in length, are inserted. The anterolateral approach provides good exposure to the cervical spine from C2 to C7. In cases of fracture-dislocation from flexion injury with severe spinal instability, immediate reduction is carried out, followed in a few days by anterior plating. Extension and compressive injuries also have been plated. For compressive injuries, only those with major neurologic lesions were operated on.

No significant complications were noted in 40 patients who underwent surgery. Plates and screws had not loosened, even several years after operation. On follow-up averaging 3 years, patients with serious neurologic involvement had results comparable to those achieved with other types of surgical treatment. Twenty-nine flexion injuries, 2 extension injuries, and 9 compressive injuries were treated. Of the 40 patients, 16 had tetraplegia, Brown-Séquard syndrome, or severe neurologic lesions.

Anterior plating of the cervical spine is a safe, effective approach to traumatic lesions of the lower cervical region. The technique also may be used after resection of bone tumor, or for instability after extensive laminectomy.

▶ Anterior plate fixation appears to be safe and highly effective for cervical traumatic instability. Anterior interbody fusion has been used for some time (Cloward RD: *J Neurosurg* 18:205–209, 1961), but the bone plug may dislodge and fusion may fail. Halo fixation has been used by some, but this involves wearing an external device for some months. Plate fixation needs further study for confirmation; however, these results are impressive.— R.M. Crowell, M.D.

Brief Notes on the Cervical Spine

Imaging Techniques

Multiplanar representation of spinal MR images can be obtained from a single high-resolution 3D acquisition (Sherry CS, et al: *J Comput Assist Tomogr* 11:859–862, 1987).

After injection of positive contrast material into the epidural space, CT of the spine can identify disk herniation and nerve root compression with high accuracy in preliminary studies (Hårdstedt C, Vucetic N: *Acta Radiol Diagn* 27:173–178, 1986).

High-dose iohexol myelography is associated with an increased rate of adverse reactions and should not be used (Simon JH, et al: *Radiology* 163:455–458, 1987).

Anterior Cervical Decompression

Among 21 patients with cervical spondylotic myelopathy, an anterior multi-level decompression with fibula dovetailed strut graft led to good stability, a high union rate, and no neurologic complications (Bernard TN, Jr, Whitecloud TS III: *Clin Orthop* 221:149–160, 1987).

Of 251 patients undergoing anterior cervical diskectomy without fusion, excellent or good long-term results were achieved in 82% of patients with radiculopathy and 55% of those with myelopathy, especially with soft disk lesions at a single level (Bertalanffy H, Eggert HR: *Acta Neurochir (Wien)* 90:127–135, 1988).

Anterior cervical decompression and fusion in 46 patients with cervical spondylotic myelopathy led to unassisted walking in 22%, improvement in 78%, stability in 13%, and disease progression in 9% (Irving GB, Strachan WE: *Paraplegia* 25:18–22, 1987).

Posterior Stabilization

From a review of 212 patients with 222 operations after cervical spinal injury, it is concluded that posterior wiring of fusion is an excellent means of stabilization that is not dependent on the integrity of the posterior ligamentous structures. Anterior cervical spinal fusion alone is accompanied by loss of reduction in a number of cases and is recommended only for cases with prior extensive laminectomy. For patients with anterior decompression, either halo vest or posterior wiring should be undertaken to prevent instability. (Capen DA, et al: *Paraplegia* 25:111–119, 1987).

During posterior spinal fusion, a posterior column injury occurred that was detected by somatosensory evoked potential monitoring but not by a wake-up test (Ben-David B, et al: *Spine* 12:540–543, 1987).

Posterior cervical fusion under local anesthesia has been recommended as the ultimate spinal cord monitor (Zigler J, et al: *Spine* 12:206–208, 1987).

In patients with thoracolumbar spine fractures and incomplete neurologic deficits, anterior decompression produced superior result as compared with posterior decompression (Bradford DS, McBride GG: *Clin Orthop* 216:201–216, 1987).

General Topics

C1-2 fusion is indicated in symptomatic atlantoaxial subluxation in Down's syndrome (Shikata J, et al: *Clin Orthop* 220:111–118, 1987).

Thoracolumbar fractures in ankylosing spondylitis are dangerous in that turning the patient may cause neurologic complications. The best treatment is reduction of displacement and stabilization with Luque rods (Trent G, et al: *Clin Orthop* 227:61–66, 1987).

Among 28 patients with psoriasis and arthritis, cervical spine involvement was present in 75% of the group with ankylosing or inflammatory characteristics and with cervical myelopathy in 3 patients (Blau RH, Kaufman RL: *J Rheumatol* 14:111–117, 1987).

Atlantoaxial fixation may be accomplished by a transcervical anterior approach (Lesoin F, et al: *Neurochirurgie* 33:239–243, 1987).

Twelve patients are described with atlantoaxial tuberculosis. Transoral biopsy and decompression is recommended, followed by halo traction and posterior fusion (Lifeso R: *J Bone Joint Surg* 69B:183–187, 1987)—R.M. Crowell, M.D.

Lumbar

MR Imaging of Lumbar Arachnoiditis

Ross JS, Masaryk TJ, Modic MT, Delamater R, Bohlman H, Wilbur G, Kaufman B (Case Western Reserve Univ, Cleveland)
AJNR 8:885–892, September–October 1987 22–6

The clinical diagnosis of spinal arachnoiditis is difficult because it has no distinct symptom complex. Surface coil MR imaging with thin slices is capable of defining the nerve roots in the thecal sac, and appears to identify arachnoiditis manifested as enlarged or clumped nerve roots in a pattern similar to that seen by CT myelography. To test the validity of these observations, a retrospective study was made of patients referred for assessment of failed back surgery syndrome.

The MR, plain-film myelographic findings and CT myelographic findings in 100 patients were reviewed. Twelve had CT and plain film myelographic changes of arachnoiditis. In 11, surface coil MR showed a pattern of nerve roots believed to be abnormal and consistent with arachnoiditis.

The correlated surface coil MR/CT myelography/plain film myelography changes were divided into 3 categories. In the first group, consisting of 3 patients, the predominant surface coil MR findings were large conglomerations of nerve roots central in the thecal sac. In the second group, which included 5 patients, surface coil MR showed clumped nerve roots attached peripherally to the meninges. One patient demonstrated characteristic findings of the first and second groups. In the third group, consisting of 2 patients, T_1-weighted surface coil MR images showed increased soft tissue signal in the thecal sac below the conus medullaris, obliterating centrally most of the subarachnoid space (Fig 22–4). One surface coil MR study was false negative: arachnoiditis seen on plain film and CT myelography was not seen on surface coil MR. Instead, MR showed inhomogeneous signal from the thecal sac with no definite empty sac or central clumping. In all cases, the abnormalities were observed at level L-3 or below. The abnormal configurations of the nerve roots in the lumbar spine were observed over at least 2 vertebral-body levels in all 11 cases.

Magnetic resonance correlates excellently with CT myelographic and plain-film myelographic findings in the diagnosis of moderate to severe arachnoiditis.

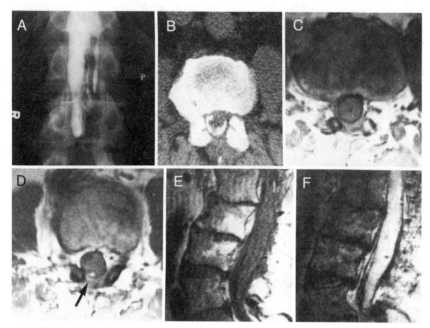

Fig 22–4.—Group 3 pattern of arachnoiditis. **A,** anteroposterior view of iohexol myelogram via C1–C2 puncture. There is block at inferior level of the L2 body, with a candle-dripping appearance of distal contrast material. Note previous laminectomy and small epidural wire from dorsal column stimulation for pain control. **B,** CT myelogram at L3 level. Soft tissue attenuation mass fills much of lumbar thecal sac. **C,** axial T1-weighted MR image (TR = 500 msec, TE = 17 msec) at same level. The thecal sac is nearly filled with mass of intermediate signal. Cerebrospinal fluid signal is present as peripheral rim about mass and in small central collection. **D,** axial T1-weighted MR image (TR = 500 msec, TE = 17 msec) at L2 level. Adherent roots are also visible at this level, as well as small area of high signal from residual Pantopaque (*arrow*). **E,** sagittal T1-weighted MR image (TR = 500 msec, TE = 17 msec). Abnormal mass of intermediate signal is present throughout lumbar thecal sac. **F,** sagittal T2-weighted MR image (TR = 2,000 msec, TE = 90 msec). High signal within dural tube does not allow distinction between normal CSF and arachnoiditis. (Courtesy of Ross JS, Masaryk TJ, Modic MT: *AJNR* 8:885–892, September–October 1987.)

▶ Magnetic resonance appears to be an effective means for diagnosis of moderate to severe lumbar arachnoiditis. In 11 of 12 cases, MR showed characteristic patterns of clumped nerve roots, roots adherent to dura or intraspinal mass. There was only one false negative. It remains to be seen whether mild arachnoiditis can be detected with this method perhaps with gadolinium enhancement. Further experience will be needed to define the precise place of MR in diagnosis of this disease process, previously diagnosable with certainty only on myelography.—R.M. Crowell, M.D.

Lumbar Spine: Postoperative Assessment With Surface-Coil MR Imaging
Ross JS, Masaryk TJ, Modic MT, Bohlman H, Delamater R, Wilber G (Univ Hosp of Cleveland, Case Western Reserve Univ, Cleveland)
Radiology 164:851–860, September 1987   22–7

The postoperative appearance of the spine following spinal surgery on magnetic resonance images (MRIs) has not been defined. Fifteen patients who were scheduled to undergo various types of lumbar spine surgery underwent preoperative, immediate postoperative (1–10 days), and late postoperative (2–6 months) MRIs to assess the postoperative changes on MRI. The MRIs were obtained with 1.0- or 1.5-T superconductive units with T_1- and T_2-weighted sequences. The MRIs of 62 patients who had undergone lumbar surgery but still had low back pain were also studied retrospectively.

In 9 of 13 patients who underwent laminectomy and diskectomy, epidural soft tissue change and mass effect mimicking preoperative findings were noted. The mass effect improved in appearance by the late postoperative period in 8 of 9 patients. The T_2-weighted sagittal images were best in demonstrating the site of annulus disruption immediately after diskectomy in 11 of 13 patients, and the rent resolved on the late images in 8 of 10 patients. Sites of foraminotomy were seen as loss of the normal fat signal. One area where the soft-tissue disruption does not impede a diagnostic study is postoperative hemorrhage. The high signal intensity of hemorrhage on T_1-weighted images allows great contrast with the intermediate-intensity epidural edema. Operative outcome could not be predicted based on the postoperative MRIs. Patients with complete or partial resolution of symptoms showed scarring involving anterior, lateral, and posterior epidural tissues.

Extensive soft-tissue changes present in the immediate postoperative period reflect the dynamic course of the normal reparative process following surgical intervention. These changes, however, severely limit the usefulness of MRI in that period for evaluating persistent or new symptoms. The exception may be postoperative hemorrhage, with its distinctive signal on T_1-weighted images.

▶ This study demonstrates the utility of MR in the early and late postoperative phase for the assessment of the anatomical effectiveness of diskectomy. It is important to note that early postoperative changes, including swelling, may resolve over the course of time. Epidural hematoma appears to be well diagnosed by the early studies. One point that has not been solved is the discrimination of late epidural fibrosis from recurrent or persistent herniated disk.— R.M. Crowell, M.D.

Back Pain and Sciatica
Frymoyer JW (Univ of Vermont, Burlington)
N Engl J Med 318:291–300, Feb 4, 1988   22–8

Low back pain is usually self-limiting, but it is a costly symptom that disables 5.4 million Americans. The author discusses back pain and sciatica. The lifetime prevalence of low back pain ranges from 60% to 90%; the annual incidence is 5%. Men and women are equally affected, although women more often report low back symptoms after age 60 years. Risk factors include involvement in occupations that require repetitive lifting, exposure to vibrations caused by vehicles or industrial machinery, and cigarette smoking.

Sciatica tends to have a more protracted course, but 50% of patients recover in 1 month. Only 10% to 20% of patients with acute low back pain can be given a precise patho-anatomical diagnosis. In most patients a history and physical examination are sufficient to begin treatment. Most patients with acute symptoms need only a nonspecific, short-term treatment regimen, which may include bed rest, analgesic medication, exercise, and education. Acute sciatica accompanying acute low back pain rarely requires surgery unless the symptoms result from massive disk rupture, epidural abscess, or tumor. These should be considered if there is a history of intractable pain, fever, or rapidly changing neurologic symptoms. In 10% of patients, low back pain persists for longer than 6 weeks, with a cause continuing to be elusive; in these patients, spinal osteomyelitis and neoplasms may have been overlooked. Patients with chronic low back pain may require a single definitive diagnostic work-up. Most patients with chronic low back pain can be treated with anti-inflammatory agents and exercise.

Simple treatment is sufficient for most patients with low back pain and sciatica. Timely surgery for a minority of patients with sciatica and neurologic claudication who do not respond to conservative care and aggressive rehabilitation for patients disabled by chronic low back pain will usually be successful.

▶ Frymoyer correctly emphasizes that the vast majority of patients with back pain are best managed conservatively. When conservative measures fail, the occasional patient will merit surgical correction of a radiographically demonstrable compressive lesion. Critical surgical selection can reduce the number of postoperative low back cripples.— R.M. Crowell, M.D.

Long-Term Follow-up of Patients With Grade-III and IV Spondylolisthesis: Treatment With and Without Posterior Fusion
Harris IE, Weinstein SL (Univ of Iowa)
J Bone Joint Surg [Am] 69A:960–969, September 1987   22–9

Although the incidence, etiology, and treatment of spondylolisthesis have been well reported, little has been written about the long-term results in patients who were not operated on, especially those who had a displacement of 50% or greater of the fifth lumbar vertebra on the sacrum, graded as a Meyerding grade III or grade IV lesion. A study was undertaken to compare the late results in patients with grade III or grade IV spondylolisthesis who did not undergo operation with those who underwent posterior interlaminar arthrodesis.

The study population included 32 patients who had been treated between 1938 and 1980 for grade III or grade IV spondylolisthesis. Of the 32 patients, 11 had been treated conservatively (group I); the other 21 patients (group II) underwent posterior interlaminar fusion.

At follow-up of an average of 18-years, 4 (36%) of 11 patients in group I were asymptomatic, 6 (55%) had mild symptoms, and 1 (9%) had significant symptoms. All 11 patients led active lives, even though 5 patients (45%) had 1 or more neurologic abnormalities. However, none of the 11 patients were incontinent, and none had made major adjustments in their life-style.

At follow-up of an average 24-years, 12 (57%) of 32 patients in group II were asymptomatic, 8 (38%) had mild symptoms, and 1 (5%) had significant symptoms. These 32 patients also led active lives, even though 9 (50%) of 18 patients who underwent a physical examination at follow-up had 1 or more neurologic findings. One patient had a pseudarthrosis, and 3 patients had progression by bending of the fusion mass; nevertheless, the patients remained asymptomatic.

In situ arthrodesis provides acceptable results in patients with grade III or grade IV spondylolisthesis and pain that is unresponsive to conservative treatment. In situ fusion is recommended for the skeletally immature patient who has disturbances of gait secondary to tight hamstrings, or for those in whom spondylolisthesis appears to be progressing.

▶ The results of this pilot controlled study suggest that fusion is helpful for patients who have grade III or grade IV spondylolisthesis together with intractable pain. Further data will be needed to confirm this initial impression.—R.M. Crowell, M.D.

Posterior Lumbar Interbody Fusion and Plates

Steffee AD, Sitkowski DJ (St Vincent Charity Hosp, Cleveland)
Clin Orthop 227:99–102, February 1988   22–10

Posterior lumbar interbody fusion (PLIF) is accepted by many as the surgical treatment for herniated disks, degenerative disk conditions, and grades I and II spondylolistheses. The PLIF is now used with newly developed segmental spine plates, using transpedicular screw fixation to enhance the osteosynthesis and success rate of interbody fusion. With these new spine plates, complete reduction with the addition of interbody fusion in grades III and IV spondylolisthesis can be done.

After decompression and excision of the disk are done, the transpedicular screws are inserted through the pedicles and into the bodies of the adjacent vertebrae, the solid bone of the sacrum, or both (Fig 22–5). Spine plates or the short, serrated, stainless steel rods are placed over the screws. Distracting the involved vertebrae is then possible, making insertion of the interbody plug easier. After allogeneic graft insertion, the plug is held in fixed, consistent compression when the screws and spine plates are tightened down.

Thirty-six patients underwent the procedure and were followed up for 6–12 months. Three continued to have chronic pain, and 2 secondary procedures were performed. Two dural tears were noted, and radiography revealed 1 instance of a broken screw. To date, 104 fusions have been done in 67 patients with no dislocations of any interbody grafts, no indications of absorption or pseudoarthrosis, and no infections. Solid fusion is achieved at about 3 months. Patients were not immobilized or confined to bed during recovery periods.

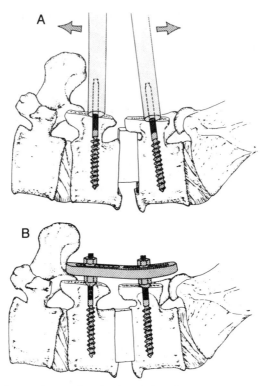

Fig 22–5.—**A,** diagram of a screw insertion through the pedicles and the role of the screw in providing distraction for easier placement of the interbody graft. **B,** interbody graft and immediate stability are achieved with application of the spine plates. (Courtesy of Steffee AD, Sitkowski DJ: *Clin Orthop* 227:99–102, February 1988.)

The PLIF is now used with newly developed segmental spine plates by using transpedicular screw fixation to enhance the osteosynthesis and success rate of interbody fusion. To date, 104 fusions have been successfully performed in 67 patients.

▶ The addition of Steffee plates to PLIF is logical and can be accomplished safely. The precise indications for PLIF (with or without plates) has yet to be established. Certainly, one cannot generally accept the author's assertion that PLIF is "the surgical treatment for herniated disc, degenerative disc conditions, and Grades I and II spondylolisthesis." The generalized adoption of PLIF and Steffee plates awaits substantial further validation by appropriately controlled clinical trials.—R.M. Crowell, M.D.

Long-Term Prospective Study of Lumbosacral Discectomy
Lewis PJ, Weir BKA, Broad RW, Grace MG (Univ of Alberta)
J Neurosurg 67:49–53, July 1987   22–11

Patients' Assessment of Results of Surgery

Result	Back Pain		Leg Pain	
	1 Yr Postop	5–10 Yrs Postop	1 Yr Postop	5–10 Yrs Postop
complete relief (%)	63	62	74	62
partial relief (%)	29	29	22	27
pain same (%)	7	5	3	7
pain worse (%)	1	4	1	4

(Courtesy of Lewis PJ, Weir BKA, Broad RW, et al: *J Neurosurg* 67:49–53, July 1987.)

The course following lumbosacral diskectomy for disk herniation was examined in a prospective series of 100 consecutive patients operated on between 1975 and 1977. None had previously had lumbar spine surgery of any type. Diskectomy was performed under general anesthesia with the patient in the lateral position. The mean patient age was 42 years, and the mean duration of leg pain preoperatively was 16 months. More than one third of patients had been hospitalized at least once.

All but 4% of 83 evaluable patients were pleased that they had undergone diskectomy (table), and more than 90% were able to return to work. Back pain was absent in 62% of patients for 5 years or longer after operation, and leg pain was relieved in the same proportion of patients. The reoperation rate was 18%; 1 patient had 2 reoperations. These procedures were performed 2 years after initial surgery on average. The repeat operative findings could not be related to the long-term outcome.

Unilateral diskectomy is a safe operation for disk protrusion in the lower spine. If a significant protrusion is removed, the period of incapacity will be substantially shortened, although similar problems may arise in the future. The long-term course in an individual patient cannot be predicted with a high degree of accuracy.

▶ Lumbosacral diskectomy gives good but not perfect results for symptomatic disk protrusion. In this nicely designed study, 90% of the patients had root pain, 82% a myelographic root defect, and 100% a disk protrusion (or extrusion) at surgery. At 5–10 years, relief of back pain occurred in 91%, with relief of leg pain in 89%. Further, 96% were pleased that they had surgery, and 93% returned to work. Although some failures were noted, this is solid scientific evidence indicating the efficacy of the procedure. Note that strict adherence to careful selection criteria (sciatica, positive myelogram) were needed to produce such good results.—R.M. Crowell, M.D.

Brief Notes on the Lumbar Spine

Radiography and Lumbar Pathology

Magnetic resonance can identify intradural disk herniation (Holtas S, et al: *J Comput Assist Tomogr* 11:353–356, 1987).

In patients with low back pain, a negative screening examination for other causes of pain, back pain with tenderness over a facet joint, and radiologic change of degenerative joint disease accurately identified facet joint disease as a significant cause for low back pain. Local injections of anesthetic and steroid may be helpful for these patients (Lewinnek GE, Warfield CA: *Clin Orthop* 213:216–222, 1986).

Disk protrusion in MR was seen in 5 of 25 asymptomatic patients aged 45–54 and in 24 of 42 patients older than 64 years. Spinal cord impingement was seen in 16% of patients under 64 and in 26% of patients older than 64 years (Teresi LM, et al: *Radiology* 164:83–88, 1987).

Magnetic resonance imaging is useful in the detection of the vacuum phenomenon, a good indicator of degeneration in a intervertebral disk (Grenier N, et al: *Radiology* 164:861–865, 1987).

Magnetic resonance is quite effective in viewing the caudate equina (Monajati A, et al: *AJNR* 8:893–900, 1987).

Computed tomography may nicely diagnose lumbosacral conjoined nerve roots (Torricelli P, et al: *Neuroradiology* 29:374–379, 1987).

Radiography After Surgery

In a group of 256 patients, CT scans were performed early on after lumbar laminectomy. These studies gave hints for the indication of early postoperative course regarding prognosis (Hammer B, et al: *Fortschr Roengenstr* 145:586–590, 1986).

Ross et al. reviewed with MRI the postoperative situation after anterior diskectomy and fusion (*J Comput Assist Tomogr* 11:955–962, 1987). Of 73 cases, they noted canal stenosis in 19 and disk herniations above or below the fusion site in 21.

Direct coronal CT scanning can diagnosis pseudarthrosis following lumbar fusion (Chafetz N, et al: *Radiology* 162:803–805, 1987).

Of 20 patients evaluated with MR for epidural fibrosis and recurrent disk herniation, morphology, epidural location, mass effect, and signal intensity correctly predicted the abnormality in 86% in whom findings were verified at surgery (Bundschuh CV: *AJNR* 9:169–178, 1988).

Magnetic resonance is superior to other methods for early detection of spinal epidural sepsis (Angtuaco EJC, et al: *AJR* 149:1249–1253, 1987).

Radiography After Chemonucleolysis

In CT scanning, chymopapain injection did not alter the size of the herniated portion of the disk during the first 3 months (Boumphrey FRS, et al: *Clin Orthop* 219:120–123, 1987).

After chemonucleolysis, there is a gradual loss of signal on MRI (Gibson MJ, et al: *J Bone Joint Surg* 68B:719–723, 1986).

Eight of 12 disks after chemonucleolysis showed clinical improvement, and there was a decrease in 1 or both dimensions of the defect in the thecal sac on lumbar MR. (Huckman MS, et al: *AJNR* 8:1–4, 1987).

Back Pain

Somatosensory evoked responses are said to be useful in the evaluation of low back pain (Perlik S, et al: *Arch Neurol* 43:907–913, 1986).

In a publication from Shanghai, 76.8% of 515 patients with protruded lumbar disks had satisfactory results from manipulative therapy (Kuo PPF, Loh ZC: *Clin Orthop* 215:47–55, 1987).

Diskography is considered an important diagnostic study in the assessment of chronic low back pain (Grubb SA, et al: *Spine* 12:282–286, 1987).

In 250 patients with low back pain and sciatica, epidural steroid injections provided a safe, cost-effective means of treatment (Hickey RF: *NZ Med J* 100:594–596, 1987).

Pain and paresis in 1 leg suggests adult diplomyelia (Wolf A, et al: *Spine* 12:233–237, 1987).

Spondylolisthesis

For grade IV spondylolisthesis, anterior vertebrectomy and fusion may be associated with pain relief and neurologic improvement (Dimar JR, Hoffman G: *Orthop Rev* 15:504–509, 1986).

In about one third of cases of spondylolysis, there is stenosis of the intervertebral foramen. Removal of the hook-like remnant of the proximal lamina is an important feature of treatment (Edelson JG, Nathan H: *J Bone Joint Surg [Br]* 68B:596–599, 1986).

Three patients underwent lateral mass fusion for spondylolisthesis. Pain was relieved (Hughes SPF, et al: *Arch Orthop Trauma Surg* 106:381–384, 1987).

Anterior interbody fusion is recommended for degenerative spondylolisthesis in patients younger than 60 years of age (Inoue SI, et al: *Clin Orthop* 227:90–98, 1988).

Staged salvage reconstruction of grade IV and V spondylolisthesis produced satisfactory results, and delayed union was the most common complication (Bradford DS, Gotfried Y: *J Bone Joint Surg* 69A:191–202, 1987).

Grade IV spondylolisthesis can be reduced and held using variable screw placement slotted plates and transpedicular screws (Steffee AD, Sitkowski DJ: *Clin Orthop* 227:82–89, 1988).

Fusions

A comprehensive system (A0) internal spinal skeletal fixation system has been described. The system involves hinged clamps and rods that can be applied to the most varied situations in the lower thoracic and lumbar spine (Ebaeb IM, et al: *Spine* 12:544–551, 1987).

Despite intraoperative awakening, postoperative quadriplegia may occur after spinal fusion for scoliosis (Diaz JH, Lockhart CH: *Anesth Analg* 66:1039–1042, 1987).

Long-term follow-up of 94 patients with lower lumbar fusions showed persistent back pain in 44%, 53% on pain medication, and 15% with repeat lumbar surgery (Lehmann TR, et al: *Spine* 12:97–104, 1987).

A plate system with hollow screws made of titanium is described for immediate interbody fusion. Bone grows into the hollow screws (Morscher E, et al: *Chirurg* 57:702–707, 1986).

Diskectomy

A comparative study of microsurgical diskectomy as compared with conventional technique in lumbar disk excision demonstrated microsurgery to be safe and nontraumatic, with good long-term results (Nystrom B: *Acta Neurol Scand* 76:129–141, 1987).

A controlled study demonstrated that small disk herniations had slightly better results with chemonucleolysis as compared with surgery, whereas patients with medium-sized or large herniations had better results with surgery (Postacchini F, et al: *Spine* 12:87–96, 1987).

In a controlled study, obese patients fared no differently from nonobese patients as regards surgical results after disk excision (Hanigan WC, et al: *Neurosurgery* 20:896–899, 1987).

Zenoderm, a porcine-treated dermis, is ineffective in preventing adhesions after laminectomy in rabbits (Boot DA, Hughes SPF: *Clin Orthop* 216:296–302, 1987).—R.M. Crowell, M.D.

Tumors

Intra-Axial Tumors of the Cervicomedullary Junction
Epstein F, Wisoff J (New York Univ Med Ctr)
J Neurosurg 67:483–487, October 1987   22–12

Radical surgical excision of intra-axial tumors in the cervicomedullary junction region has been avoided, because it is assumed that extensive dissection in this region will result in significant morbidity and mortality. Radiation therapy has been considered the treatment of choice, with progressive disability and death inevitable. Operative management of 20 intra-axial tumors of the cervicomedullary junction was reviewed.

The series included 15 children and 5 adults. The 2 distinct modes of clinical presentation were lower cranial nerve dysfunction and spinal cord dysfunction. Both patient groups commonly had indolent courses: symptoms were present for 6 months to 2 years in 75%. All patients underwent radical excision. Monitoring of brain stem-evoked potentials was a valuable surgical adjunct. The approach used was through a cervical laminectomy with or without a small suboccipital craniectomy.

Intraoperative transdural ultrasonography was used before the dura was opened; it was indispensable in defining the rostral-caudal limits of the neoplasm and the presence of associated cysts. After the dura was opened, the myelotomy was done over the entire length of the solid component of the neoplasm (Fig 22–6). Tumor excision began in the region where the tumor was most voluminous. The neoplasm was gradually debulked with the use of the Cavitron ultrasonic surgical aspirator and the surgical laser. Tumors in the medulla were also exposed through a myelotomy where the neoplasm was closest to the surface of the area postrema or the floor of the fourth ventricle. Tumors in the brain stem and spinal cord were removed from inside out until white matter was observed or brain stem-evoked potentials became disordered. There was no surgical mortality. Three patients had impaired position sense in the upper extremities after surgery; 6 had transient weakness and spasticity in the lower extremities. A 10-year-old girl moderately disabled before surgery became quadriplegic after surgery. Another patient had sleep apnea

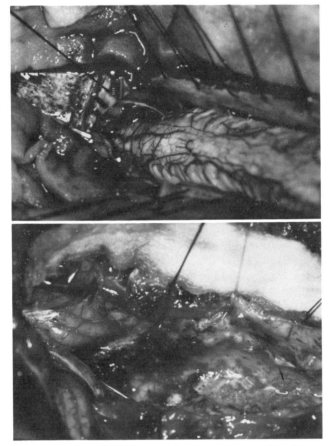

Fig 22–6.—Operative exposure before (*top*) and after (*bottom*) tumor excision. (Courtesy of Epstein F, Wisoff J: *J Neurosurg* 67:483–487, 1987.)

syndrome for 6 weeks after surgery. Postoperative neurologic recovery was directly related to preoperative neurologic status. All patients with malignant astrocytomas died of tumor progression 6 to 9 months after surgery, and 1 with a gangliogioma died of tumor progression 3 months postoperatively. Three months to 6 years postoperatively, 8 patients were alive.

Intrinsic gliomas of the cervicomedullary junction are amenable to radical excision. An aggressive surgical approach can potentially result in neurologic recovery and long-term survival.

▶ Radical excision of intramedullary cervicomedullary tumors can be achieved with low risk using modern methodology. Among 20 cases there was no mortality or a single lasting serious complication. Long-term survivals were noted in some cases with less invasive lesions. The eventual impact on the disease course is not yet known. Further experience will be required to evaluate the long-term impact of such heroic therapy, before this approach may be recommended for general use.— R.M. Crowell, M.D.

The Role of MR Imaging in Evaluating Metastatic Spinal Disease
Smoker WRK, Godersky JC, Knutzon RK, Keyes WD, Norman D, Bergman W (Univ of Iowa, Iowa City; Univ of Utah, Salt Lake City; Univ of California, San Francisco; Radiology Associates of Sacramento, Sacramento, Calif)
AJNR 8:901–908, September–October 1987   22–13

Magnetic resonance imaging (MRI) is an excellent technique for visualizing the spinal cord. The role of MRI in the evaluation of patients with spinal cord or root compression from metastatic disease was determined in 58 patients with suspected epidural metastases. Six patients were examined on 2 separate occasions. The MRIs were obtained on a 0.5-T superconductive scanner using a standard body coil; both T_1- and T_2-weighted sagittal MRIs were obtained. Twenty-two patients also underwent myelography, and the results were compared with those of MRI.

Magnetic resonance imaging was considered diagnostic in 60 of 64 studies. Most of the patients presenting with a myelopathy had spinal cord compression or at least subarachnoid space compression, which was demonstrated on MRI. Five of 22 patients presenting with back pain only in the absence of neurologic deficits had some degree of cord compression demonstrated on MRI. There was excellent correlation between the myelographic and MRIs in 19 of 22 patients who underwent both examinations. Magnetic resonance imaging provided additional information not seen with myelography in 13 of 22 patients, including demonstration of both the upper and lower extent of the lesion in 4 patients, paraspinal involvement in 3, additional areas of spinal cord compression in 2, and additional osseous spinal metastatic disease in 2. Repeat MRIs in 6 patients evaluated for new or increasing symptoms identified the progression of disease in all of them.

Magnetic resonance imaging should be the examination of choice for evaluating suspected metastatic spinal disease. The T_1-weighted images are best for demonstration of spinal cord compression, whereas the T_2-weighted images best show subarachnoid space impingement in the absence of cord compression. The main limitation to the use of MRI is primarily technical.

► Magnetic resonance imaging is extremely valuable in evaluating metastatic spinal disease. Patients with back pain only may have positive studies with cord compression. There is excellent MR correlation with myelography, and additional information, such as the upper and lower extent of the main compressive lesion, is provided in many cases. Thus, MRI is certainly the study of choice in evaluating patients with suspected spinal metastatic disease, and in most cases it can eliminate the need for myelography, with its potential hazards.— R.M. Crowell, M.D.

Luque Rod Stabilization for Metastatic Disease of the Spine

Cybulski GR, Von Roenn KA, D'Angelo CM, DeWald RL (Rush-Presbyterian-St. Luke's Medical Ctr., Cook County Hosp, Chicago)
Surg Neurol 28:277–283, October 1987   22–14

Instability of the spine from metastatic spread of primary tumors is a serious risk for spinal cord or nerve foot compression. To restore stability and relieve neural compression, several surgical techniques originally used for reduction of nonpathologic spinal fractures have been used. A technique developed mainly for correction of scoliosis was applied to the treatment of metastatic spinal fractures.

Six patients with spinal instability and neural compression from metastatic tumors underwent spinal stabilization with Luque rods, sublaminar wiring, and methyl methacrylate. The patients, 5 women and 1 man, were aged 58 to 72 years. In a representative case, plain films of the spine, myelogram, and CT scan demonstrated compression fractures at T7 and T12 and epidural blockage at T12. This patient was treated with radiotherapy for 1 week with no pain relief. A decompressive laminectomy was done at T12 with a posterolateral resection of the T12 vertebral body and decompression of the T12 nerve roots. Frozen section analysis indicated adenocarcinoma. A T5 to L3 stabilization with a contoured Luque D-ring, sublaminar wiring, and methyl methacrylate aug-

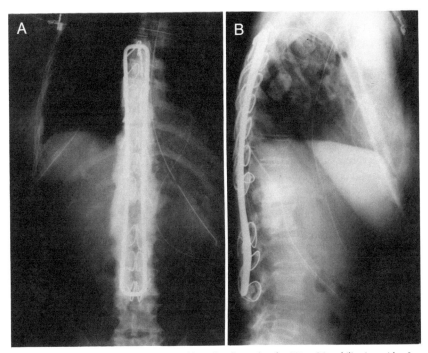

Fig 22–7.—A and **B,** anteroposterior and lateral radiographs after T5 to L3 stabilization with a Luque rod. (Courtesy of Cybulski GR, Von Roenn KA, D'Angelo CM, et al: *Surg Neurol* 28:277–283, October 1987.)

mentation was performed (Fig 22–7). This patient was ambulatory by the fourth day after surgery and enjoyed significant pain relief. Sixteen months after surgery, she is alive and well.

Restoration of stability was successful in all 6 patients, with alleviation of preoperative pain and return to full activity. No evidence of instability was noted.

This series and other small series demonstrated that Luque rod stabilization provides a valuable addition to the techniques available for stabilization of metastatic fractures of the spine. The precise role of Luque rod segmental spinal stabilization in treating metastatic disease of the spine has yet to be defined, but thus far it has proved useful in cases of multiple vertebral body involvement or instability beyond 1 vertebral level.

▶ Luque rods can provide stabilization for metastases to multiple segments of the spine. In a number of nonmalignant settings, spinal surgeons have demonstrated that Luque rod instrumentation is safe and effective for spinal stabilization. When a single level is involved, direct operation and interbody stabilization may be appropriate, but when multiple levels are involved, the Luque instrumentation is probably a superior approach. It is clear that the best results can be obtained when neurologic and orthopedic surgeons work together in this complex arena.— R.M. Crowell, M.D.

Surgical Treatment of Spinal Chordomas
Sundaresan N, Huvos AG, Krol G, Lane JM, Brennan M (St Luke's/Roosevelt Hosp Ctr, Mem Sloan-Kettering Cancer Ctr, New York)
Arch Surg 122:1479–1482, December 1987   22–15

Chordomas are rare primary tumors of the axial skeleton. Surgery may be curative, but late clinical presentation with a frequent occurrence at inaccessible surgical sites and comorbid medical conditions may deter attempts at surgery. With the availability of computed tomography and newer surgical approaches to the spine, more curative operations are now feasible.

The clinical features and results of 34 patients with chordomas treated over a 7-year period were reviewed. Twenty patients had tumors originating in the sacrum, 12 in a true vertebra, and 2 involving the base of the skull. Computed tomographic scans outlined both the soft tissue as well as the osseous involvement of the tumor. Myelography showed epidural extension in all but 2 patients with purely intraosseous tumors.

Surgical treatment consisted of wide local excision in 6 patients, marginal resection in 3, intralesional resection in 20, and biopsy in 3. Eighteen patients received external radiotherapy, and 7 patients had brachytherapy. There was no surgical mortality. Overall median survival was 60 months, and 19 patients were still alive, including 12 who were free of disease. Overall local recurrence rate was 65%, with distant metastases developing in 30% of the patients. Local recurrence occurred at a median of 20 months (range, 1–3 years) after initial treatment, and it was directly related to the extent of surgical resection.

The improvement in disease-free survivors (35% compared with the previously reported 10%) reflects both early diagnosis of even smaller tumors with computed tomography and more effective operation. The current approach to a sacral chordoma should be an attempt at curative operation at the time of first operation; for tumors involving a true vertebra, it is possible to excise all gross disease by total or subtotal spondylectomy.

▶ Sundaresan and colleagues present an interesting report regarding spinal chordomas. The results show reduction in recurrence after radical surgery. Certainly, this approach is reasonable in vertebrae, but in other locations such as sacrum and skull base, the surgeon must be guided by potential operative morbidity as he or she considers a radical excision.— R.M. Crowell, M.D.

Spinal Arteriovenous Malformations: A Comparison of Dural Arteriovenous Fistulas and Intradural AVM's in 81 Patients
Rosenblum B, Oldfield EH, Doppman JL, Di Chiro G (Natl Inst of Neurological and Communicative Disorders and Stroke, The Clinical Center, Bethesda, Md)
J Neurosurg 67:795–802, December 1987   22–16

Data on 81 patients seen between 1964 and 1985 with spinal arteriovenous malformations (AVMs) were reviewed. Twenty-seven patients, or one third of the group, had dural arteriovenous (AV) fistulas (Fig 22–8), and 54 had intradural malformations. Forty-three of the latter group had intramedullary malformations, and 11 had direct AV fistulas. The intramedullary lesions included 14 glomus AVMs and 29 juvenile malformations.

Both dural and intradural AVMs produced paresis, sensory abnormalities, sphincter disturbances, and pain. Subarachnoid hemorrhage caused initial symptoms in about one third of the patients with intradural lesions, most often glomus AVMs. Those with juvenile-type lesions or direct AV fistulas most often presented with weakness. No dural AV fistula caused subarachnoid bleeding. Most patients with dural and intradural lesions had a gradual onset and progressive neurologic deterioration. The intradural AVMs occurred more diffusely along the spinal axis than the dural AV fistulas.

Surgery was done on 96% of patients with dural AV fistulas and 80% of those with intradural AVMs. Of the former patients, 72% improved postoperatively and the rest remained stable. Half of the patients with intramedullary AVMs were unchanged after surgery, whereas one third improved and 14% became worse. One patient died during circulatory bypass after excision of an AVM.

Dural AV fistulas are consistently treatable, but some cord AVMs cannot be totally excised without unacceptable neurologic risk. Glomus lesions now may be palliated by embolotherapy with microparticulate ma-

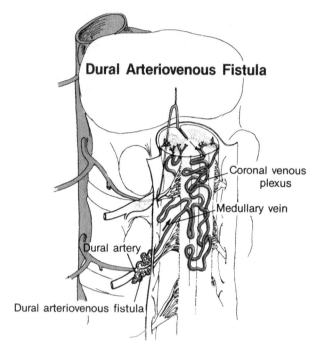

Dural Arteriovenous Fistula

Coronal venous plexus

Medullary vein

Dural artery

Dural arteriovenous fistula

Fig 22–8.—Artist's drawing of a dural arteriovenous fistula. The vascular nidus, supplied by the dural artery, is in the dural covering of the nerve root and adjacent spinal dura. The fistula is drained intradurally by retrograde flow (*arrow*) through the medullary vein and causes engorgement of the coronal venous plexus and the intraparenchymal radial veins. (Courtesy of Rosenblum B, Oldfield EH, Doppman JL, et al: *J Neurosurg* 67:795–802, December 1987.)

terial. The feeding vessels of intradural AV fistulous lesions can also be embolized.

▶ This large review of 81 cases from NIH illustrates the range of varied AV abnormalities that may be found in the spinal canal. One can now distinguish dural AV fistula, intradural AV fistula, as well as glomus and juvenile-type AVMs. Selection of appropriate embolic therapy, surgical excision, or both depends on the precise angiographic delineation of the lesions. It is clear that, to obtain best results, management of such lesions must be confined to experienced centers.—R.M. Crowell, M.D.

MR of Postoperative Syringomyelia
Barkovich AJ, Sherman JL, Citrin CM, Wippold FJ II (Walter Reed Army Med Ctr, Washington, DC; Uniformed Services Univ of Health Sciences, Bethesda, Md; Magnetic Imaging of Washington, Chevy Chase, Md; George Washington Univ)
AJNR 8:319–327, March–April 1987   22–17

Twenty-seven magnetic resonance imaging (MRI) scans of 20 patients surgically treated for syringomyelia were reviewed to define the relation between the type of surgical treatment and the various proposed pathophysiologic mechanisms of syringes. Thirteen patients had syringomyelia associated with the Chiari I malformation, 4 were posttraumatic, and 3 were idiopathic. Syringosubarachnoid and syringoperitoneal shunting, myelotomies, and foramen magnum decompressions (FMDs) were performed.

The shunt catheter was seen in 15 of 20 scans of patients in whom the syrinx cavity had been shunted. In all patients, the appearance was that of a curvilinear lucency within the subarachnoid space, substance of the cord, or syrinx cavity. When adequately treated by shunting, syringes were completely collapsed and showed no flow void. Nine patients underwent FMD; all were seen on MRI on sagittal sections through the craniocervical junction as having a widened foramen magnum with truncation of the occipital bone posterior to the normal position of the opisthion. In all patients but 1, the new opisthion was tapered in appearance. In 6 patients whose conditions were clinically improved, the syrinx was collapsed, and cerebrospinal fluid was between the bone of the foramen magnum and the cerebellum or the brain stem on at least 1 sagittal MRI image. Three patients had poor clinical results; 2 also had completely collapsed syrinx, and 1 had a syrinx markedly diminished in size but the cerebellum and brain stem were abutting the bony foramen magnum on every image. In 1 patient, the cerebellar hemisphere was frankly impressed upon the occipital bone. These cases are examples of slumping of the cerebellum into the foramen magnum, causing compression of the posterior fossa structures.

Magnetic resonance imaging is extremely valuable in the evaluation of surgically treated syringomyelia. The most important factors in the evaluation of treated syringes are diminution of syrinx size and elimination of the flow void within the cavity. If clinical symptoms persist despite adequate shunting by MRI criteria, the foramen magnum should be evaluated for compression at that level.

▶ This report nicely documents the utility of postoperative MRI for syringomyelia. The authors emphasize the importance of demonstrating syrinx collapse and the absence of flow void as signs of surgical success.—R.M. Crowell, M.D.

Brief Notes on Spinal Tumors

Evaluation of Spinal Pathology

Sonography provides good visualization of the neonatal craniocervical junction, including congenital malformations and hematomas (Cramer BC, et al: *AJR* 147:133–139, 1986).

In 68 cases of suspected pathology in the craniocervical zone, MRI is considered the imaging technique of choice, and gadolinium-DTPA is necessary in selected cases only (Fridburg H, et al: *Fortschr Roentgenstr* 145:315–320, 1986).

In the MR differentiation of intramedullary neoplasms and cysts, the combination of distinct margins and uniform signal intensity equal the CSF consistently correlated with spinal cord cyst (88%) (Williams AL, et al: *AJR* 149:159–164, 1987).

Evaluation of Spinal Tumors

Of 22 intramedullary, 17 intradural, and 20 extradural lesions, MRI with surface coil and T_1 and T_2 sequences demonstrates the pathology nicely in all cases. Gadolinium was unnecessary (Zanella FE, et al: *Fortschr Roentgenstr* 145:326–330, 1986).

Benign tumors of the spinal canal may present with isolated pain, and MRI may produce satisfactory diagnostic discrimination (Guillot M, et al: *Sem Hôp Paris* 63:1579–1581, 1987).

Magnetic resonance imaging in 68 examinations from 62 patients was helpful in detection of vertebral infiltration by a variety of tumors (Weigert VF, et al: *Fortschr Roentgenstr* 146:123–130, 1987).

Magnetic resonance imaging detects radiculomeningeal vascular malformations of the spine, including changes within the cord distal to the malformation (Masaryk TJ, et al: *Radiology* 164:845–849, 1987).

Gadolinium-DTPA improves detection of intraspinal neurinoma or meningioma (Schroth G, et al: *J Neurosurg* 66:695–700, 1987).

Extradural component of tumor was detected with CT in 21 children. Myelography seemed unnecessary, and contrast CT was deemed sufficient (Geoffray A, et al: *Ann Radiol* 29:333–338, 1986).

Non-Hodgkin's lymphoma may present with spinal epidural involvement (Epelbaum R, et al: *Cancer* 58:2120–2124, 1986).

Twenty-one cases with genitourinary neoplasm were reported with epidural cord compression. Metastases were the initial sign of malignancy in 6 cases (31.5%). Only 5 patients (26%) survived 24 months after diagnosis. Only 2 cases in this series with paraplegia had improvement to ambulation after decompression by surgery (Liskow A, et al: *Cancer* 58:949–954, 1986).

Cerebrospinal fluid myelin basic protein levels in leptomeningeal metastases provide an indicator of disease activity (Siegal T, et al: *J Neurol Sci* 78:165–173, 1987).

In 57 cases of infection and tumor of the spine, reliable differentiating criteria were developed. Infection was characterized by prevertebral soft tissue involvement, diffuse osteolytic destruction, gas in bone and soft tissue, and a process centering on a disk. Neoplasm was characterized on CT by posterior element involvement, absent soft tissue swelling, and osteoblastic alterations. (Van Lom, KJ et al: *Radiology* 166:;851–855, 1988).

Chordoma

Magnetic resonance imaging depicts chordoma as isointense or hypointense on T_1 and of moderately to extremely high intensity on T_2 with excellent delineation of extent of the tumor. Chondroit and typical lesions can be discriminated by MR, with correspondingly improved outlook for chondroit chondroma (Sze G, et al: *Radiology* 166:187–191, 1988).

Cryosurgery may be helpful in the treatment of sacrococcygeal chordoma (de Vries J, et al: *Cancer* 58:2348–2354, 1986).

In 54 patients with primary sacral tumors, nearly half of the tumors were chordomas, and the others were mostly giant cell tumors and neurofibromas. Ten percent were malignant. Preservation of upper sacral nerve roots was possible in most cases among the benign group. Ligation of both internal iliac arteries and temporary occlusion of the common iliac arteries or aorta minimized bleeding. X-ray therapy was provided postoperatively (Sung HW, et al: *Clin Orthop* 215:91–98, 1987).

Syrinx

In an MRI study, no significant relationship between neurologic function and dimensions of the syrinx could be demonstrated in 12 cases (Grant R, et al: *J Neurol Neurosurg Psychiatry* 50:1008–1014, 1987).

In a retrospective study of 32 patients with syringomyelia, a change in the caliber of the spinal cord with different positions during CT metrizamide myelography had a sensitivity of 38% and a specificity of 87%. Central cord enhancement had a sensitivity and specificity of 91% and 87%, respectively (Gates PC, et al: *Neurology* 36:1245–1248, 1986).

Shellfish allergy with medullary vascular malformation may lead to acute reversible paraplegia (Laurent A, et al: *Sem Hôp Paris* 62:3133–3135, 1986).—R.M. Crowell, M.D.

Other Topics

Relation Between Spinal Cord and Epidural Blood Flow
Shimoji K, Sato Y, Endoh H, Taga K, Fujiwara N, Fukuda S (Niigata Univ, Niigata, Japan)
Stroke 18:1128–1132, November–December 1987   22–18

From previous anatomical studies of the epidural venous plexus, it is assumed that tissue blood flow in the spinal epidural space is closely correlated with that in the spinal cord. If there is a linear relationship between spinal cord blood flow (SBF) and epidural blood flow (EBF), measurement of EBF may be warranted as a technique for monitoring SBF in clinical practice. Regional SBF (rSBF) and regional EBF (rEBF) were simultaneously and sequentially measured by the hydrogen clearance method in response to changes in arterial carbon dioxide pressure (tension) ($PaCO_2$) and mean arterial blood pressure (MAP) in rats anesthetized with pentobarbital, before a clinical study.

There were positive correlations between $PaCO_2$ and rSBF or rEBF, but there was no significant relation between $PaCO_2$ and regional muscle blood flow (rMBF). An excellent correlation was obtained between rSBF and rEBF over a $PaCO_2$ range of 27.8–66.7 torr, with minimum changes in MAP. A close correlation between rSBF and rEBF was seen in response to changes in MAP from 30–130 mm Hg, and the rate of change in both parameters was also almost the same.

That rEBF has a strikingly linear relation with rSBF in response to changes in $PaCO_2$ and MAP was demonstrated, while rMBF did not show a close correlation with either rSBF or rEBF. Although the value of rEBF was slightly lower than that of rSBF, its rate of change was very similar to that of rSBF in response to variation of both $PaCO_2$ and MAP, suggesting that rSBF and rEBF are regulated by a similar mechanism.

There are three possible interpretations for the measured values or rEBF in this study: the epidural electrode may detect purely regional blood flow in the epidural tissue distinct from that in the cord; the epidural electrode may measure the rate of clearance from the underlying spinal cord of hydrogen that diffuses through the dura to the electrode; or the epidural electrode may also measure the clearance rate of hydrogen from both the cord and epidural tissues. Nevertheless, the close relationship between rSBF and rEBF shown suggests that monitoring rSBF by the epidural catheter electrode is feasible without damaging the dura or spinal cord.

The applicability of monitoring rSBF by measuring rEBF is suggested by assuming that a similar close relationship between rSBF and rEBF exists in human beings. If measuring human SBF becomes possible by simply placing an epidural electrode in the epidural space, it would provide a new technique for monitoring rSBF during major surgeries that might affect SBF.

▶ This interesting study demonstrates a strikingly linear relationship between spinal cord and epidural blood flow. The conditions of the study, however, were confined to normal animals under a variety of levels of $PaCO_2$ and mean arterial pressure. Whether the linear relationship holds under pathologic conditions such as injury or tumor remains to be seen.—R.M. Crowell, M.D.

Brief Notes

Spinal Cord Compression

Of 611 patients with biopsy-proved adenocarcinoma of the prostate, spinal cord compression developed in 41 (6.7%). Survival following spinal cord involvement was relatively poor and unrelated to tumor differentiation. Forty-six percent of patients survived less than 6 months, and 20% lived less than 2 months. Spinal cord involvement most often occurred in the thoracic area, with 95% of patients showing radiographic evidence of osseous vertebral metastasis. Seven patients were treated with laminectomy and radiation, and 33 with radiation only. Median survival with decompression was 12 months vs. 5 months for those treated with radiation alone (Kuban DA, et al: *Urology* 28:364–369, 1986).

Anterior decompression of vertebral osteosarcomas relieved paraplegia in 2 patients, but chemotherapy and radiotherapy did not prevent painful local recurrence. (Jaffray D, et al: *Clin Orthop* 214:210–215, 1987).

Extramedullary hematopoiesis in thalassemia may lead to cord compression (Mann KS, et al: *J Neurosurg* 66:938–940, 1987).

Crohn's disease can lead to spinal extradural abscess with cord compression and paraplegia (Aitken RJ, et al: *Br J Surg* 73:1004–1005, 1986).

On electron microscopic study, myxopapillary ependymoma of the filum terminale may contain characteristic single microtubules (Specht CS, et al: *Cancer* 58:310–317, 1986).

Erections on walking may be a symptom of spinal canal stenosis (Hopkins A, et al: *J Neurol Neurosurg Psychiatry* 50:1371–1374, 1987).

Cysts

On MRI, the combination of distinct margin and uniform signal intensity equal to CSF consistently correlated in 88% with spinal cord cysts as opposed to neoplasms (Williams AL, et al: *AJNR* 8:527–532, 1987).

Thoracic epidural cyst may be detected by CT and treated effectively by cyst removal and elimination of the fistula with a subarachnoid space (D'Haens J, et al: *Surg Neurol* 27:26408, 1987).

Basic Studies

Perspective graphics can portray the distribution of radiolabeled ligands in the spinal cord with intrathecally administered ^{3}H morphine (Gregory MA, et al: *Anesth Intensive Care* 14:426–430, 1986).

In experimental spinal ischemia, hypothermic regional perfusion appears to offer significant protection (Colon R, et al: *Ann Thorac Surg* 43:639–643, 1987)—R.M. Crowell, M.D.

23 Trauma

Introduction

Magnetic resonance images correlate well with the neurobehavioral sequelae of mild and moderate head injuries (Abstract 23–1). The prospective comparative study of MR and CT indicates a clear advantage for MR in the detection of diffuse axonal injury, contusion, and subtle brain injuries (Abstract 23–2). Magnetic resonance is able to image contusion and hemorrhage within the spinal cord after injury (Abstract 23–4). Catecholamine levels appear to have great value in predicting outcome after severe head injury (Abstract 23–3). A review of data on 122 children with spinal injuries revealed a higher incidence of spinal cord injury without changes seen radiologically and more injuries at the C1–C2 level (Abstract 23–5).

Robert M. Crowell, M.D.

Magnetic Resonance Imaging and Computerized Tomography in Relation to the Neurobehavioral Sequelae of Mild and Moderate Head Injuries
Levin HS, Amparo E, Eisenberg HM, Williams DH, High WM Jr, McArdle CB, Weiner RL (Univ of Texas, Galveston)
J Neurosurg 66:706–713, May 1987   23–1

The ability of magnetic resonance imaging (MRI) and computed tomography (CT) to detect brain lesions in patients with minor to moderate closed head injuries was compared, and the findings were related to neurobehavioral sequelae. Twenty patients with non-missile-caused injuries underwent CT on the day of admission with subsequent MRI. Magnetic resonance images were obtained in the transaxial and coronal planes using 2 spin-echo sequences. Glasgow Coma Scale scores were at least 9 for all patients and did not fall below this level.

Of the 20 patients, 85% had lesions visualized by MRI but not by CT. Three patients had normal findings on both studies. Focal parenchymal lesions in the frontal and temporal lobes were impressively detected by MRI imaging. Distinctive patterns of neurobehavioral sequelae were associated with localization of brain lesions by MRI in individual patients (Fig 23–1). Neuropsychological test performance correlated better with MRI-estimated lesion size than with CT appearances. Marked reductions in lesion size seen on follow-up were associated with improved cognitive function and memory.

Further studies using MRI in the management and rehabilitation of patients with mild and moderate closed head injuries are warranted. Parenchymal lesions that resolve within 2–3 months of injury are associated

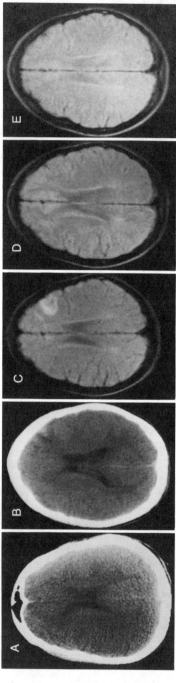

Fig 23–1.—Neuroimaging in a patient after apparently minor head injury. The MRIs in C, D, and E were spin-echo images obtained at TR, 2,000 msec, and TE, 60 msec. **A,** CT scan on admission (day of injury) at the level of the lateral ventricle bodies. The scan was interpreted as normal. **B,** baseline CT scan obtained 5 days after injury showing a left frontal lesion, seen as an area of mixed low and high density. **C,** baseline MRI, obtained 5 days after injury at the identical level as the CT scan shown in **B,** shows a left frontal lesion with heterogeneous areas relative to the brain. **D,** and **E,** MRIs obtained 1 month (**D**) and 3 months (**E**) post injury showing resolution of the frontal lesion. (Courtesy of Levin HS, Amparo E, Eisenberg HM, et al: *J Neurosurg* 66:706–713, May 1987.)

with improved performance on neuropsychological tests and with resumption of normal activities.

► Frequently, MRI demonstrates extensive frontotemporal injury after mild to moderate head trauma even when CT findings are negative. Initial and follow-up MRI correlates well with detailed neuropsychological testing in these head-injured patients. Images should be obtained by MR in patients with Glasgow Coma Scale scores of 9–13 to demonstrate objective pathology. Such data will be helpful in assessing the level of disability, so frequently an issue in these patients. The neurosurgeon is often reassured when there is no need to operate, but patients with mild to moderate head injuries frequently have great difficulty in returning to productive lives.—R.M. Crowell, M.D.

Prospective Comparative Study of Intermediate-Field MR and CT in the Evaluation of Closed Head Trauma
Gentry LR, Godersky JC, Thompson B, Dunn VD (Univ of Iowa)
AJNR 9:91–100, January–February 1988   23–2

Computed tomography (CT) has enabled early recognition and treatment of extracerebral hemorrhage in patients with head trauma. However, CT has been less beneficial in identifying other types of cerebral injury. Magnetic resonance imaging (MRI) is more sensitive than CT in detecting many diseases involving the central nervous system, but it has not been used extensively for assessing acute closed head trauma. A prospective study was done to compare the diagnostic efficacy of CT and MRI in 40 patients with closed head trauma.

Traumatic lesions were found in 38 patients. Severity of injury ranged from 3 to 14 on the Glasgow Coma Scale. The CT and MRI sensitivities were calculated for those with hemorrhagic and nonhemorrhagic intra-axial lesions, extra-axial hematomas, and diffuse hemorrhage. The CT and MRI, T_1– and T_2–weighted, studies were highly and similarly sensitive in detecting hemorrhagic intra-axial lesions. However, MRI was much more sensitive in detecting nonhemorrhagic lesions (Fig 23–2). Cortical contusions and diffuse axonal injury comprised 91.9% of all intra-axial lesions. In this group of lesions, the sensitivities of CT, T_1–weighted MRI, and T_2–weighted MRI for nonhemorrhagic lesions were 17.7%, 67.6%, and 93.3%, respectively. For hemorrhagic lesions, these values were 89.8%, 87.1%, and 92.5%, respectively. In detecting brain stem lesions, the sensitivity of CT was only 9.1%, whereas for T_1–weighted MRI and T_2–weighted MRI, it was 81.8% and 72.7%, respectively. Sensitivities for detecting extra-axial hematomas were 73.2% for CT, 97.6% for T_1–weighted MRI, and 90.5% for T_2–weighted MRI. Intraventricular hemorrhage was seen consistently with all 3 studies, but subarachnoid hemorrhage was detected much more often with CT.

Magnetic resonance imaging has clear advantages over CT in assessing closed head trauma. Although its sensitivity in detecting hemorrhagic lesions was similar to that of CT, MRI was much better than CT in detect-

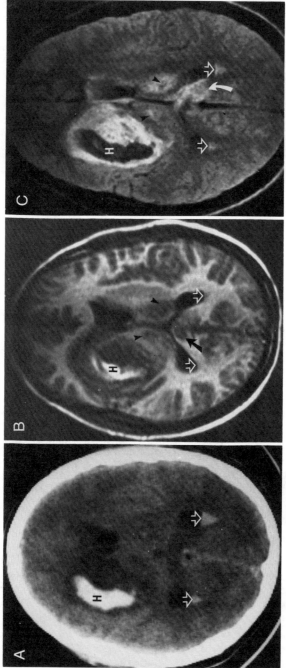

FIG 23–2.— A 19-year-old man 2 days after head trauma. **A,** axial CT scan shows large basal ganglia intracerebral hematoma (*H*) with surrounding edema as well as intraventricular hemorrhage (*arrows*). **B** and **C,** T1-weighted inversion-recovery (TR = 2,100 msec, T1 = 600 msec) (**B**) and T2-weighted spin-echo (TR = 2,300 msec, TE = 80 msec) (**C**) scans confirm hematoma and intraventricular hemorrhage (*open arrows*). Large nonhemorrhagic diffuse axonal lesion in splenium of corpus callosum (*curved arrows*) and bilateral subcortical gray matter lesions (*arrowheads*) are seen. Note—Acute hematoma is hyperintense relative to brain parenchyma on T1-weighted image and hypointense on T2-weighted image. Intraventricular hemorrhage is hyperintense relative to cerebrospinal fluid on T1- and T2-weighted scans and isointense relative to white matter on T1-weighted scan. (Courtesy of Gentry LR, Godersky JC, Thompson B, et al: *AJNR* 9:91–100, January–February 1988.)

ing nonhemorrhagic lesions, which are much more prevalent. Also, MRI was better than CT in classifying primary and secondary forms of injury and in directing treatment. However, CT allowed more rapid assessment of unstable patients who may need surgery.

▶ Magnetic resonance imaging is substantially superior to CT for evaluation of head trauma. They have similar value in the detection of extra-axial and intra-axial hemorrhage. However, MRI, especially the T–2 weighted image, is vastly superior in the detection of contusion and diffuse axonal injury, and is also much more sensitive in detecting brain stem lesions. Computed tomography, on the other hand, allows more rapid assessment of unstable patients who may require surgery for removal of intracranial hematomas.—R.M. Crowell, M.D.

The Predictive Value of Catecholamines in Assessing Outcome in Traumatic Brain Injury
Woolf PD, Hamill RW, Lee LA, Cox C, McDonald JV (Univ of Rochester)
J Neurosurg 66:875–882, June 1987   23–3

Traumatic brain injury can initiate a cascade of deleterious events that result in worsening neurologic impairment and severe metabolic and/or systemic derangements that appear to be secondary, in part, to activation of the sympathetic nervous system. These disturbances include increased cerebrospinal fluid pressure, enhanced brain oxygen requirements, and cardiac arrhythmias and necrosis, among others. Catecholamine levels reflect the severity of neurologic impairment as determined by the Glasgow Coma Scale (GCS) scores and seem to be reliable predictors of outcome. However, predicting outcome in individuals with the lowest GCS scores is difficult. Because of the central role of the sympathetic nervous system in mediating the stress response, determination of the plasma catecholamine level was explored as an endogenous marker for predicting patient morbidity and mortality.

Plasma norepinephrine, epinephrine, and dopamine levels were measured in 61 brain-injured patients within 48 hours of injury. Outcome was determined at 1 week with the GSC and at discharge with the Glasgow Outcome Scale (GOS). Levels of norepinephrine, epinephrine, and dopamine correlated strongly with admission GCS scores. In the 21 patients with GCS scores of 3 or 4 on admission, norepinephrine levels predicted the outcome at 1 week (Fig 23–3). All 6 patients with norepinephrine levels of less than 900 pg/ml improved to GCS scores of more than 11; 12 of 15 patients with norepinephrine values higher than 900 pg/ml continued to have GCS scores of 3 to 6, or died. The epinephrine and dopamine levels were not as useful. Catecholamine levels also increased significantly as the GOS score worsened. The norepinephrine and epinephrine levels were significantly higher in patients who died or remained vegetative than in those with better outcomes. For the 54 patients surviving beyond 1 week, significant correlations were noted between length of

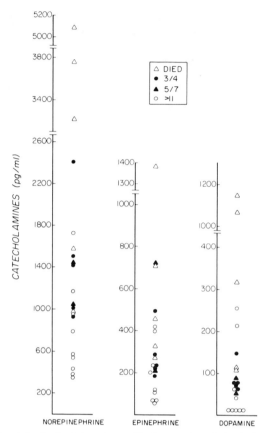

Fig 23–3.—Catecholamine levels in patients with Glasgow Coma Scale (GCS) scores of 3 or 4 vs. outcome at 1 week. *Symbols* indicate GCS scores at 1 week. (Courtesy of Woolf PD, Hamill RW, Lee LA, et al: *J Neurosurg* 66:875–882, June 1987.)

hospitalization and norepinephrine and epinephrine levels. The latter concentrations were also highly correlated with the duration of ventilatory assistance. Catecholamine levels either enhanced the reliability of the GCS scores or were independent predictors of outcome.

Changes in circulating catecholamine levels reflect the severity of the neurologic insult and provide support for the use of catecholamine measurements as a physiologic marker of patient outcome in acute and chronic phases of traumatic brain injury.

▶ This trail-blazing communication indicates that plasma norepinephrine levels correlate well with outcome in neurotrauma. Of particular importance is the fact that plasma norepinephrine levels assessed within 48 hours of injury led to a very high correlation with eventual outcome. The combination of norepinephrine values plus the GCS score appears to offer the best predictive index yet available in comatose individuals. Further confirmatory studies are required, but it seems likely that a combination of clinical, radiographic, and biochemical parameters offers the best available prognostic information after brain injury. Such information is particularly important in a time of growing concern regarding allocation of health care resources.— R.M. Crowell, M.D.

Acute Spinal Cord Injury; MR Imaging at 1.5 T
Kulkarni MV, McArdle CB, Kopanicky D, Miner M, Cotler HB, Lee KF, Harris JH
(Univ of Texas, Houston)
Radiology 164:837–843, September 1987   23–4

Surface coil magnetic resonance imaging (MRI) is useful in the evaluation of acute spinal trauma. Thirty-seven MRI studies were performed with a 1.5–T magnet and surface coils in 27 patients with suspected spinal cord injuries. Imaging was performed within 1 day to 6 weeks after injury. Three patients were examined while wearing halo vests made of MR-compatible material, 8 were examined while wearing Philadephia collars, and 1 was examined while being manually ventilated.

Spinal cord injury was demonstrated in 24 (79.2%) patients and skeletal and/or ligamentous injuries in 21 (78%). Three patterns of MRI signals were observed in spinal cord injuries. The first involved central hypointensity relative to normal spinal cord on T–2-weighted images obtained within 24 hours of injury in 5 patients. On later images obtained within 3–7 days after injury, T–2-weighted images showed a peripheral rim of hyperintensity and a central area of hypointensity. This pattern probably indicated acute spinal hemorrhage. The second pattern of injury, seen in 12 patients, was characterized by hyperintensity on T–2-weighted images obtained in the acute phase followed by rapid resolution. This pattern probably resulted from spinal cord edema and contusion. The third pattern of cord injury was seen in 2 patients and showed a mixed pattern of signal. In the acute phase, T–2-weighted images showed a central hypointensity surrounded by hyperintensity, followed by partial resolution. This probably represented injury with mixed findings from the first and second pattern. Overall neurologic recovery, as determined in 16 patients, was insignificant in those with intraspinal hemorrhage; however, patients with spinal cord edema or contusion recovered significant neurologic function.

Magnetic resonance imaging at 1.5 T is useful in the diagnosis of acute spinal cord injury and in predicting the degree of neurologic recovery.

▶ The authors point out several patterns of spinal cord image after acute spinal cord injury and correlate these patterns with outcome. The observations are of great interest, particularly in a prognostic sense. However, confirmation of the precise pathologic meaning requires pathologic verification.— R.M. Crowell, M.D.

Pediatric Spinal Trauma: Review of 122 Cases of Spinal Cord and Vertebral Column Injuries

Hadley MN, Zabramski JM, Browner CM, Rekate H, Sonntag VKH (Barrow Neurological Inst, Phoenix)

J Neurosurg 68:18–24, January 1988

23–5

Several patterns of injury were discerned in 122 pediatric patients seen from 1972 to 1986 with injury to the spinal column or cord. More than 90% of these patients were followed for a median of 44 months. Females predominated, and motor vehicle accidents were the most frequent cause of injury. Half of the patients were neurologically intact at admission and 17% had a complete myelopathy. Also, 41% had fracture of the vertebral body or posterior elements, and 33% had fracture with subluxation. Another 10% of patients had subluxation without fracture, and 16% had cord injury without radiographic signs of fracture or subluxation.

Nineteen patients underwent operation. Rigid external immobilization, usually with the halo vest, was used in 36 patients with fractures or subluxation. No patient deteriorated as a result of treatment, but 2 neurologically intact patients required delayed surgery. The results of 1 of 4 studies for posttraumatic syrinx in patients with complete lesions were positive.

Cord injury without radiologic abnormality is probably less frequent than previously thought in this setting. The prognosis for full recovery after pediatric spinal trauma is excellent except in patients younger than age 10 years and those with complete neurologic injury. Treatment should be individualized, but surgery is not often required. When early surgery is appropriate, it may be preferable to operate 2–7 days after injury.

▶ In this large experience with pediatric spinal trauma, several themes emerged. Patients to the age of 9 years had a higher incidence of spinal cord injury without radiologic abnormality and more injuries at the C1–C2 level. Except for the young patients to age 9 years and patients with complete injuries, prognosis for complete recovery is excellent in the pediatric age group. Surgical intervention is not often required, but techniques appropriate to corresponding adult injuries appear just as effective in children. In a related study, cervical spine injury could be correctly diagnosed in 58 or 59 children by performing cervical spine films in the presence of neck pain, neck tenderness, limit of neck mobility, history of neck trauma, abnormalities of reflexes, strength, sensation, and mental status (Jaffe DM et al: *Ann Emerg Med* 16:270–276, 1987).—R.M. Crowell, M.D.

Brief Notes on Trauma

Head Trauma

Hospital discharge data identified all 2,870 Rhode Island residents hospitalized with head injuries in 1979 and 1980. The incidence was 152 per 100,000 of population per year. Head injury rates in the lowest decile of median income were twice those for patients in the highest decile. Length of hospital stay and discharge to chronic care facilities increased by 20-fold with increasing age (Fife D, et al: *Am J Public Health* 76:773–778, 1986).

Experience with a head injury service since 1967 suggests that patients with a fractured skull or lower level of consciousness should be admitted to a district general hospital because of the associated 20% chance of major head injury. Patients with both fractured skull and obtundation have a 60% likelihood of major head injury and thus should be transferred immediately to a neurosurgical unit. Patients with compound or complicated skull fractures and those with neurologic impairment persisting for 4 hours or more also should be transferred to a neurosurgical unit. With these guidelines, approximately 200 patients per million will be referred to a neurosurgical center. Those with minor head injury may be sent home, with resulting reduction in the admission rate of about 60% (Brocklehurst G, et al: *Br Med J* 294:345–347, 1987).

Among 232 brain-injured patients, those treated by an aeromedical service had 31% mortality, whereas those managed by a land transport system had 40% mortality ($P < .001$) (Baxt WG, Moody P: *J Trauma* 27:365–369, 1987).

Among 545 trauma patients treated in a single institution, 104 with major blunt injury with severe brain damage (Glasgow Coma Score less than 8) had a mortality of 30.8%. Of 441 patients with major blunt trauma without severe brain injury, the mortality rate was 0.9% ($P < .0001$) (Baxt WG, Moody P: *J Trauma* 27:602–606, 1987).

Among 100 patients with acute head injury, disseminated intravascular coagulation (DIC) occurred in 24%, most frequently with acute subdural hematoma, followed by contusional hematoma and contusion. Mortality of patients with DIC was 58% (Kumura E, et al: *Acta Neurochir (Wien)* 85:23–28, 1987).

Extensive experience with head injury in the elderly from the Edinburgh Head Injury Unit indicates that there is increased mortality from head injury with increasing age as well as poor outcome in the presence of intracranial hematoma. The length of stay is increased for elderly compared with younger patients. These data suggest that the early use of CT to detect intracranial hematoma after head injury is recommended for older patients. Referral to social workers and geriatric units is likewise recommended (Pentland B, et al: *Age Aging* 15:193–202, 1986).

Studies in 17 patients with severe head injury indicate that positive nitrogen balance could be achieved only by a nitrogen intake in excess of the high protein catabolic rate (Bivins BA, et al: *J Trauma* 26:980–986, 1986).

Ventricular interleukin-I activity is elevated in patients with head injury (McClain CJ, et al: *J Lab Clin Med* 110:48–54, 1987).

Plasma cortisol and adrenocorticotropin levels are elevated in patients with head injuries as well as in those with injuries in other parts of the body (Barton RN, et al: *J Trauma* 27:384–392, 1987).

Ascending transtentorial herniation may be diagnosed by CT (Ebeling U, Huber P: *Schweiz Med Wochenschr* 116:1394–1401, 1986).

Pediatric Head Trauma

Diffuse axonal injury in early infancy may occur in the same way as in adults (Vowles GH, et al: *J Clin Pathol* 40:185–189, 1987).

Somatosensory evoked potentials are useful in the early prediction of neurologic outcome in comatose children (De Meirleir LJ, Taylor MJ: *Pediatr Neurol* 3:78–82, 1987).

In 88% of 166 children with head injury, the Glasgow Coma Scale applied in the first 24 hours was useful in predicting outcome (Wagstyl J, et al: *J Pediatr Surg* 22:127–129, 1987).

Ford EG, et al. present data on head-injured children suggesting that steroids potentiate the posttraumatic catabolic response, thus mandating aggressive nutritional support (*J Trauma* 27:1074–1077, 1987).

Spinal Trauma

Seventy-five burst fractures in radiographic characterization showed spinal canal narrowing by retropulsed fragments, marked anterior wedging, and lamina fractures near the spinous process. Nearly all burst fractures occurred from T9 to L5. Most were associated with neurologic deficit. These complex fractures are often unstable (Atlas SW, et al: *AJR* 147:575–582, 1986).

Forty-four patients with spinal cord injury complicating cervical spondylosis were recorded in a 12-year period. Initial myelopathy was complete in 10 and incomplete in 34. In those with incomplete cord lesions, partial recovery was common, however, most patients remain wheelchair dependent (Foo D: *Paraplegia* 24:301–306, 1986).

Horseradish peroxidase studies in cats indicate regeneration of supernumerary axons with synaptic terminals in spinal motoneurons after injury (Havton L, Kellerth JO: *Nature* 325:711–714, 1987).

Complete cervical spinal cord injury may be followed by recovery after rapid spinal realignment (Brunette DD, Rockswold GL: *J Trauma* 27:445–447, 1987).

Opiate receptors antagonists such as naloxone and thyroid-releasing hormone have been used with some success to improve outcome in patients with traumatic shock, spinal cord trauma, and head injury. These effects may have to do with naloxone-insensitive opiate receptors such as the k-receptor with requirement for relatively high doses of naloxone (McIntosh TK, Faden AI: *Ann Emerg Med* 15:1462–1465, 1986).

Analysis of data on 236 patients suggests that, among sacral fractures, those in the ala occasionally occur with fifth lumbar root deficit. Patients with fractures through the foramina often have sciatica, and those with fractures through the sacral canal often have saddle anesthesia and loss of sphincter function. Magnetic resonance imaging and cystometrographic evaluation are recommended. Surgical decompression appears to offer a better chance for neurologic recovery than do nonsurgical methods (Denis F, et al: *Clin Orthop* 227:67–81, 1988).

Spinal cord injury most frequently occurs in persons 15 to 20 years of age in a rate of approximately 906 per million. The average adjusted hospital charges peaked at $58,800 in 1983 (Stover SL, Fine PR: *Paraplegia* 25:225–228, 1987).

Evaluation of Spinal Trauma

Among 406 patients with head injuries, 293 had emergency cervical radiography and cervical spine injury was seen in only 5. Eight patients were clinically suspected to have associated cervical spine injury. The authors recommend that emergency cervical radiography be confined to those patients with suspicion of cervical injury among head-injured patients. In a discussion of this paper, however, it was pointed out that patients with severe head injury and a depressed level of consciousness may not provide the clinician with suspicion of cervical spine injury; therefore, such patients should certainly be evaluated with cervical spine films whether or not there is suspicion of injury in the neck (Gbaanador GBM et al: *Am J Surg* 152:643–648, 1986).

Among 28 patients with spinal cord injury, magnetic resonance imaging permitted distinct demarcation of the spinal cord with its posttraumatic lesions. It is possible that enhancers such as gadolinium may improve visualization of those lesions (Perovitch M: *Paraplegia* 25:373–380, 1987).

Thirteen patients with chronically injured cervical spinal cords were evaluated with MRI, which demonstrated intramedullary abnormalities more accurately than delayed metrizamide CT by the differentiation of myelomalacia from intramedullary cyst (Quencer RM, et al: *AJR* 147:125–132, 1986).

In a patient with central cord spinal injury, MRI showed a low signal on T–1 with a high signal on proton sequence. Myelotomy showed intense gliosis, and there was rapid postoperative improvement (Fox JL, et al: *Neurosurgery* 22:340–347, 1988).

In spinal cord injury, a routine myelogram is the most helpful test to establish the diagnosis of a herniated intervertebral disk, which is present in 0.7% of cervical spinal cord injuries and 2.3% of bilateral facet dislocations (Apple DF, et al: *Paraplegia* 25:78–85, 1987).

Anterior subluxation, lateral subluxation, and acute kyphosis demonstrated on thoracolumbar CT can identify fracture dislocations in this area (Manaster BJ, Osborn AG: *AJR* 148:335–340, 1987).

Computerized tomography is helpful in evaluating nonvisualized vertebral levels caudad to a complete block on lumbar myelogram (Herkowitz HN, et al: *J Bone Joint Surg* 69A:218–224, 1987).

Subdural Hematoma

In an elderly patient with thrombocytopenia and an acute subdural hematoma, subdural puncture with a 22–gauge spinal needle produced partial drainage of the hematoma, resulting in complete recovery (Verlooy P, et al: *J Neurol* 234:254–256, 1987).

Closed subdural drainage can be a successful means of draining subdural collections (Lesoin F, et al: *Sem Hop Paris* 63:2703–2706, 1987).

Subdural hematoma may occur in the setting of systemic lupus erythematosus, the signs of which may mimic cerebral lupus (Futran J, et al: *J Rheumatol* 14:378–381, 1987).

Magnetic resonance imaging is superior in many ways to CT for demonstration of chronic subdural hematoma (Hosoda K, et al: *J Neurosurg* 67:677–683, 1987).

Brain Death

Xenon-enhanced computed tomography demonstrated absent posterior circulation blood flow despite persistent electroencephalographic activity in a patient with brain stem infarction (Darby J, et al: *Crit Care Med* 15:519–521, 1987).

In 56 consecutive patients with the diagnosis of brain death, some electroen-cephalographic activity was present for as long as 168 hours in 11 after being declared brain dead (Grigg MM, et al: *Arch Neurol* 44:948–954, 1987).

Transcranial Doppler examinations of 24 brain-dead adult patients demon-strated persistent movement of blood within the middle cerebral arteries in 21 (Ropper AH, et al: *Neurology* 37:1733–1735, 1987).

Atlantoaxial Injuries

Atlantoaxial instability in individuals with Down's syndrome is an uncommon complication. Occasionally, symptomatic instability requires surgery for preven-tion of spinal cord injury (Pueschel SM, Scola FH: *Pediatrics* 80:555–560, 1987).

Congenital defects of the posterior elements of the axis may be treated con-servatively (Morizono Y: *Clin Orthop* 216:120–123, 1987).

Among 10 patients with atlas and 85 with axis fractures, 12% had residual symptoms in the form of local and radiating pain (Ersmark H, Kalen R: *Clin Or-thop* 217:257–260, 1987).

Cerebrospinal Fluid (CSF) Rhinorrhea

Transferrin analysis by immunofixation may be an aid to the diagnosis of CSF otorrhea (Rouah E, et al: *Arch Pathol Lab Med* 111:756–757, 1987).

Among 8 patients with posttraumatic intermittent CSF rhinnorhea examined in the nonleaking period, CT metrizamide cisternography was able to demon-strate the site of the leak in all 7 patients so examined (Fagerlund M, Liliequist B: *Acta Radiol* 28:189–192, 1987).

Head-hanging CT is an alternative method for evaluating traumatic CSF rhi-norrhea (Rothfus WE, et al: *AJNR* 8:155–156, 1987).

Rehabilitation

Rectal probe electrostimulation causes ejaculation in spinal cord-injured men (Halstead LS, et al: *Paraplegia* 25:120–129, 1987).

Division of the external urethral sphincter may be helpful in treatment of the paraplegic bladder (Ross JC, et al: *Paraplegia* 25:185–195, 1987).

Functional electrical stimulation is a promising prospect for application to the neuromuscular system in spinal cord injury, but clinical efficacy has not been demonstrated (Peckham PH: *Paraplegia* 25:279–288, 1987).—R.M. Crowell, M.D.

24 Pediatrics

Introduction

Winston has presented a lovely review of craniopagi (Abstract 24–1). For symptomatic Arnold-Chiari malformation in infants, decompressive surgery is helpful in many, but the precise mechanisms of deterioration remain obscure (Abstract 24–2). The Gardner operation is advocated for treatment of hydrosyringomyelia in childhood (Abstract 24–3). Muscular undermining is a helpful adjunct in the closure of large lumbosacral meningomyelocele defects (Abstract 24–7). Excellent results may be obtained with radical surgery for craniosynostosis (Abstract 24–4). A recent article by Gandyy and Heier (*Ann Neurol* 21:342–348, 1987) reports that MRI beautifully detects intracranial arachnoid cysts. The effects of temporary external lumbar drainage are helpful in predicting the impact of shunting in patients with normal pressure hydrocephalus (Abstract 24–9). Revascularization with encephalo-duro-arterio-syn-angio-sis (EDAS) is advocated for the surgical treatment of childhood moyamoya disease (Abstract 24–5). Intracranial arterial aneurysms occasionally occur in early childhood and must be treated with surgical obliteration (Abstract 24–6).

Robert M. Crowell, M.D.

Craniopagi: Anatomical Characteristics and Classification
Winston KR (Brigham and Women's Hosp, Harvard Univ, Boston)
Neurosurgery 21:769–781, December 1987   24–1

Craniopagi has been reported from every inhabited continent in the past 500 years. Seventy-nine published reports on craniopagi were examined. Of approximately 10.25 births of conjoined twins per million deliveries, 6.2% are craniopagi. The first 2 trimesters of the pregnancy are usually not remarkable, but in the third trimester the abdomen may be unusually large. Some evidence suggests that conjoined twinning occurs more commonly in nonwhites. The female preponderance in conjoined twinning is 3:1 and in craniopagi, 4.4:1.

Currently used classifications have no value for predicting survival and only limited value for communicating important anatomical relationships. In a proposed classification system (Fig 24–1), craniopagi can be classified according to the deepest structure shared. Craniopagi connected by scalp and subcutaneous tissues, perhaps with bony fusion, would be type A; those that share dura mater but not leptomeninges or brain, type B; those that share leptomeninges, type C; and those that have a structurally continuous nervous system, type D. The median survival for cra-

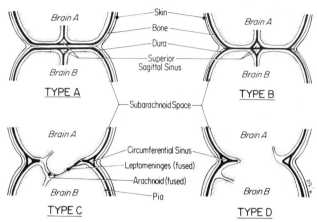

Fig 24–1.—Illustration of the classification based on extent of intersection. In type C, the arachnoid may exist as 1 fused layer or as 2 discrete entities, or may be absent between the cerebra. (Courtesy of Winston KR: *Neurosurgery* 21:769–781, December 1987.)

niopagi reportedly is 4 months; there has been only 1 report ever of a craniopagus reaching adulthood.

▶ Dr. Winston has given us a lovely and exhaustive review of the subject together with a useful classification by extent of shared structures. This review is recommended to any interested in the subject and is obviously useful for anyone faced with the management of a case.—R.M. Crowell, M.D.

Symptomatic Arnold-Chiari Malformation: Review of Experience With 22 Cases
Bell WO, Charney EB, Bruce DA, Sutton LN, Schut L (Children's Hosp of Philadelphia)
J Neurosurg 66:812–816, June 1987   24–2

Treatment of symptomatic Arnold-Chiari malformation in infants remains controversial. A review was made of experience with 22 patients who had closed myelomeningoceles, shunted hydrocephalus, and symptomatic Arnold-Chiari malformations. Seventeen of these patients were aged 2 days to 6 months (mean age, 2.1 months) and 5 were aged 3–23 years (mean age, 9 years). The infants were seen with stridor, apnea, or feeding difficulties, whereas the older patients had hemiparesis, quadriparesis, oscillopsia, nystagmus, or opisthotonos. Nineteen (86%) infants underwent posterior fossa decompression and 3 had no surgical intervention.

Fourteen infants had Arnold-Chiari decompression. Ten underwent surgery within 18 days after onset of symptoms and 4 had surgery on day 19 or later. Among the infants who had early decompressive surgery, 5 died of persistent symptoms and 5 survived, including 3 who were asymptomatic. Of the 4 patients who underwent surgery later, 2 died, 1 had lessening of stridor, and 1 was asymptomatic. Three infants had no surgical intervention; 2 died and 1 became asymptomatic. All 5 older patients underwent decompression and all had resolution of their preoperative signs and symptoms within an average of 4 months after onset.

Decompressive surgery for symptomatic Arnold-Chiari malformation is effective in children and adults but does not always improve the clinical condition of infants. This may result from the ischemic/hypoxic effects on the infant's brain stem, which may not be organized normally at birth. The fact that many infants recover brain-stem functions so slowly or not at all suggests that irreversible damage occurs to immature caudal brain-stem neurons or pathways.

▶ These results support decompressive surgery for infants with Arnold-Chiari malformation and parallel reported outcomes in other large centers (Park et al: *Neurosurgery* 13:147–152, 1983). Further investigations are needed to define the underlying pathogenesis of persistent symptoms in these infants and to establish the preferred treatment.—R.M. Crowell, M.D.

Hydrosyringomyelia and Its Management in Childhood
Hoffman HJ, Neill J, Crone KR, Hendrick EB, Humphreys RP (Univ of Toronto; Hosp for Sick Children, Toronto)
Neurosurgery 21:347–351, 1987   24–3

Syringomyelia is usually associated with the Chiari malformation. Once believed to be a degenerative disease in adults, it is now recognized as a disorder that can occur in patients of all ages. Data on 47 patients treated at 1 institution from 1977 to 1985 were reviewed.

The patients, aged 6 months to 18 years, all were presumed to have "communicating" syringomyelia, in which there was free communication of the fourth ventricle with the syringomyelic cavity. In 12, syringomyelia was associated with a Chiari I malformation. Thirty children had a Chiari II malformation and 5 had an acquired Chiari malformation. Scoliosis was present in 10 patients. Twenty-seven had upper limb weakness. Nine patients, all with a Chiari II malformation, had increasing lower limb weakness as the primary manifestation of the disorder. Dissociated sensory loss was noted in 17 patients.

Thirty-one children were treated by decompression of the Chiari malformation and plugging of the obex. Five were treated with a simple posterior fossa decompression. Nine had shunting of the syringomyelic cavity. Two were treated with combined decompression of the posterior fossa and shunting of the syrinx (table).

Of the 31 patients undergoing posterior fossa decompression with plugging of the obex, or the Gardner procedure, 25 improved. One of these patients required a second operation for late deterioration. Two patients who did not improve did so after undergoing syringopleural shunting. All patients with an acquired Chiari malformation or a Chiari I mal-

Operative Procedures and Results

Treatment	No. with Chiari I			No. with Chiari II			No. with Acquired Chiari			Total No.
	Improved	No Change	Worse	Improved	No Change	Worse	Improved	No Change	Worse	
Posterior fossa decompression with plugging of obex	5	0	0	16	6	0	4	0	0	31
Posterior fossa decompression	0	0	2	2	0	0	0	1	0	5
Syrinx shunting	3	0	0	4	2	0	0	0	0	9
Gardner procedure, syrinx shunting	1	0	0	0	0	0	0	0	0	1
Posterior fossa decompression, syrinx shunting	1	0	0	0	0	0	0	0	0	1
Total	10	0	2	22	8	0	4	1	0	47

(Courtesy of Hoffman HJ, Neill J, Crone KR, et al: *Neurosurgery* 21:346–351, 1987.)

formation improved after undergoing the Gardner procedure; 16 of the 22 patients with Chiari II malformation improved. No significant morbidity from the plugging of the obex was noted.

In this series, decompression of the Chiari malformation with plugging of the obex—the most commonly used treatment—resulted in improvement in more than 70% of the patients. Decompression alone was associated with a high incidence of failure. The results of the shunting of the syrinx were good; however, it was used only in patients with large syringomyelic cavities amenable to shunt insertion, and 2 patients subsequently required a secondary procedure of obex plugging and Chiari malformation decompression.

▶ The Gardner procedure yields good results in patients with hydrosyringomyelia, according to this report. This is particularly useful in patients with a small syrinx in whom direct syringoperitoneal shunting might be hazardous, according to the authors. Although the results are impressive, with improvement in more than 70% of the patients, the mechanism of improvement is open to question: It is quite possible that duraplasty, the lysis of arachnoid adhesions, as well as the obex plugging, may be of benefit. No radiographic evidence has been offered to support the notion that the obex plugging actually persists, and it could be that the muscle plug quickly is absent from the obex area. It is remarkable that no complications from this major cervicomedullary procedure were reported by the Toronto group.

When comunicating hydrocephalus accompanies syringomyelia, ventriculoperitoneal shunting is probably the lowest risk procedure. When there is a large syrinx, syringoperitoneal shunting is probably the safest method of treatment. When there is a small cervical syrinx and the Arnold-Chiari type II malformation, then the Gardner procedure may be generally warranted—R.M. Crowell, M.D.

Craniosynostosis: An Analysis of the Timing, Treatment, and Complications in 164 Consecutive Patients
Whitaker LA, Bartlett SP, Schut L, Bruce D (Philadelphia)
Plast Reconstr Surg 80:195–212, August 1987   24–4

The question of how to treat the infant with craniosynostosis remains unsettled. Treatment options vary from conservative observation until completion of growth to radical remodeling in infancy. Data on all patients undergoing surgery for this deformity in the past 12 years were analyzed retrospectively to clarify the timing and type of treatment needed in this complex disorder.

The series included 164 patients who were treated surgically for craniosynostosis between 1972 and 1984. The deformities were classified as either asymmetric synostosis or plagiocephaly or symmetric synostosis. Asymmetric deformities were managed with a unilateral osteotomy involving a frontal craniotomy, and a shift of approximately two thirds of the circumference of the orbit was completed (Fig 24–2). Of 92 patients undergoing surgery at less than 1.5 years of age, 62 had asymmetric synostosis, 19 had craniofacial dysostosis and variants, 8 had Apert's syndrome, and 3 had Kleebattschädel and other rare and severe deformities. Of the 35 children undergoing surgery at 1.5 to 7 years of age, 10 had asymmetric synostosis and 25 had symmetric synostosis. Of the 18 undergoing surgery between the ages of 7 to 13 years, 1 had asymmetric

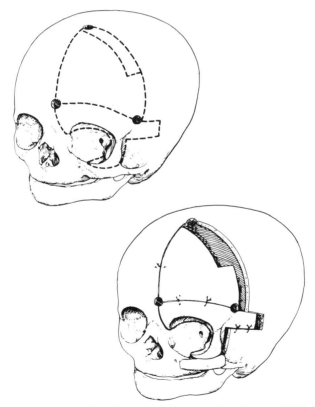

Fig 24–2.—Operative approach to the treatment of asymmetric craniosynostosis (plagiocephaly). A unilateral osteotomy of two thirds of the orbital circumference is performed; the orbit is advanced tongue-in-groove fashion and rigidly positioned with interosseous wires, and an inlay bone strut is placed at the pterion. The frontal bone is then repositioned and shaped. An onlay cranial bone graft is placed over the zygoma for symmetry as necessary. (Courtesy of Whitaker LA, Bartlett SP, Schutt L, et al: *Plast Reconstr Surg* 80:195–212, August 1987.)

synostosis and 17 had symmetric synostosis. One child with asymmetric synostosis and 18 with symmetric synostosis underwent surgery when they were older than 13 years.

Major complications with surgical implications were bony infection in 6 patients, resulting in relapse or total loss of correction in 1 and minimal alterations in the rest; hydrocephalus requiring shunt placement postoperatively in 3, and cerebrospinal fluid leakage requiring reoperation for closure in 2. Of those undergoing surgery for asymmetric stenosis, 78% needed no refinements or surgical revision, 15% needed soft tissue revisions or lesser bone-contouring revisions, 6% needed major alternative osteotomies or bone-grafting procedures, and 1% needed major craniofacial procedures, duplicating or exceeding the extent of the original surgery. The respective percentages for patients with symmetric synostoses were 16%, 20%, 37%, and 27%. Fifty of the 61 children treated when younger than 1.5 years of age needed no surgical revisions.

These data indicate that excellent results can be achieved in children with asymmetric deformities treated in infancy with a unilateral approach. For children with mild symmetric deformities, treatment by bilateral orbital advancement at this time usually gives satisfactory results. In contrast, those with more severe symmetric deformities treated in childhood have a high incidence of needed secondary major reconstructions; consideration should be given to delaying craniofacial surgery in this group until age 7 years or older, although earlier cranial surgery may be advisable.

▶ Excellent cosmetic results can be obtained with radical surgery for severe craniosynostosis. Although some patients may require multiple surgeries, the great majority of results are very satisfying to the patients and their families. It must be emphasized that an experienced team, involving neurosurgeons and plastic surgeons, is recommended to obtain the best results.

In related studies, Dufresne CR, et al. (*Plast Reconstr Surg* 79:24–32, 1987) report that volumetric quantification of intracranial and ventricular volume after cranial vault remodeling offers a more complete evaluation of preoperative pathology and documentation and prediction of projected changes. Further, a free fat transplant may prevent osseous reunion of skull defects in the treatment of craniosynostosis (Merikanto JE, et al: *Scand J Plast Reconstr Surg* 21:183–188, 1987).—R.M. Crowell, M.D.

The Surgical Treatment of Childhood Moyamoya Disease
Olds MV, Griebel RW, Hoffman HJ, Craven M, Chuang S, Schutz H (Univ of Toronto)
J Neurosurg 66:675–680, May 1987   24–5

Moyamoya disease is a chronic occlusive cerebrovascular disease of unknown etiology characterized by stenosis of the distal internal carotid artery and its branches and by compensatory enlargement of perforating

Results in 8 Patients With Moyamoya Disease Not
Treated Surgically

Case No.	Age (yrs) at Onset	Follow-Up Period	Clinical Outcome*
1	4	4 days	death
2	8	6 wks	death
3	2	14 yrs	hemiparesis, seizures, retarded
4	10	8 yrs	hemiparesis, seizures, low IQ
5	5	6 yrs	TIA's, hearing loss, IQ 68
6	½	2 yrs	mild rt hemiparesis, delayed milestones
7	4	4 yrs	dysarthria, hemiparesis, normal mentally
8	6	1 yr	mild hemiparesis, normal mentally

*IQ, intelligence quotient; TIA, transient ischemic attack.
(Courtesy of Olds MV, Griebel RW, Hoffman HJ, et al: *J Neurosurg* 66:675–680, May 1987.)

vessels at the base of the brain. In more than 75% of reported pediatric patients, the disease progressed, causing significant deficit or death during follow-up for 2 or more years. Steroid and vasodilator therapy has proved ineffective.

Fifteen of 23 children seen from 1971 to 1985 with confirmed moyamoya disease underwent revascularization procedures. The encephaloduroarteriosynangiosis (EDAS) procedure was used most frequently, and recent operations were modified to open the arachnoid beneath the transposed vascular cuff and place tacking sutures between the pia-arachnoid and the graft. Five patients underwent a superficial temporal artery–middle cerebral artery anastomosis (STA-MCA) bypass. Of the 6 surviving patients who were not treated surgically, only 1 remains neurologically intact (table). Both patients followed after only an STA-MCA operation had excellent results. Some patients had angiographic evidence of disease progression after the EDAS operation but remained clinically stable. When the arachnoid was opened, collateral channels often developed between the transposed artery and the brain within 5 months of surgery.

Untreated moyamoya disease can be expected to worsen, whereas surgery may prevent neurologic deterioration. Younger children should undergo the EDAS operation with arachnoid opening.

► Encephaloduroarteriosynangiosis led to good results in 15 pediatric patients with moyamoya disease. The operation involves placement of a segment of superficial temporal artery directly on the pia mater (Matsushima Y, et al: *Surg Neurol* 15:313–320, 1981). When the arachnoid is opened, new collateral channels to the brain may be seen on angiograms obtained within 5 months. Results of pediatric moyamoya disease without surgery are impressively poor (see table). Whereas STA-MCA bypass may be offered to older patients, younger children with moyamoya disease should undergo EDAS.—R.M. Crowell, M.D.

Intracranial Arterial Aneurysms in Early Childhood

Ferrante L, Fortuna A, Celli P, Santoro A, Fraioli B (Rome)
Surg Neurol 29:39–56, January 1988

24–6

Intracranial saccular aneurysms of noninfectious origin are rare in early childhood. Findings in 72 children younger than age 5 years were reviewed. The middle cerebral artery was involved in nearly 40%. Thirty aneurysms were classified as distal and 35 as proximal. Of the 51 patients with subarachnoid hemorrhage, 30 had a cerebral hematoma. Eighteen patients had seizures, but these were the presenting feature in only 2 patients. Thirteen children had signs of intracranial hypertension, and 6 had hydrocephalus. In 10 of 21 autopsies, associated cerebral and vascular anomalies were observed. Spasm was apparent in only 3 of 40 patients having cerebral angiography; but only 21 patients had full 4-vessel studies.

Of 42 patients undergoing surgery, in 33 the neck or supplying vessels were clipped. Removal of the aneurysmal sac was attempted in 20 instances. Operative mortality was 9.5%.

The surgical outcome appears to be better in children than in adults with saccular intracranial aneurysms. Presumably, young children withstand surgery relatively well because of their greater functional brain capacity and better vascular status. They are less susceptible to posthemorrhagic spasm, a critical prognostic factor in adults operated on for cerebral aneurysm.

▶ This communication underscores the occurrence, although rare, of typical saccular aneurysms in early childhood. Because many of the patients were operated on before the advent of modern microsurgical techniques, present-day results can be expected to be even better.—R.M. Crowell, M.D.

A New Surgical Approach to Closure of Large Lumbosacral Meningo-myelocele Defects

Ramirez OM, Ramasastry SS, Granick MS, Pang D, Futrell JW (Univ of Pittsburgh)
Plast Reconstr Surg 80:799–809, December 1987

24–7

Primary healing is important in the neurologic outcome of patients with meningomyelocele, both in preserving functioning neural tissue and preventing infectious complications. Advanced en bloc bilateral interconnected latissimus dorsi and gluteus maximus myocutaneous units, without lateral relaxing incisions or backcuts, were used to close large defects primarily. Nine patients with large thoracolumbar and lumbosacral defects not amenable to direct primary closure underwent this procedure after initial neurosurgical management (Fig 24–3). The basis for this operation is the rich anastomosis between the vasculature of the skin overlying the gluteus and latissimus dorsi muscles.

All reconstructions were completed in 1 stage without complications.

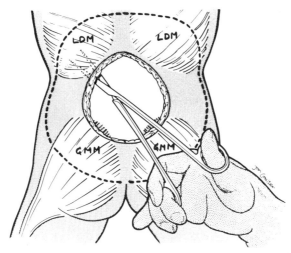

Fig 24–3.—Schematic illustration of the submuscular dissection of the latissimus dorsi and gluteus maximus myocutaneous units bilaterally. *Dotted line* indicates area of undermining at the submuscular level beneath the latissimus dorsi *(LDM)* and gluteus maximus muscles *(GMM)*. (Courtesy of Ramirez OM, Ramasastry SS, Granick MS, et al: *Plast Reconstr Surg* 80:799–809, December 1987.)

None of the flaps was lost, and no wound infections or disruptions occurred. The infants, followed for 11 months on average, had early use of both upper extremities. The average blood loss was only 20 ml. No patient has had deterioration of neurologic function.

This relatively simple procedure avoids the need for skin grafting and provides a reliable blood supply. Inclusion of the gluteus maximus facilitates closure of large deficits without tension, and it should cause no functional deficit. The use of careful dissection and electrocautery should prevent excessive blood loss.

▶ This technique of undermining beneath the latissimus dorsi and gluteus muscles permitted primary closure without relaxing incisions in 9 large thoracolumbar and lumbosacral defects without complications. Those involved in the care of myelomeningocele patients should keep this technical adjunct in mind. Anterior sacral meningocele is rare. The diagnosis rests on finding a fluid hypogastric mass attached to the sacrum together with radiologic abnormalities of the sacrum (Ozoux JP, et al: *J Chir (Paris)* 123:424–427, 1986).—R.M. Crowell, M.D.

Congenital Intraspinal Lipomas: Clinical Presentation and Response to Treatment
Lhowe D, Ehrlich MG, Chapman PH, Zaleske DJ (Massachusetts Gen Hosp, Boston)
J Pediatr Orthop 7:531–537, September–October 1987   24–8

Congenital intraspinal lipoma, a common form of occult spinal dysraphism, is often extensive and has a complex relationship to neural elements that makes spinal cord untethering difficult. Although therapy remains controversial, opinion on management of this entity appears to be changing in favor of prophylactic surgery on the lipoma itself.

Twenty-nine patients with surgically treated intraspinal lipomas were studied retrospectively to assess their manner of presentation and response to treatment. The patients had a mean age of 12.8 years at diagnosis. Only 5 patients, all less than 6 months of age, were neurologically normal by clinical examination at diagnosis. A consistent technique of resection was used for all patients. The spinal cord was freed from its dural and lipomatous attachments and the functioning neural elements were spared (Fig 24–4). Patients were followed for 32 to 103 months.

Four patients had undergone previous exploration and resection at other institutions and subsequently worsened. Of the remaining 25, 4 were neurologically intact before surgery and remained so at an average of 54 months after surgery. One patient who underwent surgery at 1 month of age and was initially thought to be neurologically intact, was found to have absent sacral nerve roots and had remained incontinent 55 months after surgery. Seven patients showed lessening of incontinence or improvement of lower extremity function or deformity an average of 63 months after surgery. Eight patients showed no clinical changes at a mean of 52 months postoperatively. Five patients worsened. Three underwent repeat exploration; 2 of these patients improved slightly, and the third showed no clinical change 24 months after the second procedure. Patient age at the time of diagnosis correlated significantly with outcome among the neurologically normal children at the average age of 5 months

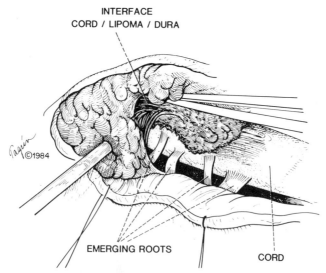

INTERFACE
CORD / LIPOMA / DURA

EMERGING ROOTS

CORD

Fig 24–4.—Diagram of the surgical approach to the dorsal lipoma. The lipoma is detached from the dorsal surface of the conus at the lateral line of fusion. The functioning neural elements, which lie ventral to this, are spared. (Courtesy of Lhowe D, Ehrlich MG, Chapman PH, et al: *J Pediatr Orthop* 7:531–537, September-October 1987.)

at operation. These children have remained stable since the operation. Orthopedic intervention was considered successful in the 11 foot procedures done after surgery on the lipoma, but in only 2 of the 5 foot procedures done before surgery on the lipoma. Consideration of intraspinal lipoma is warranted in several circumstances, including patients with foot deformity.

▶ Resection of an intraspinal lipoma can arrest progressive neurologic deterioration, as reported in this series of 29 patients. The difficulty of removing the lesions along the lateral zone of fusion with the cord and the lipoma is illustrated. Because deterioration of neurologic function (20%) was seen even in this group of patients treated by a very experienced team, this aggressive treatment should probably be restricted to centers with substantial experience. Older studies have advocated observation of intraspinal lipomas until documented neurologic deterioration warrants intervention.—R.M. Crowell, M.D.

Predictive Value of Temporary External Lumbar Drainage in Normal Pressure Hydrocephalus

Haan J, Thomeer RTWM (Univ Hospital, Leiden, The Netherlands)
Neurosurgery 22:388–391, 1988   24–9

The clinical triad of gait disturbance, dementia, and urinary incontinence is often incomplete in patients with normal pressure hydrocephalus (NPH). Radiographic images are not pathognomonic for the disease; thus it is not usually easy to establish a definitive diagnosis of NPH. Symptom improvement after lumbar puncture strongly suggests NPH but is not frequently encountered. Continuous external lumbar drainage was used to study 22 patients with NPH; the observed effects formed a basis for predicting the ultimate outcome of surgery.

Six women and 16 men aged 58–79 years were studied. Gait disturbance, dementia, and urinary incontinence were noted in 15 patients, gait disturbance and dementia in 4, gait disturbance and incontinence in 2, and gait disturbance in 1. The external lumbar drainage system was left in place for 5 days. All patients were shunted with a ventriculoatrial drain regardless of the effect of the external lumbar drainage system. Complications resulted from both lumbar drainage and shunting.

Final data were available for analysis on 17 patients; 12 patients had a good response to external lumbar drainage and 5 did not. All 12 patients who benefited from drainage also benefited from shunting; none of the 5 who did not improve after lumbar drainage improved after shunting. Thus the prediction was correct in all cases.

In this series, external lumbar drainage correctly predicted the outcome of shunting in all patients. It appears to be a safe, valuable tool for predicting the outcome of definitive shunting procedures in patients with NPH.

▶ This report demonstrates the high predictive value of temporary external lumbar drainage in normal pressure hydrocephalus. The test seems highly reliable in selecting patients for shunting procedures. Further studies may be useful in determining how long the test must be pursued and how complications may be further reduced. At this stage it seems reasonable to adopt this method for selection of patients, because shunting procedures carry a very substantial rate of complications that obviously are most undesirable in patients who cannot be expected to benefit from the treatment. An additional question raised by the study is whether lumbar-peritoneal shunt might be just as effective and less dangerous; further studies would be needed to elucidate this particular point.—R.M. Crowell, M.D.

Brief Notes on Pediatrics

Chiari Malformation

Magnetic resonance imaging is simple, accurate, and the method of choice for demonstrating Chiari II malformation (Wolpert SM, et al: *AJNR* 8:783–792, 1987).

Forty adult patients with Chiari malformation were studied over a 17-year interval. Common presenting symptoms included head and neck pain, sensory complaints, upper extremity weakness, and gait disturbance. Neurologic findings included signs of cord dysfunction, long tract signs, brain stem signs, cerebellar dysfunction, and increased intracranial pressure. Myelography and MRI were used to make the diagnosis. Thirty-three patients underwent surgery. Of these, 5 (15%) had complications. Follow-up showed 18 patients improved (55%), 10 stable (30%), and 5 deteriorated (15%), including 1 death (Eisenstat DDR, et al: *Can J Neurol Sci* 13:221–228, 1986).

Spinal Dysraphism

Magnetic resonance imaging was used in 37 infants and children in evaluation of spinal dysraphism. Results suggest that the technique is reliable, with sensitivity comparable to postmyelographic CT, although the latter has somewhat better specificity (Barnes PD, et al: *AJR* 147:339–346, 1986).

In spina bifida children, early surgery in 66 yielded a 15% 1-year mortality rate, whereas no early surgery in 126 led to a 74% 1-year mortality rate (Guiney EJ, et al: *Z Kinderchir* 41:16–17, 1986).

Hydrocephalus

Improvement in urinary incontinence after removal of 50 ml of cerebrospinal fluid by lumbar puncture is predictive of improvement after ventriculoperitoneal shunting for normal pressure hydrocephalus (Ahlberg J, et al: *J Neurol Neurosurg Psychiatry* 51:105–108, 1988).

Analysis of 21 cases confirms that when gait abnormality precedes dementia, there is a high likelihood of improvement after shunting of normal pressure hydrocephalus (Graff-Radford NR, Godersky JC: *Arch Neurol* 43:940–942, 1986).

In 14 of 19 patients with normal pressure hydrocephalus, systemic arterial hypertension was documented (Graff-Radford NR, Godersky JC: *Neurology* 37:868–871, 1987).

In 40 patients with neuropsychological examination before and after ventriculoatrial shunt operation, cognitive functions were improved in 16, unchanged in 19, and worse in 5. Improvement was seen in 80% of the patients when 3 criteria were present, including known cause, short history, low cerebrospinal fluid pressure, and small sulci or periventricular hypodensity on CT (Thomsen AM, et al: *Ann Neurol* 20:304–310, 1986).

In posthemorrhagic hydrocephalus in premature infants, the outcome of shunting procedures was poor, with 62% of shunted infants either dying or surviving with moderate or severe handicap. Routine ultrasonic screening of low-birth-weight infants is recommended to detect hemorrhage and ventriculomegaly. Placement of an external drain may be the treatment of choice once serial lumbar punctures have failed (Etches PC, et al: *Pediatr Neurol* 3:136–140, 1987).

Pumping a shunt reservoir with occlusion of the distal catheter generates microbubbles in the ventricular catheter. In children, sonography can be performed via the fontanelle to image the ventricular catheter to assess shunt patency (Widder DJ, et al: *AJR* 147:353–356, 1986).

In a series of 383 shunts there was no significant difference between ventriculoatrial and ventriculoperitoneal shunts regarding incidence of revision, operative mortality, and related morbidity (Metzemaekers JDM, et al: *Acta Neurochir (Wien)* 88:75–78, 1987).

Since 1979, 8 patients have been seen at the Toronto Hospital for Sick Children in whom, after ventriculoperitoneal shunting, the contralateral ventricle became isolated (Hubballah MY, Hoffman HJ: *Surg Neurol* 27:220–222, 1987).

The keyhole is a sign of herniation of a trapped fourth ventricle and other posterior fossa cysts (Wolfson BJ, et al: *AJNR* 8:473–477, 1987).

Transvaginal cephalocentesis for fetuses with hydrocephalus in the cephalic presentation followed by spontaneous vaginal delivery lessens maternal morbidity and is consistent with a good neonatal outcome (Silver RK, Huff RW: *Am J Perinatol* 4:16–19, 1987).

Ventricular gallbladder shunts represent an alternate procedure for hydrocephalus (West KW, et al: *J Pediatr Surg* 22:609–612, 1987).—R.M. Crowell, M.D.

25 Functional

Introduction

In the area of *pain* studies, treatment of chronic pain by deep brain stimulation has long-term effectiveness in more than half of the patients with electrodes internalized (Abstract 25–1). Several approaches to periodic migrainous neuralgia have been discussed including surgery (Abstract 25–2). The management of trigeminal neuralgia at the University of Alabama reflects the widespread utilization of percutaneous methodology and microvascular decompression for trigeminal neuralgia (Abstract 25–3). The much larger series of patients from France reports 609 percutaneous procedures and 150 microsurgical operations (Abstract 25–4).

In the field of *epilepsy,* modern methods for pediatric epilepsy surgery are reviewed by Goldring (Abstract 25–5). Magnetoencephalography may help with the identification of epileptogenic foci (Abstract 25–6).

Psychosurgery may still have a place as indicated by the good results from stereotactic cingulotomy for psychiatric illness (Abstract 25–7). When deep lesions are placed by Gamma knife methods, MRI images may detect these small lesions and are correlated to the clinical outcome in the treatment of severe anxiety disorder (Abstract 25–8).

In experimental studies of *transplantation* to the brain of hypothalamus grafts of fetal tissue, behavioral effectiveness has been demonstrated in the reversal of experimental hypothalamic deficit (Abstract 25–9). Studies of clinically implanted platinum-iridium electrodes indicates some of the basic properties that will be important in overcoming electrode-tissue interface disturbances (Abstract 25–10).

Robert M. Crowell, M.D.

Pain

Treatment of Chronic Pain by Deep Brain Stimulation: Long Term Follow-up and Review of the Literature

Levy RM, Lamb S, Adams JE (Univ of California, San Francisco)
Neurosurgery 21:885–893, December 1987   25–1

Several research teams have confirmed that electrical stimulation of the sensory thalamus and periaqueductal gray produces pain relief. The efficacy of deep brain stimulation for specific pain states and its long-term effectiveness were evaluated in 304 operations in 141 patients whose mean age was 51.2 years; the mean length of follow-up was 80 months.

Patients had experienced pain for a mean of 65 months before deep brain stimulation was attempted. All had exhausted other medical and surgical options. Pain states were characterized as being nociceptive or deafferentiation. Nociceptive pain was treated by stimulation of the peri-aqueductal or periventricular gray, and deafferentiation pain was treated by stimulation of the sensory thalamus. Eighty-four patients had deafferentiation pain, which included thalamic pain syndrome in 25, peripheral neuropathic pain in 16, anesthesia dolorosa in 12, paraplegia pain in 11, postcordotomy dysesthesia in 5, phantom limb pain in 5, thoracic neuralgia in 4, and miscellaneous pain states in 6. The 57 patients with nociceptive pain primarily had low back and skeletal pain; 6 had pain from cancer invasion.

Pain relief was achieved initially in 59% of the patients. After 80 months of follow-up, 31% continued to have significant pain relief. Some pain states, especially anesthesia dolorosa and paraplegia pain, did not respond to treatment. Major complications included wound infection in 12% of the patients and intracranial hemorrhage in 3.5%; 1 death occurred. Hardware erosion was seen in 7% of the patients, and a foreign body reaction was noted in 5%. The most common technical problems were migration of the implanted electrodes and equipment failure, which led to leakage of current and ineffective stimulation.

Deep brain stimulation can be an effective treatment for chronic, intractable pain in a carefully selected and evaluated group of patients. A review of the literature on long-term results of deep brain stimulation suggested that lasting pain relief is achieved in 47% and 60% of patients with deafferentiation and nociceptive pain, respectively.

▶ This communication shows that deep brain stimulation should be considered in the management of chronic severe long-term pain because of its substantial success rate (52.2% with electrodes internalized). There is, however, an incidence of life-threatening complications of around 5%, thus careful patient selection and meticulous electrode management must be provided by an experienced pain neurosurgeon.— R.M. Crowell, M.D.

A Review of Treatment Modalities for Periodic Migrainous Neuralgia
Wake M, Hitchcock E (Univ of Birmingham, England)
Pain 31:345–352, December 1987   25–2

Periodic migrainous neuralgia consists of unilateral pain, mainly in the ocular, frontal, and temporal areas recurring in separate bouts with daily attacks for several months, usually with rhinorrhea or lacrimation. Five men and 5 women aged 20–65 years with periodic migrainous neuralgia were treated by medical, minor surgical, and major surgical methods.

Symptoms included severe, throbbing pain in one side of the face and lasting for 3 weeks; severe left frontal pain associated with left-sided nasal obstruction, conjunctival injection, and lacrimation; right-sided facial pain and sweating that followed herpes zoster development in the first division of the trigeminal nerve; sudden onset of severe right-sided periorbital pain associated with lacrimation and right-sided rhinorrhea; severe pain in the left upper gum radiating across the face toward the left eye

Results of Treatment in 10 Patients With Periodic Migrainous Neuralgia*

Case no.	Ergotamine	Peripheral nerve block	Trigeminal ganglion block	Percutaneous rhizotomy	Trigeminal rhizotomy	Petrosal nerve section
1	+ +	−	−	−	−	−
2	Side effects	−	−	−	−	−
3	0	−	0	+ + +	−	−
4	0	−	0	−	0	−
5	Side effects	0	−	−	−	+ + +
6	+ +	−	−	−	−	+ + +
7	+ + +	−	−	−	+	+
8	+ +	−	−	−	+ + +	+
9	−	−	+	−	−	0
10	+ +	−	−	0	−	+ + +

*Dash indicates not attempted; 0, no pain relief; +, partial pain relief; + +, temporary complete pain relief; and + + +, long-term complete pain relief.
(Courtesy of Wake M, Hitchcock E: *Pain* 31:345–352, December 1987.)

and ear lasting for about 1 hour and accompanied by facial flushing; and orbital, periorbital, and frontal pain with a burning sensation associated with conjunctival injection and lacrimation. Ergotamine treatment produced long-term complete relief in 9 patients, temporary complete relief in 2, no relief in 2, and side effects in 2 (table). Other treatments included peripheral nerve block in 1 patient, without relief; trigeminal ganglion block in 3, with partial pain relief in 1; percutaneous rhizotomy in 2, with complete long-term relief in 1 patient only; trigeminal rhizotomy in 3, with some relief in 2 patients; and petrosal nerve section in 6, providing some degree of pain relief in 5 patients.

Treatment of these 10 patients with periodic migrainous neuralgia encompassed medical, minor surgical, and major surgical approaches. If medical treatment fails or severe drug side effects occur, trigeminal rhizotomy may be effective in producing long-term pain relief. If pain recurs or trigeminal rhizotomy is not effective, section of the greater and lesser superficial petrosal nerves may be useful.

▶ This report of 10 patients indicates an effective program for the treatment of periodic migrainous neuralgia: Cafergot may be effective in some cases. Percutaneous rhizotomy is occasionally beneficial, and greater superficial petrosal nerve section is usually effective when lesser treatments fail. This experience parallels that of White and Sweet.—R.M. Crowell, M.D.

The Surgical Management of Trigeminal Neuralgia at the University of Alabama at Birmingham Medical Center 1981–1986: A Comparative Study

Zampella EJ, Zeiger HE, Brock RJ, Thomas MV, Langford KH (Univ of Alabama, Birmingham)

Ala J Med Sci 24:371–377, October 1987   25–3

Surgical Treatment of Trigeminal Neuralgia:
University of Alabama at Birmingham Experience
1981–1986

Patients treated	64
Procedures:	
Microvascular decompression (MVD)	23
Percutaneous retrogasserian glycerol rhizolysis (PRGR)	34
Percutaneous retrogasserian radiofrequency rhizolysis (PRRR)	37
	94

(Courtesy of Zampella EJ, Zeiger HE, Brock RJ, et al: *Ala J Med Sci* 24:371–377, October 1987.)

The optimum treatment for trigeminal neuralgia remains elusive. Currently, the most widely used interventional treatments are percutaneous retrogasserian glycerol rhizolysis, percutaneous retrogasserian radiofrequency rhizotomy, and microvascular decompression of the trigeminal nerve root entry zone. Between 1981 and 1986, 64 patients with refractory facial pain were referred for surgical therapy. The surgical procedure of choice was selected after a careful review of the patient's history, neurologic examination, and diagnostic studies. Patients whose pain was not relieved satisfactorily by the first procedure underwent the same or a different procedure.

Ninety-four procedures were performed: 37 rhizolyses, 34 rhizotomies, and 23 microvascular decompression procedures (table). Overall, 60 (93%) of 64 patients reported satisfactory reduction in the severity of pain without medication from 6 months to 5 years after treatment. Success rates were 87%, 74%, and 73% for patients treated with decompression, rhizolysis, and rhizotomy, respectively. Late recurrence developed in 25%, 8%, and 41% of patients, respectively, at an average of 42, 19, and 34 months after initial surgical treatment.

Surgical intervention can provide long-lasting relief of symptoms among patients with trigeminal neuralgia. The rate of recurrence is high, regardless of the treatment used; however, microvascular decompression appears to be more advantageous because of the longer relief of pain. Elderly patients, patients in poor health, and those with atypical facial pain (e.g., related to multiple sclerosis) appear to benefit more from percutaneous procedures, whereas microvascular decompression appears to be advantageous for patients younger than 70 years, those with pain involving the area of the eye, and those in whom the production of an adequate lesion with either rhizolysis or rhizotomy would run the risk of producing corneal anesthesia.

► This report, which may be closer to the experience outside Pittsburgh and Zurich, reflects experience with both microvascular decompression, glycerol rhizolysis, and radiofrequency rhizotomy. Of note is the high recurrence rate and absence of anesthesia dolorosa. Surgeons should select a procedure for patients with tic douloureux based on the safety and efficacy of procedures as performed in their own clinics.—R.M. Crowell, M.D.

Neurosurgical Treatment of Trigeminal Neuralgia: Direct Approach Versus Percutaneous Method?

Sindou M, Keravel Y, Abdennebi B, Szapiro J (Hôpital Neurologique Pierre-Wertheimer, Lyon, Hôpital Henri-Mondor, Créteil, France)
Neurochirurgie 33:89–111, 1987   25–4

A comparison was made of the advantages and disadvantages of percutaneous and microsurgical therapeutic techniques in the treatment of trigeminal neuralgia based on experience with 609 percutaneous rhizotomies and 150 microsurgical procedures. After a follow-up ranging from 1 to 10 years, results in the patients who underwent percutaneous rhizotomy in treatment of refractory trigeminal neuralgia were excellent in 390 (64%), satisfactory in 183 (30%), and poor in 36 (6%). No immediate surgical failures occurred. Although 43 patients (7%) had homolateral and 10 patients (1.6%) contralateral recurrence of trigeminal neuralgia, these rates are considerably lower than those reported in the literature.

Other percutaneous techniques include cisternal glycerol injection, a technique developed by Håkanson of the Karolinska Institute in Sweden, who reported good results but a relapse rate of more than 18%. Percutaneous balloon compression of the gasserian ganglion, a technique developed by Mullan, reportedly had an immediate success rate of 98.5% but a relapse rate of 15%.

Microvascular decompression in 113 patients who were followed for 1 to 6 years resulted in complete resolution of all symptoms of trigeminal neuralgia in 93 (83.2%), partial resolution in 4 (3.5%), significant improvement in 3 (2.7%), slight improvement in 3 (2.7%), immediate failure in 5 (4.4%), and recurrence in 4 (3.5%). One (0.8%) patient died of the operation.

Each technique for the treatment of trigeminal neuralgia has advantages and disadvantages and none is clearly superior to another. The decision of which technique to use in a given patient should be made on the individual circumstances.

▶ Sindou et al. report an extensive experience in the neurosurgical treatment of trigeminal neuralgia. Among 609 percutaneous rhizotomies, a large proportion were reported as having a satisfactory or excellent outcome (94%). However, dysesthesia dolorosa occurred in a substantial number of patients (29%) after gasserian coagulation, with choreokeratitis in 6%. Because of such serious complications, Sweet has recently advocated utilization of glycerol as a safer percutaneous technique. The results of microvascular decompression were excellent in 83%, with a single death. The authors advocate the use of these techniques on the basis of a case-by-case selection.—R.M. Crowell, M.D.

Brief Notes on Pain

Pain measurement instruments have been used to characterize the dysesthetic pain syndrome in patients with spinal cord injury (Davidoff G, et al: *Pain* 29:39–48, 1987).

Thirty-four sympathectomies were performed for causalgic pain, with satisfactory relief in 94%, temporary neuralgia in 40%, and a low complication rate (Mockus MB, et al: *Arch Surg* 122:668–672, 1987).

In a double-blind study, trazodone was not effective in the treatment of dysesthetic pain caused by traumatic myelopathy (Davidoff G, et al: *Pain* 29:151–161, 1987).

Recurrent sympathetic dystrophy may respond to contralateral sympathectomy after unsuccessful unilateral sympathectomy (Munn JS, Baker WH: *Surgery* 102:102–105, 1987).

Posterior fossa decompression of the root-entry zone of the facial nerve was carried out in 5 patients with intractable cluster headache. Two patients had good relief, the effect was indeterminate in 1, and failure occurred in 2 (Solomon S, Apfelbaum RI: *Arch Neurol* 43:479–482, 1986).—R.M. Crowell, M.D.

Epilepsy

Pediatric Epilepsy Surgery
Goldring S (Washington Univ)
Epilepsia 28:S82–S102, 1987

25–5

Both frequent convulsions and their treatment can have serious effects on children's education, behavior, and psychosocial development. Cortical excisions are more feasible now that implantable arrays of epidural electrodes are available for extraoperative electrocorticography and functional localization in the waking state. Simultaneous electrocorticography and video monitoring during symptomatic seizures provide additional localizing information.

The results of monitoring in 75 children were reviewed. Most had seizures of an extratemporal, nonneoplastic origin (table). After the brain was exposed and the sensorimotor region identified, the dura was closed and a template of electrodes was sewn in epidurally, spanning the area of suspected epileptogenicity. Monitoring led to resection in 53 patients.

Forty-nine patients were followed for an average of 6 years, and 65% had good results. Sixteen patients were free of seizures. Seven of 9 children with chronic encephalitis improved significantly. Five of 7 with infantile hemiplegia no longer have seizures. Good results were obtained in patients with mesial temporal sclerosis, but not in patients with extratemporal focal sclerosis. Two of 4 children with focal cortical dysplasia did well. Few complications resulted from surgery.

Surgery has an important role in the management of selected children with intractable focal seizures. In addition to those with benign causes of epilepsy, those with gliomas often respond well to extirpation. Long-term survival may follow excision and, when indicated, irradiation.

Surgical Experience With Focal Seizure Disorder in Children, 1967–1986*	
Managed with extraoperative epidural recording electrodes	
Extratemporal origin (nonneoplastic)	66
Temporal lobe origin (nonneoplastic)	9
Tumors	1
Managed with intraoperative electrocorticography	
Nonneoplastic	3†
Managed without intra- or extraoperative recording	
Tumors	16
Total	95

*All but 3 were managed since 1971.
†Managed before 1971.
(Courtesy of Goldring S: *Epilepsia* 28:S82–S102, 1987.)

▶ Dr. Goldring presents his extensive experience with epilepsy surgery in the pediatric age group. With the use of implantable epidural electrodes, identification of epileptogenic tissue in the waking state permits safe and effective excision of the excitable focus. Implementation of this approach on a large-scale basis in selected centers appears appropriate for control of a substantial pediatric neurologic problem.— R.M. Crowell, M.D.

Magnetoencephalography and Epilepsy Research

Rose DF, Smith PD, Sato S (Natl Inst of Neurological and Communicative Disorders and Stroke, Bethesda, Md)
Science 238:329–335, Oct 16, 1987   25–6

Magnetoencephalography detects across the surface of the head the magnetic field distribution generated by neuronal discharges within the brain. It is used to localize epileptogenic regions in preparation for removing them. The spontaneous magnetic fields are measurable with a superconducting quantum interference device (SQUID) (Fig 25–1). The orientation of the current dipole is a critical factor affecting measurements of magnetic fields outside the head. The gradiometer cancels distant fields, but local background magnetic noise in the hospital setting remains a problem. A magnetically shielded room is best for clinical magnetoencephalography.

One of the chief problems in data analysis is the small area measured by the magnetometers relative to the area that has to be scanned to produce a magnetic map. If each spike or sharp wave in the electroencephalogram is carefully examined, the variability inherent in the epileptogenic region probably is preserved. It also is possible to average the magnetic signals or examine windows of electroencephalograms using the fast Fourier transformer for frequency peaks.

Advances in instrumentation should allow the prediction of current source sites during the onset and propagation of seizures in a larger num-

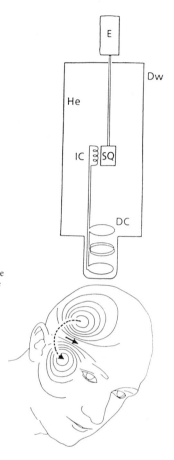

Fig 25–1.—Schematic of a SQUID gradiometer and the magnetic field of an idealized intracranial current source. The gradiometer is maintained perpendicular to the head surface during the recording sessions. The component of the magnetic flux perpendicular to the head, passing through the loops of the detection coil *(DC)*, induces a current that is transferred by the input coil *(IC)* to the SQUID *(SQ)*. The SQUID electronics *(E)* then convert the signal to a voltage proportional to the magnetic flux at the detection coil. Liquid helium *(He)* maintains the inside of the Dewar *(DW)* at superconducting temperatures. The *solid arrow* represents an idealized intracranial current source oriented tangentially to the scalp surface. The *dotted arrow* represents the magnetic flux that encircles the current dipole and is oriented at a right angle to the direction of the current dipole. The concentric lines represent isoflux contours on the head surface (magnetic field map). (Courtesy of Rose DF, Smith PD, Sato S: *Science* 238:329–335, Oct 16, 1987.)

ber of patients. Eventually, magnetoencephalography may become a clinically useful noninvasive means of localizing epileptogenic regions. Study of seizure propagation may help to elucidate paths of seizure spread.

▶ More sophisticated instrumentation and satisfactory magnetic shielding have greatly improved the ability of magnetoencephalography to detect epileptogenic discharge. Magnetoencephalography could well become clinically useful in the preoperative evaluation of patients for excision of epileptogenic foci. At the moment, however, specialized evaluation, often including study with implanted electrodes, remains important in the crucial delineation of the discharging focus.—R.M. Crowell, M.D.

Brief Notes on Epilepsy

Among 26 patients subjected to temporal lobectomy for complex partial seizures resistant to any convulsant control, 50% were completely free from seizures and in 38% seizures were reduced by at least 75% in follow-up for 5–17 years (Cutfield RG, Wrightson P: *N Z Med J* 100:163–166, 1987).

Among 58 patients who underwent temporal lobectomy for seizure control, a good outcome was more likely if a definite lesion was removed. Ammon's horn sclerosis was strongly related to a history of prolonged childhood convulsions (Duncan JS, Sagar HJ: *Neurology* 37:405–409, 1987).

Surface electroencephalography of seizure onset in patients with temporal lobe or focal cerebral epilepsy may provide false lateralization, indicating the need for depth electrodes (Sammaritano M, et al: *Ann Neurol* 21:361–369, 1987).

Cranial computed tomography was used for the diagnosis of medial temporal lesions before surgery for epilepsy. Intrathecal metrizamide was useful in a number of patients, and axial views parallel to the temporal fossa also were helpful (El Gammal T, et al: *AJNR* 8:131–134, 1987).—R.M. Crowell, M.D.

Psychiatric

Treatment of Psychiatric Illness by Stereotactic Cingulotomy
Ballantine HT Jr, Bouckoms AJ, Thomas EK, Giriunas IE (Massachusetts Gen Hosp; Harvard Univ, Boston)
Biol Psychiatry 22:807–819, 1987

25–7

The results of stereotactic cingulotomy were assessed after a mean follow-up of 8.6 years in a prospective series of 198 psychiatrically disabled patients or patients with chronic pain. Overall, 70% of the group had psychiatric diagnoses, most frequently affective disorders; 21% had chronic pain syndromes, and 9% had intractable cancer pain. The radiofrequency technique was used. No deaths occurred in 696 cingulotomies. Two hemiplegias resulted from intracerebral hematoma after ventricular needle insertion. One percent of the patients had postoperative seizures that were controlled by phenytoin.

Thirteen percent of the psychiatrically disabled patients recovered fully and were stable at follow-up. Patients with major affective disorders and anxiety disorders did the best, whereas those with schizophrenia, obsessive-compulsive disorder, or personality disorder improved less predictably. Nearly one fourth of the psychiatric patients functioned normally but continued to require psychiatric supervision and medication; another fourth remained psychiatrically disabled but were much improved.

Stereotactic bilateral anterior cingulotomy is a safe procedure that is effective in patients with major psychiatric illness who are refractory to all other measures. Substantial improvement was observed in more than 60% of the psychiatrically disabled patients in the present series.

▶ Stereotactic cingulotomy should be considered for medically intractable patients with affective disorders (or chronic pain). Although psychotropic medication is often effective, there remains a significant group of disabled patients unresponsive to medication. The general aversion to "lobotomy" should not obscure the useful role of stereotactic cingulotomy for such patients. Performed by an experienced surgical team, the method is safe (zero mortality,

0.3% morbidity). Follow-up psychiatric evaluation indicated normal function in 72 of 198 patients (36.4%) and improved, noninstitutionalized function in 50 (25.3%).—R.M. Crowell, M.D.

Magnetic Resonance Images Related to Clinical Outcome After Psychosurgical Intervention in Severe Anxiety Disorder

Mindus P, Bergström K, Levander SE, Norén G, Hindmarsh T, and Thuomas KÅ (Karolinska Hosp, Stockholm; Univ Hosp, Uppsala, Sweden)
J Neurol Neurosurg Psychiatry 50:1288–1293, October 1987   25–8

It is difficult to verify radiosurgical lesions in the white matter postoperatively using computed tomography (CT). It was possible, however, to demonstrate lesions in patients undergoing gamma capsulotomy for anxiety disorder using magnetic resonance (MR) imaging. Seven consecutive patients were studied before and 7 years after operation by psychiatrists not involved in treatment, using several rating scales. The patients had been repeatedly previously hospitalized because of anxiety disorders resistant to conventional measures. The median age at operation was 42 years. Lesions were produced by cobalt irradiation.

In all patients, MR imaging demonstrated a radiosurgical lesion most clearly on T1-weighted images, in which it appeared as a low-signal intensity area. Some patients had distinct bilateral lesions in the internal capsule. Computed tomography failed to show evidence of lesioning in 2 patients, and lesion size and site were better appreciated on MR images. Symptom scores decreased significantly after operation; 5 patients had a satisfactory outcome. Magnetic resonance imaging showed bilateral internal capsule lesions in all patients who benefited, but not in the 2 with an unsatisfactory outcome.

Magnetic resonance imaging is more accurate than CT in detecting lesions in patients undergoing psychosurgery in management of anxiety. The study might prove useful in determining a clinically effective radiation threshold estimate for radiosurgical lesions, as well as in following patients after surgery on the limbic system.

▶ This paper documents the effectiveness of bilateral radiosurgical capsulotomy in patients with severe anxiety disorder. The presentation suggests that, despite the disuse of such an approach in the United States, radiosurgical capsulotomy may have clinical value in selected patients. In addition, MR imaging is clearly the best method to reveal these tiny lesions. It may also be that MR imaging can detect deep radiation effects after stereotactic radiosurgery in other interventions for arteriovenous malformations and tumors. The detection of radionecrosis in such patients will be of particular interest. Early experience suggests that a high-intensity signal on T2 is common in the area of radiation focus, even in the absence of symptoms or signs. It has also been suggested that such T2 abnormality may vanish after a time. Further experience is needed to elucidate these matters.—R.M. Crowell, M.D.

Other Topics

The Effect of Fetal Hypothalamus Grafts on Weight Gain Resulting From Lesions of the Ventromedial Hypothalamus
Erickson RK, Brown FD, Schaible KL, Wollmann RL (Univ of Chicago)
J Neurosurg 68:112–116, January 1988   25–9

Interest in neural transplantation in mammals has increased with the finding that functioning central nervous system (CNS) grafts may survive long term. An attempt was made to determine whether grafts of fetal rat hypothalamic tissue placed in the third ventricle can alter the course of a lesion in the ventromedial hypothalamus. This is the classic lesion site producing an obese hyperphagic animal. Bilateral lesions produced hyperphagia and rapid weight gain.

Average daily weight gain decreased significantly 4–12 weeks after placement of fetal hypothalamic grafts; fetal cortical tissue had no such effect. Examination of the grafts 12 weeks after placement showed neurons, ependymal clusters, and axonal processes that appeared to infiltrate the adjacent hypothalamic parenchyma (Fig 25–2, p. 390). Six of 7 hypothalamic tissue grafts survived for the 3 months of observation. Weight gain was about halved, compared with that in control rats given cortical tissue grafts.

This model, while applicable to research in appetite control, may prove useful in studying CNS transplantation in general. Rat fetal CNS grafts survive over the long term in the third ventricle, and measurements of function are relatively convenient.

► Stimulated by reports of the clinical effectiveness of adrenal transplants to the caudate in treatment of parkinsonism, neurosurgical researchers are investigating a wide array of transplantation possibilities. A major problem in this field has been relevance of animal models to clinical problems. This communication from the University of Chicago demonstrates the ingenious utilization of a rat model to learn about the process of graft and host interaction, but the specific model remains distant from the clinical arena.—R.M. Crowell, M.D.

Electrical Characteristics of Chronically Implanted Platinum-Iridium Electrodes
McCreery DB, Agnew WF, McHardy J (Huntington Med Research Insts, Pasadena; Hughes Aircraft Co, El Segundo, Calif)
IEEE Trans Biomed Eng 34:664–668, November 1987   25–10

Although it is known that neural damage may be produced by prolonged electrical stimulation, the mechanism of such damage is unclear. Accurate knowledge of the electrode potential is essential for assessing the safety of a particular stimulation protocol. The potential of a working electrode is measured against a standard reference electrode in simple experimental systems, such as $Ag/AgCl$, Hg/Hg_2Cl_2 or $H_2/H+$. In

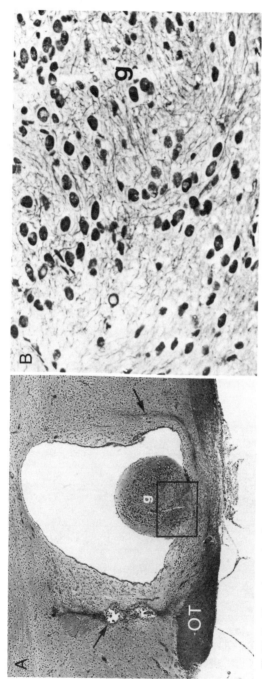

Fig 25–2.—Photomicrographs of a section from a treatment group animal. A, bilateral lesions (*arrows*) and graft of hypothalamic tissue (*g*) attached to the floor of the third ventricle (*V III*). *OT* = optic tract. Bodian stain, original magnification, ×20. B, enlargement of the area outlined by the rectangle in A, showing the interface of the hypothalamic tissue graft (*g*) and the floor of the third ventricle. (Courtesy of Erickson RK, Brown FD, Schaible KL, et al: *J Neurosurg* 68:112–116, January 1988.)

chronic experiments, however, toxicity and other concerns usually preclude or limit the use of a reference electrode. The high current densities used for stimulation with microelectrodes introduce a large ohmic component into the measured electrode voltage. If not computed with high accuracy, this introduces significant error into the estimate of the relative electrode potential. An approach was developed that overcomes these difficulties by using reproducible features of the voltage-time transients as potential markers.

Microelectrodes, fabricated from platinum 30% iridium wire, were implanted in the sensorimotor cortex of adult cats. A pure platinum counter electrode having a surface area several thousand times that of the microelectrodes also was implanted beneath the muscle adjacent to the craniectomy. The microelectrodes were pulsed using charge-balanced, symmetrical, cathodic-first, controlled-current pulse pairs 3 weeks or longer after implantation.

During charge-balanced pulsing at high current densities, the charge capacity of chronically implanted platinum iridium microelectrodes is less than when measured in vitro in 0.9% normal saline. However, from the inflections of the time derivative of the induced voltage transient displayed against the transient voltage itself, it is possible to determine objectively if the electrode potentials reached during the stimulus pulses are excessive. Because they are independent of the stimulus current over a wide range, the downward inflections, or knees, marking recruitment of hydrogen evolution during the cathodic pulse and oxygen adsorption during the anodic phases seem to be useful markers.

Several factors complicate the use of markers such as hydrogen evolution and oxygen adsorption knees as a means of predicting whether hazardous electrochemical reactions will occur during pulsing, because factors other than the electrode potential may affect their reaction rates. However, some guidelines can be drawn from extant studies of the safety of certain stimulation protocols. Findings suggest that for platinum-iridium microelectrodes of approximately the size tested in this study, excursions of the electrode potential reaching approximately 250 mV beyond the oxygen adsorption knee (about 50 mV with respect to the chronically implanted platinum counter electrode) do not recruit oxidation reactions that produce toxic products or destroy vital substrate at a rate sufficient to engender neural damage.

▶ This study suggests that measurements of the induced voltage transient indicating recruitment of hydrogen evolution or oxygen absorption are useful markers of excess stimulus applied by a clinical implanted electrode. Substantial advances in electrode technology, together with enhanced understanding of the electrode tissue interface, are needed for the successful chronic utilization of implanted electrode systems for neural augmentation. In studies of electrode stimulation of paralyzed muscles, among 1,025 electrodes implanted in 6 patients during a 38-month period, 35% failed within 4 months; of these, 75% resulted from electrode movement (Marsolais EB, Kobetic R: *J Rehabil Res Dev* 23:1–8, 1986).—R.M. Crowell, M.D.

Brief Notes

Neural Implantation

In 2 instances, adrenal medullary grafts to the putamen resulted in transient beneficial effects in patients with severe Parkinson's disease (Lindvall O, et al: *Ann Neurol* 22:457–468, 1987).

Fine has nicely reviewed the current status of neurons transplanted into the central nervous system (CNS) (Fine A: *Sci Am* 255:52–63, 1986). In rats, grafts of embryonic brain tissue can be functionally incorporated into the adult CNS, particularly in rich vascular areas, e.g., the choroid plexus. Survival is enhanced when transplantation is done with multiplying and migrating embryonic neurons. Rejection of the graft does not occur. Such transplanted cells may produce neurochemicals such as dopamine. The behavioral effects of central lesions may be reversed by ingrafting embryonic cells.

In vitro release of acetylcholine can be demonstrated from the growing embryonic neuron (Sun YA, Poo MM: *Proc Natl Acad Sci USA* 84:2540–2544, 1987).

Successful utilization of fetal nerve cell grafts in animal models of neurodegenerative disease has prompted the first clinical attempts in Parkinson patients in at least three countries (Sladek JR, Gash DM: *J Neurosurg* 68:337–351, 1988).

In rats with prefrontal cortex lesions, transplantation of embryonic neocortex leads to functional benefits that are short lasting and attributable to diffuse influences rather than a reconnection of damaged circuitries (Dunnett SB, et al: *Behav Neurosci* 101:489–503, 1987).

It is reported that 5-HT neurons have been implanted successfully in the olfactory bulb of the adult rat (Mansour H, et al: *Neurochirurgie* 32:514–518, 1986).

Rejection of fetal neocortical neural transplants by H-2 incompatible mice suggests that the central nervous system is not unconditionally privileged as a transplant site or transplant source (Nicholas MK, et al: *J Immunol* 139:2275–2283, 1987).

Functional Surgery

During posterior fossa surgery in patients with hemifacial spasm, electrical stimulation of portions of the facial nerve resulted in responses from muscles outside the direct innervation of those branches. This suggests that hyperexcitability of the facial motor nucleus and facilitation of cross transmissions to other fascicles of the nerve are associated with hemifacial spasm (Møller AR, Jannetta PJ: *Exp Neurol* 93:584–600, 1986).

Hemifacial spasm may be caused by a cerebellopontine angle lipoma (Levin JM, Lee JE: *Neurology* 37:337–339, 1987).

Tabet and colleagues describe almost 400 operative procedures for central hyperhidrosis (Tabet JC, et al: *Cleve Clin J Med* 53:83–88, 1986). Bilateral T2 ganglionectomy is done through a midline upper thoracic incision with costotransversectomy.

In spasmodic torticollis, vestibular stimulation modulates neck electromyography (Bronstein AM, et al: *J Neurol Neurosurg Psychiatry* 50:580–586, 1987).—R.M. Crowell, M.D.

26 Peripheral Nerve

Introduction

Computed tomographic scanning is advocated for brachial plexopathy, but magnetic resonance imaging may eventually supersede (Abstract 26–1). Tumors of the brachial plexus may be excised with good results, especially neurofibromas (Abstract 26–2). Early microsurgical reconstruction has posted impressive results for birth palsy victims (Abstract 26–3). Silicone splints are said to aid fiber regeneration after peripheral nerve repair (Abstract 26–4).

Robert M. Crowell, M.D.

Radiographic Evaluation of Brachial Plexopathy
Armington WG, Harnsberger HR, Osborn AG, Seay AR (Univ of Utah, Salt Lake City)
AJNR 8:361–367, March–April 1987   26–1

The neurologic signs and symptoms of brachial plexopathy can be confusing, making clinical localization of disease along the length of the brachial plexus difficult. The most direct radiographic approach to diagnosing and anatomically delineating the cause of brachial plexopathy was determined, using the clinical and radiographic records of 43 patients who had features referable to the brachial plexus and who underwent computed tomography (CT) or myelography.

Ten had sustained traumatic injuries and 25 had malignant tumors. The remaining diagnoses included benign tumor, syrinx, brachial neuritis, and postoperative brachial neuropathy. In the nontrauma group, 26 lesions were palpable or nonpalpable. All 12 nonpalpable lesions were seen as clinically "silent" areas on CT; 10 of these were infiltrating, with only 2 displaying a focal mass on CT. Also in the nontrauma group, 31 patients underwent CT, complete CT examinations being done in 20. In 3 patients the disease process responsible for symptoms was missed because of incomplete CT evaluation; in 4 others there was a significant delay in diagnosis because of inadequate CT assessment.

All 11 patients with posttraumatic brachial plexopathy were evaluated with myelography initially. Two also had CT examinations, and 1 underwent magnetic resonance imaging (Fig 26–1). Ten patients had nerve root avulsions, and 1 had a dural tear associated with a bone fragment impinging on a cervical nerve root.

Trauma patients with brachial plexus symptoms should have cervical myelography first, rather than CT. Nontrauma patients should be classified according to clinical findings as having central or peripheral disease.

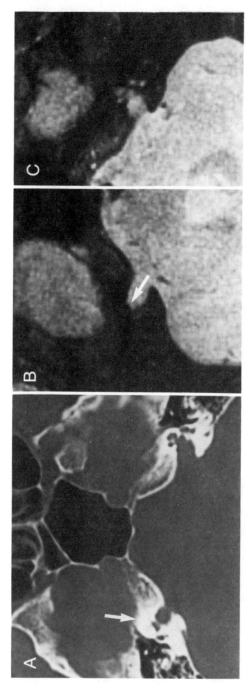

Fig 26–1.—Images of man aged 63 with a history of meningitis with subsequent profound bilateral sensory nerve hearing loss. **A,** thin-section axial CT scan at the level of the internal auditory canal shows ossification of the cochlear structures of the right temporal bone (*arrow*). **B,** long TR/long TE axial MR image of the cochlear regions shows that the left cochlea has 2 fluid-filled turns; the right cochlear turns cannot be identified because they have been replaced by bone. *Arrow* indicates modiolus. Diagnosis: labyrinthine ossificans. (Courtesy of Armington WG, Harnsberger HR, Osborn AG, et al: AJNR 8:361–367, March–April 1987.)

If the abnormality is central, myelography should be used first; if it is peripheral, CT should be used first. If disease extends beyond the anatomical compartment suggested clinically, the other technique should be used for further assessment.

▶ This interesting contribution offers an algorithm for selection of the most useful initial study in patients with brachial plexopathy. Magnetic resonance is likely to be helpful here.—R.M. Crowell, M.D.

Tumors of the Brachial Plexus
Lusk MD, Kline DG, Garcia CA (Louisiana State Univ; Charity and Ochsner Hosps, New Orleans)
Neurosurgery 21:439–453, October 1987   26–2

The incidence of brachial plexus tumors is low, and surgical management can be difficult. A precise understanding of pathologic variation is required, and each specific plexus element involved by tumor must be identified. Plexus tumors are more likely to be symptomatic than are those involving a more peripheral nerve; thus relatively early surgical management may be required. Fifty-six patients were treated for 57 tumors involving the brachial plexus.

The patients were seen in a 17-year period. The 40 neural sheath tumors included 26 neurofibromas, 8 schwannomas, 4 malignant neural sheath tumors, 1 fibrosarcoma, and 1 meningioma. Nine neurofibromas

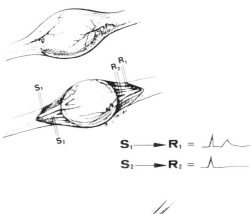

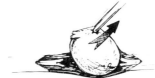

Fig 26–2.—Drawing of usual method of resection of a globular, nonplexiform neurofibroma. Fascicles entering and leaving the center of this tumor were not functional. (Courtesy of Lusk MD, Kline DG, Garcia CA: *Neurosurgery* 21:439–453, October 1987.)

were associated with von Recklinghausen's disease, and 2 were regionalized neurofibromas characterized by involvement of 1 limb with extension along the course of 1 or more plexus elements. Of the 17 tumors not of neural sheath origin, 7 were benign and 10 were metastatic malignant tumors compressing or invading the plexus.

Patients with benign neurofibromas and malignant sheath tumors almost always had pain or functional neural deficit. In patients with schwannomas a palpable mass was usually the only symptom initially. Patients with solitary neurofibromas were significantly older, often female, and more likely to have tumor on the right side than patients with schwannomas, malignant neural sheath tumors, or neurofibromas associated with von Recklinghausen's disease. Solitary neurofibromas usually could be resected totally without added deficit by sacrificing fascicles entering and exiting the tumor that were determined to be nonfunctional by intraoperative nerve action potential recordings. In contrast, a significant new deficit sometimes resulted from resection of neurofibromas associated with von Recklinghausen's disease (Fig 26–2). Schwannomas and benign nonneural sheath tumors were usually extirpated without damage to plexus elements (Fig 26–3). Forequarter amputation was advised for malignant intrinsic tumors that involved distal plexus elements, even when gross total resection seemed feasible.

In this series, the most common tumor was the neurofibroma, and 9 of the 26 neurofibromas were associated with von Recklinghausen's disease. Tumors in patients with this disease usually were plexiform and involved varying lengths of plexus elements.

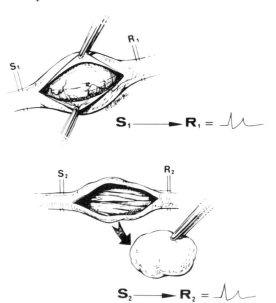

Fig 26–3.—Drawing of schwannoma resection. Because fascicles envelop the usual tumor mass, resection can always be achieved with minimal or no loss of function. (Courtesy of Lusk MD, Kline DG, Garcia CA: *Neurosurgery* 21:439–453, October 1987.)

▶ This series of brachial plexus tumors, the largest yet published, defines the state of this complex problem. Surgical resection emphasizing anatomical principles and use of action potentials intraoperatively is fundamental to appropriate management. The approach to patients with von Recklinghausen's disease and malignant plexus tumors remains controversial. Accumulation of further numbers of well-studied patients is required to sharpen understanding and improve management of these difficult cases.— R.M. Crowell, M.D.

Early Microsurgical Reconstruction in Birth Palsy
Kawabata H, Masada K, Tsuyuguchi Y, Kawai H, Ono K, Tada K (Osaka Univ, Osaka, Kagawa Med School, Kagawa, Japan)
Clin Orthop 215:233–242, February 1987   26–3

Some infants with birth palsy from plexus lesions fail to recover spontaneously. Early surgical nerve reconstruction might offer a means of improving the functional prognosis in such cases. Six infants referred at an average age of 3.7 months with unilateral involvement were operated on. Three had upper plexus and 3 had whole plexus lesions. Two of the former infants were breech presentations.

Exploration was carried out about 6 months after birth when signs of recovery in the shoulder and elbow were absent. Metrizamide myelography and computed tomographic myelography were carried out preoperatively, along with the histamine axon reflex test. Root sensory evoked potentials, nerve action potentials, and evoked muscle responses were recorded intraoperatively to plan microsurgical nerve repair, rather than relying only on macroscopic appearances (Fig 26–4). Neurolysis was carried out for lesions in continuity, and postganglionic rupture was managed by nerve graft transplantation. Neurotization was added if more than 2 completely ruptured or avulsed nerve roots were present.

After a follow-up averaging 28 months, all evaluable patients had

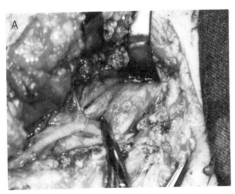
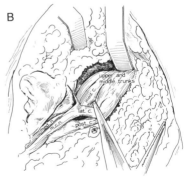

Fig 26–4.—**A**, macroscopic findings of brachial plexus lesion. The upper plexus is damaged more than the lower plexus (**B**), *med. c.*, indicates medial cord; *lat. c.*, lateral cord; *post. c.*, posterior cord; *med. n.*, median nerve; and *m.c.n.*, musculocutaneous nerve. (Courtesy of Kawabata H, Masada K, Tsuyuguchi Y, et al: *Clin Orthop* 215:233–242, February 1987.)

more than 90 degrees of forward flexion of the arm. External rotation of the arm was excellent in 3 patients and good in 2. Four patients had excellent and 1 had good elbow flexion. Finger motion remains unsatisfactory, however.

The results of early microsurgical reconstruction of the brachial plexus in infants with refractory birth palsy have not been disappointing. Intraoperative electrodiagnosis is an important aspect of the procedure.

▶ The results are encouraging, but aggressive surgery for birth palsy caused by brachial plexus lesions needs more study before it can be recommended. Application of established principles for brachial plexus surgery, aided by intraoperative electrodiagnostics, is essential.—R.M. Crowell, M.D.

Extent of Fiber Regeneration After Peripheral Nerve Repair: Silicone Splint vs. Suture, Gap Repair vs. Graft

Ashur H, Vilner Y, Finsterbush A, Rousso M, Weinberg H, Devor M (Hadassah Mt Scopus Univ Hosp, Hebrew Univ of Jerusalem)
Exp Neurol 97:365–374, August 1987   26–4

One of the main goals of nerve repair is to maximize the number of fibers that regenerate past the suture line. A simple, quantitative electrophysiologic method, which compares the size of nerve responses evoked by stimulation distal and proximal to the anastomosis, allows measurement of the degree of nerve regeneration past the suture line. The ratio of the potential evoked by stimulating distal and proximal to the anastomosis was calculated in 5 different repair procedures using rat sciatic nerves. In procedure A, a simple end-to-end suture anastomosis was performed. In procedure B, the nerve suture was covered with a thin-wall polyester fiber-reinforced silicone sheath with a narrow longitudinal slit. In procedure C, the nerve ends were approximated but not sutured, and a silicone sheath was applied so that its 2 anchoring sutures prevented nerve separation. Procedure D was similar to procedure C, except that a 5-mm gap was left between nerve ends and covered with a silicone sheath. In procedure E, the nerve was cut twice at a 5-mm interval; the isolated nerve segment was lifted out and immediately replaced and sutured at both ends; the region of the autograft was covered with a silicone sheath.

After simple anastomosis, about 40% of the severed parent fibers regenerated past the suture line. However, regeneration was significantly improved to 63.4% when the suture line was ensheathed in silicone (procedure B); these results were comparable to those of procedure C, indicating that the presence or absence of suture thread at the point of anastomosis had no effect on nerve regeneration. Regeneration across a 5-mm gap ensheathed in silicone was better (67%) than regeneration through a 5-mm autograft (45%).

Application of a pliable thin silicone sheath provides a simple and useful supplementary treatment for a variety of peripheral nerve repairs. Contrary to previous reports, the extent of regeneration is not affected by the presence or absence of suture material at the point of anastomosis. Most encouraging is the relatively successful regeneration across a 5-mm gap, largely as a result of the use of the slit silicone sheath as well.

▶ This interesting report suggests that a silicone sheath improves penetration of fibers across a gap in peripheral nerve repair. These results are counter to unfavorable results previously obtained in neurosurgical investigations. The results were validated in the present study by an interesting electrophysiologic technique but not with long-term anatomical or clinical implants; these would be needed to validate this method before clinical application.—R.M. Crowell, M.D.

Brief Notes on Peripheral Nerve Topics

Brachial Plexus

Myelography with postmyelographic computed tomographic scanning provides excellent diagnostic accuracy in the demonstration of root avulsion after brachial plexus injury (Marshall RW, Desilva RGD: *J Bone Joint Surg* 68B: 734–738, 1986).

Scapulothoracic dissociation is associated with severe brachial plexus injury and an unreconstructable, nonfunctional upper extremity that may require amputation and fitting for prosthesis (Kelbel JM, et al: *Clin Orthop* 209:210–214, 1986).

Tumors

Immunocytochemical techniques have been used to demonstrate calcineurin in human nerve cell tumors (Goto S, et al: *Cancer* 60:2948–2957, 1987).

Technetium-99m pertechnetate effectively localizes and sizes peripheral nerve tumors, even when clinically occult (Koch KJ, et al: *J Nucl Med* 27:1713–1716, 1986).

Twenty-five limb schwannomas were treated microsurgically, with grafting required only occasionally, with mixed nerves being affected and associated neurologic deficit (Lebreton E, et al: *Sem Hop Paris* 62:3267–3273, 1986).

Magnetic resonance imaging correctly identified all 15 tumors involving the brachial plexus, and in 25 patients with no neurologic signs or symptoms correctly identified tumor outside the brachial plexus (Castagno AA, Shuman WP: *AJR* 149:1219–1222, 1987).

Excision of a malignant schwannoma of the sciatic nerve was followed by recovery with a 20-year follow-up (Duplay J, et al: *Sem Hop Paris* 62:3555–3557, 1986).

A sciatic neurilemoma can cause sciatica. Computed tomographic scanning can be diagnostic. Surgical removal may be followed by normal neurologic function (Prusick VR, et al: *J Bone Joint Surg* 68A:1456–1458, 1986.)

Nerve Regeneration and Grafting

Laminin-coated filament can provide in vivo guidance of regenerating nerve axons (Yoshii S, et al: *Exp Neurol* 96:469–473, 1987).

After reinnervation of rat muscle, there is evidence for dissociation of physiologic and histochemical properties (Gillespie MJ, et al: *J Neurophysiol* 57:921–937, 1987).

Results in adult monkey experiments demonstrate that either a distal nerve stump or a nerve graft will act as a specific target for regenerating primate proximal nerve stump (Mackinnon SE, et al: *J Hand Surg* 11A:888–894, 1986).

Rayment et al. studied 8 patients with cross-facial nerve transplantation (Rayment R, et al: *Br J Plast Surg* 40:592–597, 1987). They found useful voluntary movement after this approach in patients even 15 years after onset of the palsy, with a number of patients more than 2 years after palsy.

Peripheral nerve regeneration with entubulation repair is dependent on the composition of the tubular prostheses and varies according to the time of survival of the experimental animals (Madison RD, et al: *Exp Neurol* 95:378–390, 1987).

Astrocytes block axonal regeneration in mammals by activating the physiologic stop pathway (Liuzzi FJ, Lasek RJ: *Science* 237:642–649, 1987).—R.M. Crowell, M.D.

27 Neuroscience

Introduction

Among the torrent of clinically relevant reports in basic neuroscience, a few deserve special attention. The status of *information storage* via biochemical mechanisms has been reviewed by Black and colleagues at Cornell (Abstract 27−1). The extraordinarily important brain *calcium channels* have been characterized by immunologic techniques (Abstract 27−2). Radioimmunoassay and genetic techniques have been used to visualize and characterize *interleukin-1 receptors* in the brain (Abstract 27−3). *Atrial natriuretic factor* has been identified in the brain and may have important implications for water and electrolyte metabolism (Abstract 27−4).

Robert M. Crowell, M.D.

Biochemistry of Information Storage in the Nervous System
Black IB, Adler JE, Dreyfus CF, Friedman WF, LaGamma EF, Roach AH (Cornell Univ)
Science 236:1263−1268, June 5, 1987   27−1

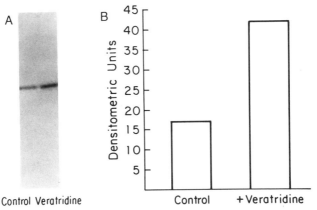

Fig 27−1.—Results of immunoblot analysis performed with ^{125}I-labeled protein A and a specific antiserum against tyrosine hydroxylase (TH) to quantitate enzyme protein after depolarization. The TH molecule number was increased by depolarization, suggesting that impulse activity may increase the number of enzyme molecules in brain neurons. **A**, visualization of immunoreactive TH protein extracted from locus ceruleus cultures grown for 1 week and then exposed to control nutrient medium *(C)* or veratridine-supplemented nutrient medium *(V)* for an additional week. **B**, densitometric analysis. Density of bands is expressed in arbitrary densitometric units. (Courtesy of Black IB, Adler JE, Dreyfus CF, et al: *Science* 236:1263−1268, June 5, 1987.)

Functionally critical molecules in the peripheral and central nervous systems now are known to encode and store environmental information over time. Memory no longer is regarded as being localized to restricted cell populations in the brain. Storage over time in the peripheral sympathetic system regulates cardiovascular function, whereas storage in the locus ceruleus system of the brain is important in arousal and attention.

Long-term induction of tyrosine hydroxylase (TH) by relatively brief stimuli is mediated by a rise in TH messenger ribonucleic acid (mRNA) and increased biosynthesis of TH. Environmental stimuli, through altering steady-state levels of mRNA species-encoding neurotransmitters, can alter synaptic and neuronal functions over time. Altered impulse activity and membrane depolarization are followed by selective changes in the expression of specific transmitter genes. The precise intracellular mechanisms involved remain to be determined.

Biochemical mechanisms of information storage may be discerned in diverse peripheral and central neuronal populations (Fig 27–1). The potential for mnemonic function may be widely distributed in the nervous system. Increased understanding of the molecular plasticity of synapses may help to elucidate mnemonic functions at the molecular, cellular, and system levels.

▶ Rudimentary memory traces may be stored in single neurons in the central or peripheral neurons systems. This discovery gives support to molecular strategies to improve memory, as in Alzheimer's disease. Such approaches might include intraventricular drug infusions or transplantations.—R.M. Crowell, M.D.

Identification of an α Subunit of Dihydropyridine-Sensitive Brain Calcium Channels

Takahashi M, Catterall WA (Univ of Washington, Seattle)
Science 236:88–91, Apr 3, 1987   27–2

The voltage-sensitive calcium channel is a key factor in the control of calcium-linked cellular functions, e.g., action-potential generation, muscle contraction, and hormone and neurotransmitter secretion. Because of the importance of Ca^{2+} channels in neurons and the many functional differences between Ca^{2+} channels in neurons and skeletal muscle, it is of interest to determine the molecular properties of dihydropyridine-sensitive Ca^{2+} channels in the brain. The polyclonal antibodies (PACs) that recognize the α subunits of the purified skeletal muscle Ca^{2+} channel were identified and used to mark and compare a corresponding polypeptide component of the dihydropyridine-sensitive Ca^{2+} channels in the brain.

Polyclonal antibodies (PAC–2) against the α subunits of purified rabbit skeletal muscle calcium channels immunoprecipitated those channels labeled with the dihydropyridine PN200–110 from skeletal muscle and brain. The immunoreactivity of PAC–2 with the skeletal muscle channel was greater than that with the brain calcium channel and was absorbed

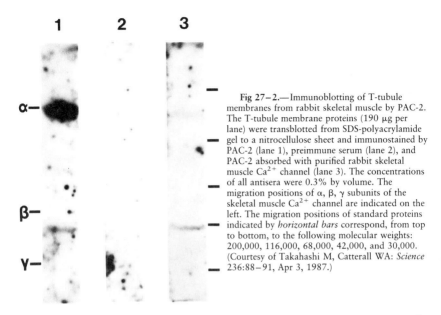

Fig 27–2.—Immunoblotting of T-tubule membranes from rabbit skeletal muscle by PAC-2. The T-tubule membrane proteins (190 μg per lane) were transblotted from SDS-polyacrylamide gel to a nitrocellulose sheet and immunostained by PAC-2 (lane 1), preimmune serum (lane 2), and PAC-2 absorbed with purified rabbit skeletal muscle Ca^{2+} channel (lane 3). The concentrations of all antisera were 0.3% by volume. The migration positions of α, β, γ subunits of the skeletal muscle Ca^{2+} channel are indicated on the left. The migration positions of standard proteins indicated by *horizontal bars* correspond, from top to bottom, to the following molecular weights: 200,000, 116,000, 68,000, 42,000, and 30,000. (Courtesy of Takahashi M, Catterall WA: *Science* 236:88–91, Apr 3, 1987.)

partially by treatment earlier with the brain channel (Fig 27–2). Polyclonal antibodies could specifically recognize a large peptide in synaptic plasma membranes of rabbit brain with an apparent molecular size of 169,000 daltons. This protein resembles an α subunit of the skeletal muscle calcium channel in apparent molecular weight, antigenic properties, and electrophoretic behavior after reduction of disulfide bonds.

The dihydropyridine-sensitive calcium channel of rabbit brain has an α subunit that is homologous, but not identical, to those of the skeletal muscle calcium channel. The different functional properties of these channels may result from minor variations in structurally similar components.

▶ In this lovely work, immunologic techniques were used to discriminate the molecular properties of various types of Ca^{2+} channels in various tissues. Further characterization of the anatomical and physiologic properties of calcium channels are likely to lead to improved understanding of these critical pores, which have emerged as so crucial to a number of cellular functions, e.g., neurotransmitter secretion. In a related study, Wendling and Harakel (*Stroke* 18:591–598, 1987) report that verapamil and nifedipine block calcium uptake through various channels in bovine middle cerebral arteries.—R.M. Crowell, M.D.

Visualization and Characterization of Interleukin 1 Receptors in Brain
Farrar WL, Kilian PL, Ruff MR, Hill JM, Pert CB (Natl Cancer Inst, Frederick, Md; Hoffman-LaRoche, Nutley, NJ; Natl Insts of Health, Bethesda, Md)
J Immunol 139:459–463, July 1987   27–3

Although best known for its effect on the central nervous system (CNS) to cause fever, interleukin-1 (IL-1) also influences cell growth, food intake, and slow-wave sleep. The neuroanatomical distribution of IL-1 receptors in rat brain was examined. A binding assay for ^{125}I-labeled recombinant murine IL-1 that was developed was highly specific. Affinity cross-linking studies indicated that the rat brain IL-1 receptor has a molecular weight of approximately 80,000, which is similar to the previously described recognition molecule on T cells and fibroblasts.

Throughout the rat brain, ^{125}I-IL-1 binding was widespread and detectable, using autoradiographic techniques, in numerous discrete brain areas. The binding was most evident in neuron-rich regions, e.g., the granule cell layer of the dentate gyrus, the pyramidal cell layer of the hippocampus, and the granule cell layer of the cerebellum, as well as the hypothalamus, and is almost the same as the pattern achieved by staining brain sections for Nissl with classic methods.

That both the binding of IL-1 and neuron-stained sections are most dense in regions where cell bodies are clustered suggests that IL-1 binding might occur in neurons throughout the brain. Where neurons are dense, binding is dense; where neurons are sparse, binding is pale. Several features of the IL-1 binding pattern differ from those of a cell stain pattern, supporting the idea that the receptors are localized on only a subset of neurons. Although the IL-1 binding pattern is similar to that of a cell stain typically used to identify the boundaries of nuclei, the possibility that IL-1 is bound to neuron-associated glial cells in these regions cannot be excluded.

Two potential binding proteins that may represent binding proteins of heterogeneity or possible degradation products typical of this form of analyses were revealed by affinity cross-linking of ^{125}I-IL-α to rat brain, but the 2 species discerned are in accordance with described binding proteins for T lymphocytes, fibroblasts, and B lymphocytes. Both species are believed to bind to the same receptor, as well as generating febrile responses.

These data provide a unique example of a common receptor for a cytokine produced by both the immune system and the central nervous system. The biologic role of IL-1 may be distinctive in the respective systems, although a similar receptor is identified in both physiologic systems. Autoradiography allows quantitative and qualitative evaluation of receptor distribution, which may provide clues to physiologic behavior and neuroendocrine activities of IL-1 previously not appreciated.

▶ This exciting study combines radioautography and the monoclonal antibody technique for visualization and characterization of IL-1 receptors in brain. This is a unique example of a common receptor for a cytokine produced both by the immune system and the central nervous system (CNS). Further studies are underway to characterize this group of receptors, which may have important functions in CNS physiology as well as in immunologic control of tumors.— R.M. Crowell, M.D.

Regulation of Brain Water and Electrolyte Contents: The Possible Involvement of Central Atrial Natriuretic Factor

Dóczi T, Joó F, Szerdahelyi P, Bodosi M (Univ Med School; Biological Res Ctr, Szeged, Hungary)

Neurosurgery 21:454–458, October 1987   27–4

Atrial natriuretic factor (ANF)-like immunoreactive cells have been found in human and rat brain. Because a central neuroendocrine system has been hypothesized to regulate brain tissue ion and volume homeostasis, a study was conducted to determine the role of ANF in the control of brain water and electrolyte balance in rats. Synthetic rat ANF (syn rANF), 2 µg, sequence 101–126 of the precursor, was administered into the right lateral ventricle after intravenous infusion of a hyposmolar fluid load (2.5% dextrose in water). Rats without intravenous fluid load served as controls.

Administration of a hyposmolar fluid load alone increased brain water content significantly because of a water intoxication mechanism. Intraventricular administration of syn rANF prevented water accumulation in the hemispheres induced by a systemic hyposmolar fluid load. In addition, there was a significant loss of sodium from the nervous tissue, but the potassium content remained unchanged. This effect of syn rANF was not mediated by systemic changes, as syn rANF administration had no effect on serum osmolality and ion content. Administration of syn rANF to rats not treated with a hyposmolar fluid load caused no significant change in the water, potassium, or sodium content of the brain.

It appears that centrally administered ANF prevents water accumulation in the brain after systemic water intoxication. These data support the hypothesis that a central neuroendocrine system regulates brain ion and volume homeostasis. The possible role of ANF in the management of cerebral edema should be considered.

▶ This initial attempt to demonstrate a physiologic role in the central nervous system for ANF opens an interesting new chapter for homeostasis. Although the authors suggest that the results indicate that ANF acts directly on the cerebral capillaries to prevent brain water accumulation, there are methodologic objections to this conclusion, including the use of an unphysiologic vehicle (0.9% sodium chloride) and the use of a 2.5% glucose solution without determining its effect on blood pressure or cerebral blood flow. We await further studies in this exciting new area that address the various methodologic problems inherent in such difficult experiments.— R.M. Crowell, M.D.

Brief Notes on Neuroscience Topics

Neurogenetics

Members of a nicotinic acetylcholine receptor gene family are expressed in different regions of the mammalian central nervous system (Goldman D, et al: *Cell* 48:965–973, 1987).

In the proteolipid protein gene, an alternative splice site selection can determine the product of a specific cellular gene. This is critical in the development of central nervous system myelin assembly (Nave KA, et al: *Proc Natl Acad Sci USA* 84:5665–5669, 1987).

Cloning of complementary DNA for GAP-43, a neuronal growth-related protein, has recently been reported (Karns LR, et al: *Science* 236:597–600, 1987).

Other Topics

Radioimmunoassays have been used to characterize a variety of dynorphins, opioid peptides in the rat brain, and the spinal cord (Xie GX, Goldstein A: *J Neurosci* 7:2049–2055, 1987).

A digoxin-like natriuretic factor is released in response to subarachnoid hemorrhage, probably as a result of hypothalamic damage (Wijdicks EFM, et al: *Br Med J* 294:729–732, 1987).—R.M. Crowell, M.D.

28 Miscellaneous Topics

Introduction

Patients with acquired immunodeficiency syndrome often require non-neurosurgical interventions, including abdominal and thoracic surgery (Abstract 28–1). Modern investigations have permitted improved understanding of intracranial hemorrhage in infective endocarditis and appropriate management of these patients (Abstract 28–2). Magnetic resonance imaging (MRI) and computed tomography (CT) have complementary utilization in the diagnosis of neurocysticercosis (Abstract 28–3). Epidermoid cyst of the brain may now be readily recognized by CT and MRI (Abstract 28–4).

Robert M. Crowell, M.D.

Surgery in Patients With Acquired Immunodeficiency Syndrome
Robinson G, Wilson SE, Williams RA (Univ of California at Los Angeles)
Arch Surg 122:170–175, February 1987   28–1

A review was made of data on 21 patients with acquired immunodeficiency syndrome (AIDS) on whom 31 operations were performed at 2 centers in 1982–1985. Skin, lymph node, and endoscopic biopsy speci-

Infections and Neoplasms Found at Surgery*

Condition	No. of Cases
Infections	
Cytomegalovirus	
Colon	2
Lung	1
Epididymis	1
Toxoplasmosis	
Central nervous system	2
Candida	
Gallbladder	1
Staphylococcus	
Pericardium, botryomycosis	1
Ameba (Hartmannella-Acanthamoeba group)	
Central nervous system	1
Neoplasms	
Kaposi's sarcoma	
Small bowel and colon	1
Cystic duct	1
Lung	1
Poorly differentiated gastrointestinal lymphoma	
Stomach and duodenum	1

*(Courtesy of Robinson G, Wilson SE, Williams RA: *Arch Surg* 122:170–175, February 1987.)

mens were not included in the series. The 20 men and 1 woman had a mean age of 36 years. All patients met the Centers for Disease Control case definition for AIDS. There were 8 major elective operations, 16 minor elective operations, and 7 emergency procedures in the series. Four emergency operations were tube thoracostomies and 2 were celiotomies for cytomegalovirus (CMV) colitis. Elective thoracotomy with open-lung biopsy was done on 4 occasions. Five patients underwent elective abdominal operations.

The pathologic findings included CMV colonic perforation, disseminated Kaposi's sarcoma of the bowel, cystic duct obstruction by Kaposi's sarcoma, *Candida* acalculous cholecystitis, staphylococcal botryomycosis of the pericardium, and pulmonary Kaposi's sarcoma. The most common infective agent was CMV (table). Operative mortality was 57% after emergency surgery and 48% overall. Deaths usually were secondary to progressive opportunistic infection or malignancy.

About half of all surgically treated patients with AIDS in this series died within 30 days of surgery. High operative mortality usually was associated with progression of opportunistic infection, most often CMV, or malignancy.

▶ Neurosurgeons should be aware of the non-neurologic aspects of AIDS. The central nervous system is commonly involved, but Kaposi's sarcoma or opportunistic infection may affect the lung, pericardium, bowel, or gallbladder. Because infected body fluid may spread the virus to the surgical team, double gloves and protective glasses are recommended for all procedures, as well as extraordinary care to avoid needle sticks.—R.M. Crowell, M.D.

Mechanisms of Intracranial Hemorrhage in Infective Endocarditis
Hart RG, Kagan-Hallet K, Joerns SE (Univ of Texas, San Antonio)
Stroke 18:1048–1056, November–December 1987   28–2

About 5% of patients with infective endocarditis sustain intracranial hemorrhage. This is usually ascribed to a ruptured mycotic aneurysm, but septic erosion of the arterial wall also may be responsible. Data on 17 patients with active infective endocarditis and intracranial hemorrhage were reviewed. Hemorrhage was diagnosed from a noncalcific computed tomography density or xanthochromic spinal fluid. Eight percent of patients with infective endocarditis had intracranial hemorrhage, which was present at admission in 7 of the 17 patients.

Six patients were intravenous drug abusers. About half were infected with *Staphylococcus aureus*. Five patients received anticoagulation or had a bleeding diathesis at the time of hemorrhage. Ten patients (59%) died. Seven patients had endocarditis caused by *S. aureus*, with onset of intracranial hemorrhage during uncontrolled infection. All 3 studied had septic arteritis (Fig 28–1). Two others had secondary hemorrhagic transformation in association with anticoagulation; 2 nonanticoagulated pa-

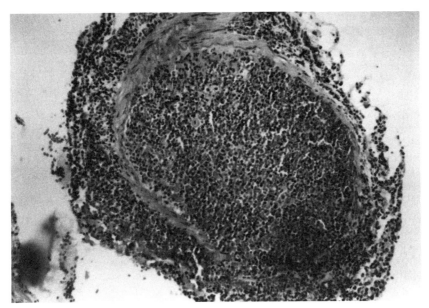

Fig 28–1.—Septic embolus in middle cerebral artery with pyogenic arteritis. (Courtesy of Hart RG, Kagan-Hallet K, Joerns SE: *Stroke* 18:1048–1056, November–December 1987.)

tients had a similar disorder. Only 2 patients had a proved mycotic aneurysm.

Intracranial hemorrhage complicating infective endocarditis can result from acute pyogenic necrosis or an aseptic aneurysm that ruptures some time after bacteriologic cure. True mycotic aneurysms are uncommon in this setting. *Staphylococcus aureus* most often underlies symptomatic intracranial bleeding. These hemorrhages usually occur during the stage of uncontrolled infection.

▶ New data assists the neuroclinician in the management of neurologic aspects of bacterial endocarditis. Computed tomographic (CT) scanning can diagnose intracranial hemorrhage even when it is asymptomatic. Therefore, patients with bacterial endocarditis should have a CT scan with and without contrast enhancement. Although the frequency of bacterial aneurysm in intracranial hemorrhage from endocarditis is low, patients with such hemorrhage should have cerebral angiography when their condition stabilizes. It may also be argued that patients with sudden focal deficit, even in the absence of intracranial hemorrhage, should undergo angiography. Intravenous antibiotic therapy is the mainstay of management in all of these patients, because most of the aneurysms will thrombose on this program. Only with enlarging aneurysms despite antibiotic therapy is surgical excision recommended.

In a related study, Panzer et al. (*Arch Intern Med* 145:1800–1803, 1985) used multivariant statistical analysis to help with clinical differentiation of hemorrhage from infarct. Coma on arrival was present in 60% of the patients with hemorrhage. Marked hypertension, unrecognized hypoglycemia, and warfarin therapy are common with hemorrhage. If 3 or more of these predictors were present, the probability of hemorrhage was more than two thirds. If all of these predictors were absent, the probability of hemorrhage was less than 5%. Nonetheless, to be sure a CT scan will be needed.—R.M. Crowell, M.D.

MRI and CT Patterns of Neurocysticercosis

Rodiek SO, Rupp N, von Einsiedel HG (Städtisches Krankenhaus München-Bogenhausen und Institut für Räntgendiagnostik; Techn Univ München, West Germany)
Fortschr Röntgenstr 146:570–577, 1987   28–3

Neurocysticercosis is a parasitic disorder that is caused by infestation of a larval pork tapeworm. Transmission is usually via fruits or vegetables that have been fertilized with contaminated pig manure. The small oncospheres penetrate the intestinal mucosa and are quickly carried to target organs such as the brain and muscles where lesions start to develop within 2–3 months. Neurocysticercosis commonly causes multiple lesions, but the morphology of such lesions depends on the stages of the parasite's life cycle and can include the presence of vital cysticerci, inflammatory parenchymatous reactions to degenerating cysts, and calcified granulomas. A previous study showed that computed tomography (CT) accurately diagnosed cysticercosis in 97% of the cases. Five patients with cysticercosis were examined by CT; 4 were also examined by magnetic resonance imaging (MRI).

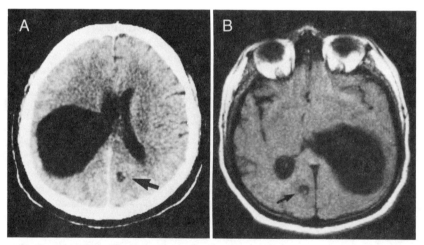

Fig 28–2.—**A,** native CT. Large parieto-occipital cysticercus cyst. Displacement of the midline structure toward the contralateral side. Small cysts with peripheral scoleces are visible in the occipital lobe (*arrow*). **B,** axial MR (SE: TR 0.5/TE 35). Scolex of the cyst in the paramedial occipital lobe appears larger than on CT. Fluid in the large cysticercus shows signal similar to that of cerebrospinal fluid. (Courtesy of Rodiek SO, Rupp N, von Einsiedel HG: *Fortschr Röntgenstr* 146:570–577, 1987.)

Man, 30, originally from Yugoslavia, was hospitalized because of increasingly severe one-sided headaches of 4 weeks' duration and one-sided weakness and paresthesias. Five years earlier, while visiting his homeland, he had passed a tapeworm. While the patient was in the hospital, acute symptoms of cerebral decompensation and vascular constriction developed; he became comatose and stopped breathing. The CT and MRI examinations of the brain showed a large, parieto-occipital cyst on the left side (Fig 28–2). He underwent emergency operation for removal of the cyst. The patient was fully coherent on the first postoperative day and recovered without any neurologic sequelae.

A comparison of CT and MR imaging showed that, whereas CT can identify small calcifications that are usually missed by MRI, the latter technique is superior in showing morphological details of the cyst wall and scolex. The 2 diagnostic techniques are complementary methods that together provide a high degree of specificity in the diagnosis of neurocysticercosis.

▶ This communication shows how MRI and CT can be complementary in the diagnosis and management of neurocysticercosis. Although praziquantel is frequently effective, occasionally surgical intervention (particularly for intraventricular lesions) will be needed, as shown in this presentation.— R.M. Crowell, M.D.

Atypical Epidermoid Cyst of the Brain
Naim ur-Rahman (King Saud Univ, Riyadh, Saudi Arabia)
Neurosurgery 22:122–124, 1988   28–4

Epidermoid and dermoid cysts of the brain typically appear as low-density mass lesions on computed tomography (CT). Few hyperdense lesions have been described. Because CT attenuation values depend on chemical composition as well as on the physical state of density, the fluid in certain dermoid and epidermoid cysts may have such a high attenuation value that it is indistinguishable from that of a solid tumor of similar shape and location. A patient was seen with an epidermoid cyst of the brain erroneously diagnosed as meningioma on CT.

Man, 60, had been treated for epilepsy and intermittent headache for 20 years. He began to have gradually increasing morning headache and weakness in an arm and a leg. Plain CT showed a large, sharply defined, uniformly hyperdense tumor occupying most of the right middle cranial fossa. A marked midline shift was noted. Contrast administration did not change this picture. The clinical findings, in addition to the CT findings, led to a diagnosis of meningioma, although angiography showed an avascular, infrasylvian mass with marked upward displacement of the middle cerebral artery. A large right temporal craniotomy was done with the expectation of finding a solid tumor. A large cyst was encountered and 120 ml of viscid, yellow fluid was aspirated. A postoperative scan showed total removal of the cyst. Rapid, complete resolution of neurologic symptoms followed surgery.

Because there is considerable overlap in the attenuation values of various fluid and solid lesions, a definitive diagnosis is not always possible on the basis of CT results alone. Correlation must be made with the results of other diagnostic tests, particularly angiography.

▶ This case report demonstrates that an epidermoid cyst may show up on CT with hyperdensity. Appropriate depiction by magnetic resonance can often help make the diagnosis (bright on T1 and T2), although occasionally angiography may be necessary.—R.M. Crowell, M.D.

Clinical and Magnetic Resonance Features of Primary Intracranial Arachnoid Cysts

Gandy SE, Heier LA (New York Hosp-Cornell Med Ctr, New York, NY)
Ann Neurol 21:342–348, April 1987   28–5

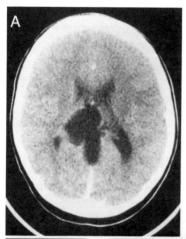

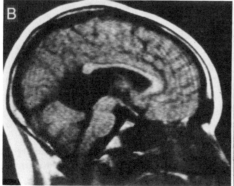

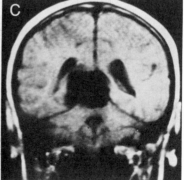

Fig 28–3.—Computed tomographic scan (**A**) and magnetic resonance images (MRI) (**B** and **C**) of a 24-year-old man with nystagmus and truncal ataxia. The CT scan shows a hypodense mass lesion of the quadrigeminal cistern, revealed by MRI to be an arachnoid cyst distorting the superior cerebellum. (Courtesy of Gandy ES, Heier LA: *Ann Neurol:* 21:342–348, April 1987.)

The clinical findings were reviewed concerning 33 patients with primary intracranial arachnoid cysts seen in 1979–1984. Nine patients underwent magnetic resonance imaging with multiple spin-echo techniques. All patients but 4 had neurologic syndromes referable to the cyst.

Computed tomography (CT) showed 22 cysts to be exclusively supratentorial, 9 were subtentorial, and 2 extended above and below the tentorium. Magnetic resonance imaging was especially helpful in localizing subtentorial and temporal fossa lesions and in the multiplanar definition of complex cysts (Fig 28–3). Magnetic resonance also was useful in distinguishing arachnoid cysts from other lesions that are hypodense on CT scans. Surgery was carried out in 11 patients with symptomatic brain compression, 8 with hydrocephalus, and 2 with cranial nerve palsies. The outcome was uniformly good, but mild focal weakness and seizure disorders persisted in some patients. All patients maintained the premorbid level of neurologic functioning.

Surgery is indicated for patients with primary intracranial arachnoid cyst when disability results from either brain compression or obstruction of cerebrospinal fluid flow. Appropriately managed patients can expect to have an excellent clinical outcome.

▶ Multiplanar magnetic resonance imaging is the best diagnostic examination for suspected arachnoid cyst. Usually, depiction is adequate to permit management without contrast studies. When cyst compression is symptomatic, cyst-peritoneal shunting is indicated. When hydrocephalus is symptomatic, ventriculoperitoneal shunting is indicated. The relatively benign course and good results of shunting are strong arguments against radical cyst removal or marsupialization into cisterns.— R.M. Crowell, M.D.

Brief Notes on Miscellaneous Topics

AIDS

Cerebral mucormycosis has been reported in patients with acquired immunodeficiency syndrome (Cuadrado LM, et al: *Arch Neurol* 45:109–111, 1988).

Nocardial cerebral abscess in patients with acquired immunodeficiency syndrome may require complete surgical excision (Adair JC, et al: *Arch Neurol* 44:548–550, 1987).

Genetic variation of human immunodeficiency viruses in the central nervous system can lead to distinctly different cellular invasions (Koyanagi Y, et al: *Science* 236:819–822, 1987).

Intracranial Infections

Cerebral aspergillosis in 4 patients was diagnosed by surgical biopsy and treated with antifungal drugs intravenously; the mortality rate was 75% (Hajjar J, et al: *Neurochirurgie* 33:142–147, 1987).

Magnetic resonance imaging of intraventricular cysticercosis is superior to computed tomography (Rhee RS, et al: *J Comput Assist Tomogr* 11:598–604, 1987).

Intraventricular therapy of cryptococcal meningitis by a subcutaneous reservoir in combination with systemic therapy with amphotericin seems beneficial and relatively safe in patients with meningitis and a poor prognosis (Polsky B, et al: *Am J Med* 81:24–28, 1986).

In 10 patients symptomatic intracranial tuberculoma developed during the treatment of tuberculosis (Teoh R, et al: *Q J Med* 63:449–460, 1987).

Spinal Infections

Magnetic resonance images tuberculous spondylitis with particular clarity in the coronal plane (de Roos A, et al: *AJR* 147:79–82, 1986).

In 30 reported patients, gas within the vertebral body or disk space is associated with spinal infection (Bielecki DK, et al: *AJR* 147:83–86, 1986).

Postlaminectomy disk space infection has been reported in 125 patients to date. Recurrent pain after initial relief and muscle spasm, fever, and positive straight leg raising are the most common signs. An increased sedimentation rate is almost always present. Radioisotope and computed tomography scan abnormalities may appear within 1–2 weeks, but plain films require several weeks before abnormal findings appear. Needle biopsy and aspiration under image intensification increases the frequency of bacteriologic diagnosis. Conservative management with bed rest and antibiotics is the treatment of choice. Occasionally, early surgery may be required; late surgical intervention is facilitated by an anterior approach (Fernand R, Lee CK: *Clin Orthop* 209:215–218, 1986).

Among 12 patients with neurologic complications of vertebral osteomyelitis, good results were obtained in 8, with poor results in 2, and 2 deaths. Diagnosis was facilitated by myelography and postmyelographic computed tomography. Treatment of anterior compression was carried out by costotransversectomy. Diffuse abscesses were treated with laminectomy (Abramovitz JN, et al: *Spine* 11:418–421, 1986).

Experiments with sheep indicated that diskitis is initiated by infection, although bacteria were difficult to isolate 3 weeks and later after initial inoculation (Fraser RD, et al: *J Bone Joint Surg* 69B:26–35, 1987).

In lumbar spinal surgery, wound infection was accessed by opening of the wound packing and delayed resuture after antibiotic therapy (Prosser AJ, Waddell G: *J R Coll Surg Edinb* 31:296–299, 1987).

In the February 6, 1987, number of *Morbidity and Mortality Weekly Report* from the Centers for Disease Control, a patient with Jakob-Creutzfeldt disease is described in whom the disease was presumably transmitted by use of a graft of human dura mater processed in Germany in 1982. Presently known procedures to sterilize dura mater are not sufficiently effective to inactivate the agent completely. In light of this occurrence, the *FDA Drug Bulletin* (17:3–4, April 1987) invites surgeons to consider the use of temporalis fascia, fascia lata, or synthetic substitutes as alternatives, or at least to verify that their sources follow stringent selection and processing criteria such as those promulgated by the American Association of Tissue Banks.

Cysts

Among 18 patients with posterior fossa epidermoid cysts, most appeared as hypodense areas on computed tomography (with 3 hyperdense areas); all but 2 showed no enhancement on contrast administration (Salazar J, et al: *Acta Neurochir (Wien)* 85:34–39, 1987).

A mobile intraventricular cyst of the third ventricle was treated successfully with stereotactic puncture (Ericson K, et al: *Acta Radiol Diagn* 27:501–503, 1986).

Magnetic resonance shows intracranial arachnoid cysts like cerebrospinal fluid on both T1- and T2-weighted images (Wiener SN, et al: *J Comput Assist Tomogr* 11:236–241, 1987).

Spontaneous rupture of an intracranial dermoid cyst is reported with diagnosis by computed tomographic scanning (Boissonnot L, et al: *J Radiol* 67:917–919, 1986).

Magnetic resonance imaging can demonstrate intraspinal epidermoid cysts. These can be low intensity, intermediate intensity, or bright on T1-weighted images (Phillips J, Chiu L: *J Comput Assist Tomogr* 11:181–183, 1987).

Neuroanesthesia

Low-dose synthetic narcotic infusions (fentanyl or sufentanil) may be used for cerebral relaxation during craniotomy (Bristow A, et al: *Anesth Analg* 66:413–416, 1987).

A high concentration of isoflurane reduces the amplitude of visual evoked potentials in patients (Chi OZ, Field C: *Anesthesiology* 65:328–330, 1986).

Regional anesthesia and general anesthesia produce similar perioperative hemodynamic and surgical outcomes, but regional anesthesia results in a shorter hospital stay and less cardiovascular morbidity (Muskett A, et al: *Am J Surg* 152:691–694, 1986).

In animal studies, tertatolol, a noncardioselective beta-adrenergic drug, acts as a potent blocking agent but differs from propranolol by preserving renal perfusion (Leeman M, et al: *J Hypertens* 4:581–587, 1986).

Other Topics

Perforation of the gastrointestinal tract is a less well-recognized complication of steroid therapy than is gastrointestinal bleeding, although it occurs more frequently, is more difficult to diagnose, and is far more serious. Prevention of constipation may help to avert this complication, and early diagnosis improves the outcome (Fadul CE, et al: *Neurology* 38:348–352, 1988).

In the Departments of Neurology and Neurosurgery at Bowman Gray School of Medicine, neurosurgical nurse clinicians trained through a 6-month program with a 2-month practical internship. These nurse-clinicians have served in the Department of Neurosurgery and are believed to make a significant contribution to the educational efforts of the residents. These trained nurses carry out many activities of a routine nature including suture removal, ordering radiographic studies, securing social services, and the like, thus freeing the residents to study, read, do research, write, and participate in the operating room (Alexander A Jr: Branch CL Jr: *Surg Neurol* 27:590–592, 1987).

Intravenous ^{133}Xe measurements of cerebral blood flow (CBF) made in 15 patients in the sitting position showed that mean supine CBF rose from 43 ml/100 gm/minute to 62 ml/100 gm/minute and remained there throughout surgery (Nelson RJ, et al: *J Neurol Neurosurg Psychiatry* 50:971–975, 1987).

Indomethacin is effective against neurogenic hyperthermia after trauma or surgery (Benedek G, et al: *Can J Neurol Sci* 14:145–148, 1987).—R.M. Crowell, M.D.

Subject Index

A

Acoustic
neurilemoma, incompletely excised,
radiotherapy for, 199
neurofibromatosis, bilateral, 253
pathogenetic mechanism for three
types of, 254
neuroma (*see* Neuroma, acoustic)
Acquired immunodeficiency syndrome (*see*
AIDS)
Acromegaly
surgery, growth hormone and
somatomedin C to predict benefit
of, 240
Adenocarcinoma
of ethmoid sinus, combined ENT and
neurosurgical approach in,
232
Adenoma
pituitary (*see* Pituitary, adenoma)
prolactin-secreting, bromocriptine and
surgical outcome in, 241
Adrenal
medullary graft to putamen, 84
Aged
parasomnia in, 24
Parkinson's disease, management
strategies, 143
AIDS
encephalomyelitis of, subacute, 95
neurological complications of, 97
neuropathological findings in, 99
surgery of, 407
Alcohol
fetal alcohol syndrome, neurological
findings, 62
stroke and, 42
Alzheimer's disease
clinical features, 35
differentiation from vascular dementia,
11
early-onset, predictors of
institutionalization and death, 36
familial, genetic defect on chromosome
21, 36
incidence rates, 35
twin pair study, 37
vacuolar change in, 33
Amaurosis
fugax in teenagers, 9
Amitriptyline
in migraine, 90
Amnesia
transient global, secondary to triazolam,
24

Amphotericin B
in meningitis, cryptococcal, 104
Amyotrophic lateral sclerosis
cerebral glucose utilization lowered in,
131
motoneuron loss in, natural history of,
130
plant excitant neurotoxin in, 129
Anaplastic
astrocytoma, resection and survival in,
217
Aneurysm
basilar artery fusiform, case review,
302
carotid, unclippable, common carotid
occlusion for, 298
cerebral
giant, etomidate, arterial occlusion
and angiography in, 296
ruptured, cerebral blood flow in, 292
intracranial
arterial, in early childhood, 371
fusiform, clinicopathology, 303
saccular, collagen type III deficiency
in, 300
saccular, ruptured, immune
complexes and complement after,
301
unruptured familial, IV digital
subtraction angiography in, 291
mycotic, and infective endocarditis, 50
occlusion by intrasaccular injection of
fibrin sealant (in rabbit), 196
supratentorial, early surgery in, and
mortality, 295
Aneurysmal
subarachnoid hemorrhage, vasospasm
and methylprednisolone, 293
Angiography
cerebral, in infective endocarditis, 50
in cerebral aneurysm, giant, 296
digital subtraction IV, in familial
intracranial aneurysms, 291
magnetic resonance, of peripheral,
carotid and coronary arteries, 168
neuroangiography (*see*
Neuroangiography)
Angioma
cavernous, MRI appearance, 315
Angioplasty, transluminal
percutaneous, of subclavian arteries,
190
of vertebral and basilar arteries, 141
Anomalies
(*See also* Malformations)
arteriovenous (*see* Arteriovenous,
malformation)

417

Author Index

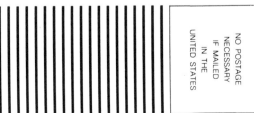

TO ORDER: DETACH AND MAIL

Please enter my subscription to the journal(s) and/or Year Book(s) checked below:
(To order by phone, call toll-free 800-622-5410. In IL, call collect 312-726-9746.

	Practitioner (approx.)	Resident	Institution
Current Problems in Surgery® (1 yr.)	___$55.00	$29.95	$72.00
Current Problems in Pediatrics® (1 yr.)	___$44.00	$29.95	$65.00
Current Problems in Cancer® (1 yr.)	___$49.95	$29.95	$65.00
Current Problems in Cardiology® (1 yr.)	___$55.00	$29.95	$72.00
Current Problems in Obstetrics, Gynecology, and Fertility® (1 yr.)	___$49.95	$29.95	$65.00
Current Problems in Diag. Radiology® (1 yr.)	___$55.00	$29.95	—$72.00
Current Problems in Dermatology® (1 yr.)	___$49.95	$29.95	$65.00
Disease-A-Month® (1 yr.)	___$44.00	$29.95	$65.00

Binder ___ $14.95

	Practitioner	Resident
1989 Year Book of Anesthesia® (AN-89)	___$45.00	$30.00
1989 Year Book of Cancer® (CA-89)	___$47.00	$30.00
1989 Year Book of Cardiology® (CV-89)	___$47.00	$30.00
1989 Year Book of Critical Care Medicine ® (16-89)	___$45.00	$30.00
1989 Year Book of Dentistry® (D-89)	___$46.00	$30.00
1989 Year Book of Dermatology® (10-89)	___$48.00	$30.00
1989 Year Book of Diagnostic Radiology® (9-89)	___$47.00	$30.00
1989 Year Book of Digestive Diseases® (13-89)	___$45.00	$30.00
1989 Year Book of Drug Therapy® (6-89)	___$45.00	$30.00
1989 Year Book of Emergency Medicine® (15-89)	___$47.00	$30.00
1989 Year Book of Endocrinology® (EM-89)	___$48.00	$30.00
1989 Year Book of Family Practice® (FY-89)	___$45.00	$30.00
1989 Year Book of Geriatrics and Gerontology (GE-89)	___$42.00	$30.00
1989 Year Book of Hand Surgery® (17-89)	___$45.00	$30.00
1989 Year Book of Hematology® (24-89)	___$42.00	$30.00
1989 Year Book of Infectious Diseases® (19-89)	___$42.00	$30.00
1989 Year Book of Medicine® (1-89)	___$44.95	$30.00
1989 Year Book of Neurology and Neurosurgery® (8-89)	___$47.00	$30.00
1989 Year Book of Nuclear Medicine® (NM-89)	___$47.00	$30.00
1989 Year Book of Obstetrics and Gynecology® (5-89)	___$42.95	$30.00
1989 Year Book of Ophthalmology® (EY-89)	___$47.00	$30.00
1989 Year Book of Orthopedics® (OR-89)	___$47.00	$30.00
1989 Year Book of Otolaryngology-Head and Neck Surgery® (3-89)	___$45.00	$30.00
1989 Year Book of Pathology and Clinical Pathology® (PI-89)	___$47.00	$30.00
1989 Year Book of Pediatrics® (4-89)	___$45.00	$30.00
1989 Year Book of Perinatal/Neonatal Medicine (23-89)	___$42.00	$30.00
1989 Year Book of Plastic and Reconstructive Surgery® (12-89)	___$49.00	$30.00
1989 Year Book of Podiatric Medicine and Surgery®(18-89)	___$42.00	$30.00
1989 Year Book of Psychiatry and Applied Mental Health® (11-89)	___$45.00	$30.00
1989 Year Book of Pulmonary Disease® (21-89)	___$45.00	$30.00
1989 Year Book of Rehabilitation® (22-89)	___$42.00	$30.00
1989 Year Book of Sports Medicine® (SM-89)	___$45.00	$30.00
1989 Year Book of Surgery® (2-89)	___$50.50	$30.00
1989 Year Book of Urology® (7-89)	___$47.00	$30.00
1989 Year Book of Vascular Surgery (20-89)	___$45.00	$30.00

*The above Year Books are published annually. For the convenience of its customers, Year Book enters each purchaser as a subscriber to future volumes and sends annual announcements of each volume approximately 2 months before publication. The new volume will be shipped upon publication unless you complete and return the cancellation notice attached to the announcement and it is received by Year Book within the time indicated (approximately 20 days after your receipt of the announcement). You may cancel your subscription at any time. The new volume may be examined on approval for 30 days, may be returned for full credit, and if returned Year Book will then remove your name as a subscriber. Return postage is guaranteed by Year Book to the Postal Service.

Prices quoted are in U.S. dollars. Canadian orders will be billed in Canadian funds at the approximate current exchange rate. A small additional charge will be made for postage and handling. Illinois and Tennessee residents will be billed appropriate sales tax. All prices quoted subject to change.

NAME_____ACCT.NO._____

ADDRESS_____

CITY_____STATE_____ZIP_____

Printed in U.S.A.

DF1

Year Book Medical Publishers
200 North LaSalle Street Chicago, Illinois 60601